HIGH-RISK
INTRAPARTUM NURSING

HIGH-RISK INTRAPARTUM NURSING

Edited by
Lisa K. Mandeville, R.N., M.S.N.
Nan H. Troiano, R.N., M.S.N.

Division of Maternal Fetal Medicine
Vanderbilt University
Nashville, Tennessee

With 20 Contributors

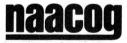

The Organization for Obstetric, Gynecologic, & Neonatal Nurses

J. B. LIPPINCOTT COMPANY
Philadelphia   New York   London   Hagerstown

Sponsoring Editor: David P. Carroll
Production Supervisor: Lori Bainbridge
Production: Till & Till, Inc.
Compositor: The Composing Room of Michigan, Inc.
Printer/Binder: R. R. Donnelley & Sons Company

6 5 4 3 2

Library of Congress Cataloging-in-Publication Data

High-risk intrapartum nursing / edited by Lisa K. Mandeville, Nan H.
   Troiano ; with 20 contributors.
      p. cm.
   Includes bibliographical references and index.
   ISBN 0-397-54811-7
   1. Obstetrical nursing.   2. Pregnancy, Complications of—Nursing.
3. Labor, Complicated—Nursing.   I. Mandeville, Lisa K.
II. Troiano, Nan H.
   [DNLM: 1. Critical Care—nursing.   2. Maternal-Child Nursing.
3. Pregnancy Complications—nursing.   WY 157.3 H638]
RG951.H537   1992
610.73′678—dc20
DNLM/DLC
for Library of Congress   91-42091
                                                                      CIP

Any procedure or practice described in this book should be applied by
the health-care practitioner under appropriate supervision in accordance
with professional standards of care used with regard to the unique circumstances that apply in each practice situation. Care has been taken to
confirm the accuracy of information presented and to describe generally
accepted practices. However, the authors, editors, and publisher cannot accept any responsibility for errors or omissions or for consequences from
application of the information in this book and make no warranty, express
or implied, with respect to the contents of the book.

Every effort has been made to ensure drug selections and dosages are
in accordance with current recommendations and practice. Because of
ongoing research, changes in government regulations, and the constant
flow of information on drug therapy, reactions, and interactions, the reader
is cautioned to check the package insert for each drug for indications,
dosages, warnings, and precautions, particularly if the drug is new or
infrequently used.

C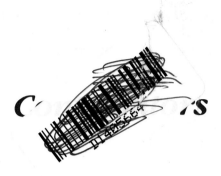s

Abbe Bendell, RN, BSN, MBA-HA
Assistant Director of Nursing
Women's Hospital Center
Jackson Memorial Hospital
Miami, Florida

Victoria Cahill Bockman, RN, MS
Perinatal Clinical Nurse Specialist
Women and Children's Care
Saint Joseph's Hospital and Medical Center
Phoenix, Arizona

Mary Ellen Burke, RN, MS
President, Perinatal Resources
Clinical Teaching Associate,
Brown University School of Medicine
Providence, Rhode Island

Gay M. Chisum, BA, RN, CD
Director, Perinatal Addiction Consultants
Clinical Consultant to Perinatal Wellness
   Program,
Northwestern Memorial Hospital
Chicago, Illinois

Jane B. Daddario, RN, MSN
Assistant Professor for the Practice of Nursing
Vanderbilt University School of Nursing
Senior Consultant
Harvey, Troiano & Associates
Nashville, Tennessee

Joan Drukker Dauphinee, RNC, MS
Director of Nursing, Obstetrical Services
Magee-Womens Hospital
Pittsburgh, Pennsylvania

Linda K. Davis, RNC, BSN
Staff Nurse, Labor and Delivery
The Women's Center
University Community Hospital
Tampa, Florida

Karen Dorman, RN, MS
Coordinator, Maternal Transport Service
Department of Obstetrics & Gynecology
Baylor College of Medicine
Houston, Texas

JoNell Efantis-Potter, RN, MSN, ARNP
Instructor
Department of Obstetrics & Gynecology
University of Miami
Miami, Florida

Carol J. Harvey, RNC, MS
Project Director
The Center for High Risk and Critical Care
  Obstetrics
Department of Obstetrics and Gynecology
The University of Texas
Medical Branch
Galveston, Texas

Gayle Johnson, RN, BSN, CCRN, EMT
Flight Nurse
Vanderbilt LifeFlight
Vanderbilt University Medical Center
Nashville, Tennessee

Marian F. Lake, RNC, MPH
Instructor, Department of Obstetrics
  & Gynecology
Division of Maternal Fetal Medicine
University of Medicine and Dentistry
  of New Jersey
Robert Wood Johnson Medical School
New Brunswick, New Jersey

Lisa K. Mandeville, RN, MSN
Administrative Coordinator
Division of Maternal Fetal Medicine
Assistant in Obstetrics
Department of Obstetrics and Gynecology
Vanderbilt University
Nashville, Tennessee

Katharyn A. May, DNSc, RN, FAAN
Associate Professor and Chair
Department of Family and Health Systems
  Nursing

Vanderbilt University School of Nursing
Nashville, Tennessee

A. Diann Neal, RNC, MS
Director, Women and Children's Care
Saint Joseph's Hospital and Medical Center
Phoenix, Arizona

Susan Pozaic, RNC, MS
Director of Perinatal Services
Children's Hospital Home Care
Children's Hospital of Buffalo
Buffalo, New York

Melissa Sisson, RN, MN
Director of Labor and Delivery
  and Perinatal Diagnostic Center
Northside Hospital
Atlanta, Georgia

Karen L. Starr, RN, MSN, NCAC II
Clinical Nurse Specialist
Vanderbilt Institute for Treatment of Addiction
Vanderbilt University Medical Center
Nashville, Tennessee

Nan H. Troiano, RN, MSN
Co-Director, Critical Care Obstetrics
Division of Maternal Fetal Medicine
Assistant in Obstetrics
Department of Obstetrics and Gynecology
Vanderbilt University
Nashville, Tennessee

Bonnie Wiltse, RN, BS, MPH
Vice President Nursing Practice
  and Maternal Child Health Program
Saint Luke's Regional Medical Center
Sioux City, Iowa

Contents

Foreword

As we move toward the 21st century, the challenge for perinatal nurses is to continue to gain expertise in caring for intrapartum patients and their families. While the past 50 years have seen dramatic changes in the delivery of intrapartum care, we are constantly reminded that pregnancy and childbirth are natural physiologic events. In the late 1950s and early 1960s, the movement toward "natural childbirth" began in the United States. Prenatal care as we know it today was established, and education programs began to help couples prepare for birth. Gradually, we made the transition from the amnesia of "twilight sleep" induced by scopolamine and fortified by general anesthesia, to newer, safer methods of pain management that enabled mothers to participate in the delivery.

By the mid 1970s, most labor units permitted fathers to be present during labor and delivery. By the 1980s, with the move toward single-room maternity care, entire families, support persons, and even friends and neighbors witnessed the birth. Since World War II, the average hospitalization for postpartum patients has decreased from 15 days to less than 24 hours. Because of less time spent in the health care system, much of the emphasis of perinatal nursing now focuses on educating parents and families as well as on humanizing the birth experience.

Over the past 50 years, much has been learned about pregnancy and the birth experience for women with normal, healthy pregnancies; however, perinatal nurses will always have to care for a percentage of pregnant women whose pregnancy is life threatening. Fortunately, advances in scientific knowledge and biomedical technology have given new hope to women who previously would not have survived childbirth, or for whom pregnancy would have certainly been synonymous with increased morbidity and mortality.

These technological advances, when combined with the art and science of nursing, have propelled nurses into a new era of care for pregnant women at the highest risk: critical care obstetrics, the newest frontier for perinatal nurses. *High-Risk Intrapartum Nursing* is written for nurses and other health care workers who care for mothers and infants at risk. This book combines the nursing specialties of critical care and high-risk obstetric nursing to help nurses provide optimum care for mothers and infants at risk. Extensive coverage is given to current topics in the care of critically ill pregnant women or pregnant women whose life-style places them at increased risk. In addition, the book also emphasizes areas such as psychosocial care, quality assurance, and risk assessment. The text is supplemented with numerous sample procedures and protocols, as well as documentation flowsheets and forms to assist nurses in the daily practice of high-risk perinatal nursing.

As readers will quickly recognize, this book provides the foundation and the force for continuing to improve the future of high-risk intrapartum care. The editors, Lisa Mandeville and Nan Troiano, are recognized experts who have carefully chosen contributors for their knowledge, experience, expertise, and reputations in specific areas of high-risk obstetric nursing. The resulting product is a resource nurses will use in providing quality care and in improving outcomes.

Ann L. Ropp, RN, MS
1991 President
NAACOG

I

FOUNDATIONS FOR PRACTICE

1
◆ ◆ ◆

Introduction

Lisa K. Mandeville
Nan H. Troiano

The nature of obstetric health care practice is changing and with it the role of the perinatal nurse. Historically, obstetric patients have been treated as one homogeneous group. However, a recognizable dichotomy has emerged with respect to the patient population. On one hand, the majority of patients are without identified risk factors and proceed through pregnancy, labor, delivery, and the postpartum period without complications. The unique challenge posed by this group is to provide individualized care within a wellness-oriented framework. When this concept was first introduced, it appeared simple and straightforward; now however, implementation has proved complex and dynamic, often requiring adaptation of facility, personnel, and care protocols. On the other hand, a new at-risk population may be readily identified. This group is more ill and has a greater variety of illnesses than ever before. For this obstetric population, the primary challenge is to integrate new technology and expand the knowledge base in the obstetric health care setting.

In view of these issues, the question of how to adequately plan and provide nursing care for a diverse patient population arises. One approach is to assume that all perinatal nurses possess knowledge and skills commensurate with any patient situation. Another is to create and encourage the development of perinatal nursing subspecialization. At present, the first approach is chosen most often, largely by facility administration or other factions instead of nursing. Nurses, in fact, passively have allowed others to make critical decisions in health care planning and ultimately in the role of the nurse. This approach is incongruous with the state of perinatal nursing development. As nursing emerges as a self-governing profession, prerequisites for clinical practice clearly fall within nursing's responsibility. Practice competence is determined and validated by preparation, orientation, and continuing education. In almost all areas of the country each of these components is designed, implemented, and evaluated by and for nursing with joint responsibility between administration and the individual clinician.

Inherent in the discussion of competence is the issue of nursing standards of practice. Knowledge and use of standards are measures of practice competency and make up another prerequisite for clinical practice. Standards for clinical practice are promulgated by and for general and specialized nursing services and are independent of medical practice. Unlike the areas of preparation, orientation, and continuing education, these standards are not used by many practicing nurses in their daily work. Standards are written by representatives within national professional organizations and are designed in consideration of the activities of the clinical nurse. They exist to provide a fundamental guide for nursing practice and to encourage implementation of a minimal acceptable level of care. In addition to national organizations, these standards are influenced by facility policy and protocol which further refine and interpret the national word. The practicing nurse (and oftentimes nursing administration) may not be aware of sources for practice standards. This may occur because although some standards are written, others are implicit and determined by a national practice trend. They are, however, no less governing of appropriate practice. Furthermore, standards are reflective of changes in nursing roles and practice and therefore are constantly evolving. As practice is in large part dictated by these standards, they are further determined and refined by changing practice. A firm foundation of nursing practice facilitates integration of nursing care within a multidisciplinary framework. Achievement of competent individual practice without the guidance and incorporation of standards often leads to practice based on tradition (*e.g.,* "We've always done it this way") or on a medical model determined and enforced by medical staff or hospital administration.

In returning to the original question of how to plan and provide care for the patient population, it is clear that nursing must determine the role and pace of practice development. Practice following validation of competence and based on national standards is mandatory. The choice between generic perinatal nursing and subspecialization traditionally has been made by hospital administrators and is usually based on facility constraints. In lieu of these processes, nursing schemes must be developed based on patient subgroup and individual needs. Care of the critically ill patient requires a practicing nurse with current and sufficient intensive care knowledge and skills. The patient without apparent risk who desires a homelike birth experience also deserves a competent nurse prepared to meet her health care needs. Thus, subspecialization seems a reasonable choice but may be constrained by issues of continuity of care which need to be addressed.

There are many instances where nursing has proactively influenced the direction and content of health care for pregnant women, fetuses, and newborns. For example, perinatal nursing has implemented practices addressing home health care, substance abuse, battering, and critical care, in strides often surpassing medicine. Such activities demonstrate an accountability to the patients and to the profession and provide a model for continued development of perinatal nursing practice.

2

Promoting Quality Nursing Care

Bonnie Wiltse

Nature and Importance of Quality Nursing Care

In today's health care environment, quality nursing care is not just a goal of the nursing profession: It is also an expectation of the public. The increasingly well-informed consumer, concerned with health care costs, expects and demands quality from all health care providers. Because of their unique position within the health care system, nurses can be a vital force in promoting quality. Because nurses interact with all health care providers, quality nursing care standards can serve as a model for other providers.

Historical Perspective

The very foundation of nursing is quality care. Florence Nightingale founded the nursing profession in response to the conditions she witnessed during the Crimean War in the 1850s. Her belief that care by trained persons could improve patient outcome led to the development of nurse training programs. She not only established the first schools, but also is credited with developing the first nursing quality-assurance program by establishing measurements to demonstrate the improved results obtained when trained personnel and clean facilities and supplies were used.[1]

In the 1960s, the American Nurses Association began to promote baccalaureate education for entry into practice, not only to improve the educational preparation of the nurse and therefore the quality of nursing care provided, but also to provide more credibility to nursing as a profession. At the same time, nursing leaders began to recognize the need for nursing to monitor the quality of practice. In the past, the focus had been simply to provide "good nursing care" as defined by the nurse responsible for a specific patient or unit. Now the focus became how to objectively measure that care to ensure that good nursing care was truly being provided. These trends—the push to recognize nursing as a profession and to increase educational requirements for practice—and the need for nurses to ensure quality supported each other. Professions must be accountable to the public for services provided. This accountability can only be demonstrated through an effective quality-assurance program.

A major concern in initiating quality-assurance programs was the need for standards against which practice could be measured. Three types of standards were identified: structure, process, and outcome. Originally, most of the standards used were structure standards established by licensing or accrediting agencies such as the Joint Commission on Accreditation of Hospitals Organization (JCAHO). In 1973, NAACOG published the first edition of *Standards for Obstetrical, Gynecologic, and Neonatal Nurses.* This was followed in 1974 by statements that defined structure, process, and outcome standards, with examples for their use in quality-assurance programs. During the 1980s JCAHO set the agenda for quality assurance in health care organizations. Although the procedure and terminology have varied from routine chart audits to problem-focus reviews to the current emphasis on monitoring and evaluation and the future use of clinical indicators, the overall objective of improved patient care has been consistent. A major portion of the JCAHO accreditation process is a review of nursing practice. No other service within the organization is scrutinized as closely. This scrutiny is a result of the recognition of nursing care's importance in the overall operation of the organization and its impact on patient outcome.

NAACOG has continued to play a major role in promoting quality obstetric, gynecologic, and neonatal nursing care. As a participant in the voluntary quality review committee with the American College of Obstetricians and Gynecologists, NAACOG members participate in reviews and evaluation of obstetric services on request. NAACOG has developed many practice resources and educational programs as well as revisions to the standards manual that have helped in establishing quality standards for obstetric, gynecologic, and neonatal nursing practice.

Now, in the 1990s, the focus on quality nursing care is even more crucial. The shortage of nurses and other health care professionals and the advanced, costly technologies that require not only highly knowledgeable and skilled nurses but nurses able to adapt to rapidly changing environments and stresses emphasize a need for quality control as an essential component of operations. The publication of mortality data by the federal government generated many questions on quality from the public. The development of JCAHO's clinical indicators and their future use in hospital accreditation decisions are under much discussion within professions as well as organizations.

Quality must be defined from both the clinical and the organizational perspective, and correlates of quality are cost, productivity, and risk.[2] Beyers believes that the concepts are interrelated and that nursing has a major role in defining these relationships so that patients receive appropriate care.[2] No longer is it appropriate for each service or health care provider within an organization to work independently. The focus must be on the total outcome for the patient, not the outcome of one individual service. This requires interdepartmental collaboration as well as patient involvement.

Beyers further discusses Garvin's evolution of quality within the United States as "four quality eras: inspection, statistical quality control, quality assurance, and strategic quality management."[2] Nurses, as well as most other health care providers, currently operate in the era of quality assurance. To move to strategic quality management involves the recognition that quality is essential to the success of any service or business and must be integrated into overall operations. This is particularly true for nursing. The future of the nursing profession may well rest on how well quality is integrated into the delivery of nursing care. Quality should be at the forefront as nursing care standards are developed, new nursing care delivery systems implemented, and new services planned.

Health care organizations are beginning to look to businesses as examples of quality assurance in action. These organizations recognize that those who have made quality a top priority and incorporated that commitment into all activities of the business have become the industry leaders. These leaders, such as IBM with their total quality management program,[3] have also recognized that an essential ingredient of quality is the ability to maintain close relationships with their customers and to encourage active involvement of personnel in the operations of their business. By integrating these concepts into health care, organizations can begin to improve the quality of their services.

In health care, involvement of patients will ensure that service truly meets the "customer's" needs and expectations. Issues of productivity, cost, and risk cannot be ignored. Interdisciplinary collaboration will be essential. As the largest provider of health care, nurses have an opportunity to provide leadership into the fourth era of quality, clearly demonstrating a professional commitment to excellence. Quality is truly the focus of the 1990s.

Factors Influencing Quality Care

The many settings in which health care is provided and the large number and variety of health care providers and suppliers involved can make attempts to improve overall quality difficult. In addition, the public's demand for health care as a basic right and the reluctance to acknowledge the possibility of unfavorable outcomes without negligence, or even to accept the inevitability of death, put additional pressure on the system.

The major factors that influence the quality of health care can be divided into three general categories: people, organizations, and national policies and economics.

People

Nurses, as the largest group of health care providers, have the greatest opportunity to influence quality; however, their success depends on their ability and desire to make quality nursing care a priority. Nurses need a strong educational base to provide theoretical knowledge and clinical skill, develop interpersonal and communication skills, as well as to develop creative solutions to old, as well as new, problems. As the health care providers who are most closely connected to the patients, nurses need to involve the patients in the evaluation of their care. Many nurses are reluctant to openly question patients as to their perception of the care provided. For many years, nursing leadership promoted the nurse as the patient's advocate. If this was truly operational, there would be many fewer quality issues in health care today.

As the shortage of nurses and other health care providers grows, nurses must learn to delegate and supervise other workers in order to ensure that nursing care is available to all. Many nurses are reluctant to accept the idea that other persons can assist in providing basic care as long as the nurse assesses, plans, and evaluates that care. Their education has not prepared them to coordinate care—only to provide it. By failing to recognize this, nurses are continuing to subject themselves to excessive workloads, long hours, and increasing frustration as they see patient care suffer. Nurses not only owe it to their patients but to themselves to look for new methods to ensure the quality that is so much a part of nursing.

To attempt to identify all types of providers who make up the health care team is almost impossible. Within nursing there are staff nurses, specialty nurses, nurse practitioners, nurse midwives, educators, administrators, and nurse anesthetists, just to mention a few. Physicians are specialized and subspecialized. Every body system has professional and technical specialists who perform many of the functions originally performed by the staff nurse and family practice physician. While this type of specialization has lead to many improvements in health care, the problems associated with communication and coordination among all providers have increased enormously. Much of this responsibility has fallen to nursing and is seldom recognized as having an impact on nursing productivity.

As specialties have developed, territories have been staked out and, in most instances, guarded with vigor. The turf battles that ensued have consumed time and energy, thus detracting from the main objective of providing the best possible outcome for patients. Within any health care organization, the providers—as a group—must first focus on defining the desired patient outcome and then identify the problems or variances that can negatively influence this goal. Once this is accomplished, roles, responsibilities, and systems should be redesigned to eliminate the problems and achieve the desired goals. Multidisciplinary planning is key to this effort.

The relationship between the nurse and the physician is of special significance. Mutual respect with open communication and cooperation will enhance relationships and, very possibly, patient outcomes. One study of patients in intensive care units in major medical centers indicates that the relationship between nurses and physicians within these units is a major factor influencing positive patient outcomes.[4] This is not a surprise to most nurses.

The public should play a major role in both maintaining their own health and in ensuring that quality health care is provided. Within the past decade, many people have recognized their responsibility for their own health and have changed their lifestyles to reduce their risk of cardiovascular disease. However, many others still play a dependent role and assume little to no responsibility for their own health. This group expects health care providers to correct or control the diseases brought on by harmful lifestyles. Compliance to prescribed treatment protocols is sketchy or nonexistent.

While the public places great value in health care, there has been little participation by the public in setting health care standards or other measures to ensure quality. This has been left to the professionals who have been slow to recognize the need for public input, especially because the public has not demanded it. The rapid rise in medical malpractice litigation in the past 10 years indicates that the public has begun to question quality of care and has found it lacking. As frequently happens in times of rapid change, some have gone from one extreme to another, from assuming all care is excellent to assuming all care is suspect. Today, proof of innocence is required when outcomes are unfavorable. This overreaction can reduce the availability of health care and increase its cost, rather than increase its quality. It is time for health care providers to encourage public participation in setting quality standards and for patients to become active participants in monitoring and evaluating that care.

Organization

Much of the current literature on organizations focuses on quality or excellence as the necessary ingredient for competitive and economic success. While this would seem to be self-evident, studies show this clearly is not universal.[5,6] Businesses and health care organizations in the United States are now looking to Deming, who is recognized for his work in improving Japanese production and quality, as they struggle to regain competitive advantages, both nationally and internationally.[7]

All of these experts focus on the importance of a strong, unswerving commitment to quality by top management as the key to quality production or service. The emphasis is on doing things right the first time. Philip Crosby states, "Quality is free. It's not a gift, but it is free. What costs money are the unquality things— all the actions that involve not doing the job right the first time."[8] He lists four key principles of quality management for managers to understand: conformance to requirements, deficit prevention rather than inspection, standards of zero defects, and recognition that the costs of poor quality can amount to 40% of the operating costs in a service agency. The Crosby Quality Management Maturity Grid (Figure 2-1) can be used to assess the level of perception of quality by management within an organization.[9] The grid identifies five stages to quality maturity. The first is uncertainty where problems are dealt with as they occur, followed by awakening. This occurs when a quality assurance team is developed to begin investigation about lack of quality. The third stage is enlightenment where corrective action is instituted and management becomes committed to quality. The fourth stage is wisdom and occurs when potential problems are identified early by employees. This requires an openness to suggestions for improvements and change. The last stage is certainty where the majority of problems are prevented, except in unusual situations.

Many health care organizations have developed quality-assurance programs,

Quality Management Maturity Grid

Rater _____   Unit _____

Measurement Categories	Stage I Uncertainty	Stage II Awakening	Stage III Enlightenment	Stage IV Wisdom	Stage V Certainty
Management understanding and attitude	No comprehension of quality as a management tool. Tend to blame quality department for quality problems.	Recognizing that quality management may be of value but not willing to provide money or time to make it all happen.	While going through quality improvement program learn more about quality management: becoming supportive and helpful.	Participating. Understand absolutes of quality management. Recognize their personal role in continuing emphasis.	Consider quality management an essential part of company system.
Quality organization status	Quality is hidden in manufacturing or engineering departments. Inspection probably not part of organization. Emphasis on appraisal and sorting.	A stronger quality leader is appointed but main emphasis is still on appraisal and moving the product. Still part of manufacturing or other.	Quality department reports to top management all appraisal is incorporated and manager has role in management of company.	Quality manager is an officer of company effective status reporting and preventive action. Involved with consumer affairs and special assignments.	Quality manager on board of directors. Prevention is main concern. Quality is a thought leader.
Problem handling	Problems are fought as they occur: no resolution, inadequate definition, lots of yelling and accusations.	Teams are set up to attack major problems. Long-range solutions are not solicited.	Corrective action communication established. Problems are faced openly and resolved in an orderly way.	Problems are identified early in their development. All functions are open to suggestion and improvement.	Except in the most unusual cases problems are prevented.
Cost of quality as % of sales	Reported: unknown Actual: 20%	Reported 3% Actual: 18%	Reported: 8% Actual: 12%	Reported: 6.5% Actual: 8%	Reported: 2.5% Actual: 2.5%
Quality improvement actions	No organized activities. No understanding of such activities.	Trying obvious motivational short-range efforts.	Implementation of the 14-step program with thorough understanding and establishment of each step.	Continuing the 14-step program and starting make certain.	Quality improvement is a normal and continued activity.
Summation of company quality posture	We don't know why we have problems with quality.	Is it absolutely necessary to always have problems with quality?	Through management commitment and quality improvement, we are identifying and resolving our problems.	Defect prevention is a routine part of our operation.	We know why we do not have problems with quality.

Figure 2-1. Quality Management Maturity Grid. *Source:* Crosby PB. *Quality is Free.* New York, New American Library, 1979, 32–33.

more in response to JCAHO requirements than an administrative commitment to quality. The varied successes of these programs may well be due to the presence or absence of this commitment. In addition, for quality to be operational, there must be an organizational environment that recognizes the need for active employee involvement in the quality process. Quality occurs at the employee level. Unless employees are involved in establishing standards, identifying solutions, and participating in the rewards, there will be little quality in the organization.

It is not enough to tell employees that they are to be members of the quality team. Employees need education and mentoring if they are to understand how to contribute and what the program can mean to their own job satisfaction. Some hospitals have begun implementation of employee empowerment programs that focus on encouraging employees to become business partners with administration in the operation of the organization. Educational programs are provided to acquaint the employee with the business aspect of the organization and introduce the idea of entrepreneurship, as well as the process the employee can use to assume both authority and responsibility for solving problems within the work area. These programs are intended to change the culture of the organization by eliminating territoriality, improving open first-party communication, and allowing those individuals most knowledgeable of the situation to solve problems. Employees are encouraged to identify methods of increasing quality and productivity, reduce costs, and develop creative ideas for new programs or services. Some organizations have also included incentive compensation programs for employees to share in financial successes.

Health care organizations have a major advantage as they begin to understand the need for commitment to quality and begin to implement quality management programs. Health care professionals, by education and vocation, are committed to quality and can provide leadership in this endeavor. The key is getting professionals to recognize that quality needs to be improved and that it *can* be improved. Many professionals believe they individually provide quality care, but that they are unable to change the system or other providers who impede quality. The professionals, including physicians and nurses, are often individualists; getting them to commit to active interdisciplinary involvement is not easy, especially in view of the current malpractice concerns. By focusing on prevention of error and the importance to the patient of doing it right the first time, they may be more willing to participate.

National Policy and Economics

The quality of the health care of the nation is a direct reflection of national priorities and policies. A nation that places health care as a top priority provides a system that ensures that all people receive basic health care. In the United States, while health care consumes a growing percentage of the gross national product, there are areas of medical need. Medicare and Medicaid programs were established to assist the elderly and the poor. However, state funded programs vary widely with differing priorities. The inability of the American public to prioritize care has resulted in vast sums spent for advanced technology with basic health care unavailable or limited for many.

Health care has become an expensive commodity with health insurance almost unattainable for those individuals who are not part of employers' health plans. In the past, health insurance was a primary employee benefit, with employers frequently paying all or most of the costs. Now, as organizations struggle with mounting health costs, employers are attempting to increase the employee's share of health care costs. The philosophy behind this move is that until employees share the costs of health care, they will not become knowledgeable consumers and costs will continue to escalate. Additional efforts are aimed at health care providers with Medicare and increasing numbers of private insurance companies moving from charge reimbursement to diagnosis related groups (DRGs) or fixed-payment fee schedules.

The nation is increasingly concerned with the future of health care in the United States. Legislators as well as business leaders are looking to other health care systems, the Canadian system in particular, and there are ongoing debates as to the directions that should be taken. The issues are many and are not likely to be resolved quickly. Unmet health care needs will continue to be a national as well as a professional concern for some time with the danger that cost will be the priority rather than accessibility and quality.

Components of Quality Assurance

The implementation of a quality-improvement approach within nursing has the potential to revitalize the profession as well as increase the quality of nursing care. Nurses need to believe they make a difference and that their performance is recognized as having a direct impact on patient outcomes. Nursing studies for over 20 years have pointed out the need for a change in the work environment in order to attract and retain nurses. Unless organizations and nursing departments in particular are willing to change the environment and culture within the organization, the problem of an adequate supply of qualified nurses will persist.

Organizational Commitment

Just as the chief executive officer must demonstrate a commitment to quality for the organization, the nurse executive must demonstrate this same commitment within nursing practice. This commitment can be demonstrated in many ways beginning with the nursing practice philosophy and selection of an appropriate nursing theory on which to base practice at that organization. Most nursing departments have a written philosophy, but few have spent the time and effort to research, select, and implement nursing theory into their practice. Without a theory upon which all nursing activities can be based, there will be disagreement concerning priorities and directions for nursing practice within that organization. Once a theory is selected, integration into all aspects of practice can begin. This includes orientation of staff, development of standards and practice protocols, and implementation of nursing process and quality-assurance activities, as well as performance standards and reviews. The nurse executive is key in articulating this vision of quality and must demonstrate this commitment through selection of qualified managers and staff who understand and demonstrate this principle. Rewards and recognition for quality service and performance are essential. The nurse executive as a member of the senior management team can be influential in promoting incentive systems that reward these efforts.

Since quality occurs at the point of service, nursing managers must have a thorough understanding and commitment to quality and their role in its achievement. A major focus of the manager must be on orientation of new employees. If doing it right the first time is the goal, the manager must be assured the employee knows how to do it right. For many nurse managers, much time is spent correcting problems. There needs to be a reassessment of priorities with focus on the prevention of problems rather than correction. The importance of patient involvement in assessing quality must be recognized. Too often, the maternalistic attitude prevails. If quality is defined as meeting patients' expectations, it is obvious that the patients must be involved. In some instances, assisting patients to develop realistic expectations of health care will be necessary.

Just as the first line manager must be committed and involved, so must the staff. An environment that values staff as active contributing members of the organization will do much to enlist their cooperation. The nurse manager's role will change from the primary focus of directing and managing unit activities to one of developing staff through role modeling, coaching, teaching, and mentoring. This presents challenges for all managers and involves risk taking as more practice decisions are placed in the hands of the practitioner. Implementation of shared governance is becoming widespread and represents an effort not only to give practicing professional nurses more authority for practice but also to increase their accountability. With privileges come responsibilities, and this must be recognized by all involved.

In order to provide quality nursing care, standards of both practice and performance must be identified. Professional nursing standards can either be set as a result of research or by consensus of nurse experts. In nursing practice most standards have been identified by consensus, although nursing research is increasing and will provide valuable input in the future. Standards must be objective and measurable to enhance understanding and communication among practitioners as well as to provide a workable tool for monitoring and evaluating activities. Standards of practice not only identify how nursing is to be practiced but also serve as a base for staff orientation, education, and evaluation, as well as development of policies, procedures, and protocols. In addition, standards provide a basis for the legal definition of nursing practice and professional accountability to the public.

Nursing Practice and Performance Standards

Professional nursing organizations are responsible to set practice standards for their members and to assist them in implementing these standards into their practice settings. This is the most important function of a professional nursing organization: to assist its members in providing quality care to the public—the mission of nursing. Individual organizations are responsible to assist nurses by providing a climate and setting that is conducive to quality practice. The organizational nursing policy, procedures, and protocols should reflect the professional nursing standard and be developed jointly by administration and nursing.

Standards can be divided into three types: structure, process, and outcome. Structure standards form the framework within which nursing is practiced.

Smith-Marker identifies structure standards as "elements from physical and environmental issues to philosophical and administrative issues," and further states, "They encompass all aspects of a nursing system except the process of giving care and its desired outcomes."[10] Examples of structure standards include requirements for facilities and equipment, licensure, and mandatory continuing education. Most of the standards for nursing developed by JCAHO relate to structure and are intended to ensure a setting conducive to quality care.

Process standards are those related to the practice of nursing and identify how nursing is performed. There are several types of process standards including nursing care standards, procedures, protocols, position descriptions, and performance standards. There is frequently confusion as to what is a structure standard and what is a process standard. A structure standard may state that there shall be procedures to guide nursing staff and nursing practice. The procedure itself, however, is a process standard as it outlines how to perform a certain task. As a general guide, anything that identifies what nurses do in performing care or in fulfilling their professional roles can be considered a process standard. They are the "doing part" of nursing.

Nursing care standards are another type of process standard and are developed for groups of patients, usually by medical diagnosis or nursing diagnosis. For example, a nursing care standard by medical diagnosis of the patient who had a normal vaginal delivery would identify all nursing activities required from admission to discharge. A nursing standard by nursing diagnosis would relate to the management of a patient who had a normal vaginal delivery but who also has a knowledge deficit.

Outcome standards focus on results. This is one of the more difficult standards for nurses to identify as the tendency is to focus on the provision of care rather than the achievement of specific outcomes. Unless the desired outcome of care is clearly identified and communicated, ritual nursing care will be provided with little ongoing evaluation to see if the goal is being achieved. Process becomes the major focus. Outcome standards frequently relate to education and self-care as well as the desired physiologic status. Experienced nurses know when their patients are ready for dismissal and with guidance can begin to identify the specific outcomes necessary to be achieved. Focusing on outcomes brings a different mindset to practice and has the potential to identify problem areas more readily, as well as to anticipate the potential problems that could arise. The use of outcome standards can become helpful in areas other than direct patient care. Identifying outcome standards in orientation programs, for example, will more likely result in qualified staff than if the focus is only on the orientation process.

Monitoring and Evaluation

Once there is administrative commitment to quality and practice and performance standards have been developed, the monitoring and evaluation process can be initiated. The first question to be answered is, Who is responsible to coordinate the quality-improvement process? While the nursing administrator is ultimately responsible for the quality of nursing care provided, the coordination of day-to-day activities is usually delegated, either to one individual or to a committee. Either system is workable as long as it is clearly understood that the responsibility of the individual or committee is coordination, not monitoring and evaluation. If quality in nursing occurs at the bedside, the provider of that care must be involved in monitoring and evaluating the quality of care provided.

The next task is to develop an overall quality-improvement plan for the nursing department, which will outline responsibilities and the process of monitoring and evaluating. While the coordinator or committee may actually write the plan, input from managers and staff should be solicited. In addition, the nursing department quality-improvement plan must be coordinated with the organization's quality-improvement plan and should support the organization's mission, as well as the nursing department's philosophy or theory of practice.

The monitoring and evaluation model outlined in the JCAHO publication, *Examples of Monitoring and Evaluation in Special Care Units* (1988) provides detailed step-by-step instructions that can be used as a guide, both in writing and implementing the plan.[11] While it is not necessary for each unit to have its own plan, once the nursing department's plan is developed, consideration may be given for its use as a guide in assisting managers in the development of a similar plan for their units. This could be done as an educational workshop with the managers actually developing the plan as each step is described. Then at the end of the workshop, the plan would be completed. This would ensure that the managers understood the monitoring and evaluation process and would provide them with a completed document. It is difficult for managers to find time to develop these types of projects on their own because of many other demands made on them.

First, the plan must define the responsibilities of the vice president of nursing, the coordinator or committee, and each member of the nursing staff. Professional, technical, and clerical staff all influence quality and should each have a clear understanding of their responsibility in the monitoring and evaluation process. The next step would be to define the scope of nursing practice provided within the organization. For the department, the description would be global, for example, specifying services or specialties, levels of care, outreach activities, and type of nursing care delivery system.

Third, the aspects of care to be monitored and evaluated must be identified. This could include areas such as medication administration, patient safety, readmission, high-volume or high-risk patients, problem-prone patients or nursing care activities, or patient satisfaction. The plan should specify the number of aspects of care to be monitored at any one time. It is better to select one or two important aspects of care and concentrate efforts rather than attempt too much and be ineffective. Additionally, monitoring and evaluation activities take time, and it is important that staff participate without feeling frustration due to increased workload.

The fourth step in the plan is to define indicators and their selection process. Indicators are measurable elements of care; they may relate to structure, process, or outcome. Structure elements may be equipment, policies, or other resources used to provide patient care. Process elements relate to the provision of care; they include those functions which are carried out when care is provided, such as assessments, education, tests, or medication administration. Outcome elements are the results achieved; they may be either positive or negative. The indicators chosen should only be those that significantly influence or demonstrate quality outcomes; otherwise there will be little commitment by staff to making improvements to eliminate variances. It is also important that indicators not focus primarily on documentation, but involve patient feedback as well as staff observations.

The fifth step requires that thresholds or levels of compliance be established for each indicator. Thresholds are the desired level of compliance and are high for positive indicators such as "nursing assessments completed within one hour of admission" and low for negative indicators such as "infections in the Neonatal ICU." When positive thresholds are not met, or negative thresholds are exceeded, extensive review and evaluation are conducted to determine the cause. Thresholds may differ for each indicator depending on the importance of that indicator to the patient's well-being. As a general rule, positive indicators should never be lower than 80%, preferably 90%, while negative thresholds should be under 5%. There may be times when 100% or 0% are appropriate. If an indicator is so serious as to be critical to the welfare of the patient, 100% or 0% thresholds would ensure that all variations are evaluated.

The sixth and seventh steps in the plan are data collection and analysis. The data collection process includes identifying data resources, forms for documentation, sample size, and length of time to gather data and monitor a specific indicator. The most frequently criticized aspect of quality-improvement programs is the lack of focus on analysis of data. Many programs focus on data collection and reporting rather than analysis and corrective action. If the data show variations, a complete analysis will show that the variation will fall into one of three categories: knowledge, behavior, or system variances. It is essential the plan require that this step be completed as it is the basis for the eighth step.

The eighth step explains how to implement actions that will correct variations. The most frequent type of corrective action is education. While this is appropriate in many situations, the plan should assist in recognizing the ineffectiveness of implementing actions that do not relate to the true cause of the variation. Frequently, variations believed to be due to knowledge or behavior are really system problems. The plan should emphasize the need for multidisciplinary efforts to correct system problems as nursing cannot correct these alone. Included in this step is the need for assigning specific time frames for implementation and follow-up review, as well as identifying responsibility for implementing the actions.

The ninth step defines how to assess the effectiveness of corrective actions, including how long monitoring and evaluation should continue once the action is implemented and the process to follow if the action taken did not resolve the variation. The last step in the nursing quality-assurance plan addresses the communication process. Communication should occur on all appropriate levels, including the unit or units involved, the nursing department as a whole, and then the organization's quality-improvement program. From there, the information eventually is reported to the board of directors who hold final accountability for care provided within the organization. Various forms should be provided to ensure complete documentation of the monitoring and evaluation process. However, it is important that the documentation be streamlined, easy to follow, and yet clearly demonstrate quality improvements.

Implementation of Unit-Based Quality Improvement

For unit-based quality improvement to be operational, the nurse manager must demonstrate knowledge and commitment to quality as an ongoing process, not a program that is put in place to appease reviewers. The nurse manager must demonstrate this commitment through expectations of staff performance and a determination to identify and correct any problem that negatively influences the care provided to patients on that unit. The nurse manager who is skilled in problem-solving techniques will have little difficulty in implementing a unit-based quality-improvement plan.

It is crucial to the success of the quality-improvement process for unit staff to understand that the focus of nursing quality improvement is on nursing practice, not medical practice. This is also an important factor organization-wide as each professional group begins quality-improvement activities. It is also necessary that nurses be involved in the planning as well as the implementation of quality improvement. Nurses do not want to provide poor care. A thorough understanding of the quality-improvement process will assist them to recognize the need to evaluate quality and assist them in discovering areas for change that will benefit patients. The focus must be on improving care rather than checking documentation or punitive actions for variances.

For staff who have never participated in quality-improvement activities, there may be some reluctance to spend the time and effort required. Some may state that care is good and such a program is a waste of time—time that could better be spent providing care, especially with staff shortages. A helpful exercise to stimulate discussion and demonstrate the purpose and need for quality improvement could be to discuss a specific patient situation that could have been prevented or specific recurring problems that detract from quality outcomes. In order to recognize the value of quality improvement, staff need to first recognize a need for improvement.

Some staff may view quality improvement as a responsibility of the nurse manager. If someone is always available to check the staff's work, they may not develop the professional's sense of accountability. It is important to emphasize the individual's responsibility to see care is provided correctly the first time. In preparing staff for involvement in quality improvement, the nurse manager may need to change management style in order for staff to begin developing more of a sense of autonomy and accountability.

Education of the staff should include terminology as well as procedure and individual responsibility. As with any concept, terms such as *indicators, thresholds,* and *data collection* must be defined with examples so that there is no mystery about the process.

Unit-Based Quality-Assurance Process

If the nursing department determines that each unit develop a unit-specific quality-improvement plan, the format should mirror the nursing department plan, but the content would be specific to that unit. The scope of practice would identify patient types, treatment modalities, educational programs, and nursing care delivery systems utilized on the unit, as well as bed capacity and staff mix. For example, patient elements to include on a postpartum service would be patients with vaginal and cesarean section deliveries and sterilizations. If mother and baby care are practiced, newborns would be added. If the unit provides care to high-risk and antepartum patients, they would be included. A gynecologic service may include patients from medical and surgical gynecology areas, perhaps gynecologic oncology. Treatment modalities could include chemotherapy or hyperalimentation. Usually this information can be contained in one paragraph and simply provides an overview of the unit. Responsibilities relating to quality improvement for each level of staff should be identified with the nurse manager responsible to ensure quality care is provided, monitored, and evaluated. The coordination can be delegated to a unit coordinator or a unit committee. It is important that the coordination responsibility be rotated among the staff to provide equal opportunity and responsibility for participation. The plan would then describe how the quality-improvement process is carried out on the unit.

Important Aspects of Care

With or without a written unit-based quality-improvement plan, there should be a clearly defined procedure to determine the important unit-specific aspects of care to be monitored and evaluated. While the nursing department may define department-wide care aspects such as medication administration, which all units would monitor and evaluate, these should be limited in number and spread over time; the time frame is usually one year, so that each unit can also select areas unique to that service. The staff need to be involved in developing a list that should include patient diagnoses—those that are high-volume, high-risk, and problem-prone patients or nursing activities.

To identify high-volume patients, review the discharge statistics over the past year to determine which patient types are most frequently cared for on the unit. Memory is not always reliable, and an actual count from the medical records department will be helpful. From this list of diagnoses staff can also identify those patient groups that are at high risk for complications. In selecting high-risk patients for review, the staff should concentrate on those in whom nursing plays a major role in the quality outcome. While this may seem true for all patients, some will be more so than others. Other areas to review could be infection rates, transfers to intensive care units, or readmissions. From these resources, several patient groups can be identified to represent the high-volume, high-risk, or problem-prone patient for possible quality-improvement review.

The staff must also review nursing practice to determine specific skills or practice responsibilities that have significant impact on quality patient outcomes. In the labor and delivery unit, this might include interpreting fetal monitor strips. In the neonatal intensive care unit, it may be a technical skill such as insertion of umbilical catheters or an educational responsibility such as teaching cardiopulmonary resuscitation skills to parents of infants discharged on apnea monitors. Several areas of nursing practice should be identified and added to the quality-improvement list.

There should also be some thought given to patient involvement in the quality-improvement process. Staff can identify the types of patient or family complaints most frequently expressed either verbally or through written questionnaires. These may range from lack of timely response to call lights, lengthy waits for pain medication, or complaints on visitor limitations. Nursing is a service profession and patient satisfaction with that service is important to the profession as well as to the organization. One or two of the most frequent complaints can then be added to the list. Once these areas have been explored, the staff can review the list and add any other aspect of care they intuitively believe may be a concern. Many times these additions are the most important. Nurses on the unit know where deficiencies are once they become alert to the quality-improvement process.

There should also be discussion with physicians who admit patients to the unit to determine their perceptions of the nursing care provided on the unit. They may have specific areas of concern that can be included in the quality-improvement process. Involving them not only communicates nursing's commitment to quality, but will encourage joint discussions on patient concerns which will benefit both patients and staff. Additionally, physicians may be more willing to participate in those educational programs determined to be needed.

When this list is complete, the staff need to prioritize the items. Prioritization is important as it forces nurses to make a choice. Too often, nurses have difficulty prioritizing activities or concerns and are unable to focus their efforts to be most effective. The top priorities should be those the staff believe have the most impact on the overall quality of the unit or those patient types they believe are having less than quality outcomes.

Initially it may be difficult for staff to identify these important aspects of care and prioritize them. In these situations, short-term concurrent reviews may be conducted on high-volume patients to assist the staff in determining if there are quality concerns. A quick method to use in conducting these studies is to use the nursing standard of care for that particular patient group, select four to six major indicators from the standard, set a threshold, and review the next 10 to 15 patients to see if the threshold is met. This can be done during the patient stay or at time of discharge. If there is inconsistency or a major lack of compliance noted, that patient type would require further monitoring and evaluating. If not, another diagnosis or nursing activity could be reviewed. This is a useful screening process to prevent monitoring and evaluation activities on inappropriate aspects of care. As staff become more knowledgeable of the quality-improvement process, they will be able to identify possible quality concerns in their daily activity.

Some nursing departments require units to develop a yearly calendar of quality-improvement activities. The calendar shows which aspects of care are to be monitored and evaluated, in which months of the year, and for how long. While this may be necessary to ensure a variety of areas are monitored and evaluated, there should be flexibility allowed. A preferable method is to prioritize the aspects of care, choose the first two, and initiate monitoring and evaluation activities for one to three months during which time various corrective actions can be instituted. If there is an aspect of care that is shown to have serious quality deficits and requires more effort to correct, a longer period of time may be necessary to resolve the concern. Efforts in this aspect of care should continue rather than be given to another topic or result in double work. The major reason for a calendar is to eliminate lengthy monitoring and evaluation activities that do not result in resolution of the problem or to monitor and evaluate areas in which no real problems are demonstrated.

Indicators and Threshold

Once the important aspects of care are prioritized, indicators and thresholds need to be defined. An important aspect of care may be the high-volume vaginal delivery patient. The indicator might be, "All patients will verbalize understanding of infant care prior to discharge." Indicators should be limited to the two to three major elements that truly influence quality for that group of patients. Each indicator would have a threshold or level of compliance established. The overall nursing department plan should provide guidance in selecting appropriate thresholds.

Indicators should be selected from preexisting sources that are available and familiar to nursing staff. Sources can include nursing care standards, policies, procedures, or position descriptions. Department protocols are an important resource. Protocols are frequently developed to provide a guide for nursing practice in high-risk areas of practice and for new treatment modalities. Smith-Marker states, "Protocols define appropriate nursing action for effective management of common patient care problems. . . . Protocols differ from procedures in that procedures are task-oriented while protocols relate to ongoing nursing management of patient care problems."[10] She further identifies five areas for protocols: managing patients both on invasive and noninvasive equipment; diagnostic, therapeutic, or prophylactic interventions requiring nursing care; physiologic states; psychologic states; and selected nursing diagnoses. Protocols can be of three different types: independent, dependent, or interdependent. Independent protocols are those that are developed by nurses and outline independent nursing activities that are initiated on nursing judgment. An example of areas for independent protocols would be nursing diagnoses or noninvasive equipment or testing. Dependent protocols are those requiring a physician

order before initiation and those containing medical orders. These are frequently used in intensive care units or to cover emergency management of
patients. Interdependent protocols are those that contain both independent and
dependent nursing activities. These protocols also require a physician order to
initiate because of the medical orders involved. Interdependent protocols are
developed jointly by physicians and nurses. Both dependent and interdependent
protocols frequently become a departmental standard approved by the appropriate medical department and are followed on all patients unless a physician
orders otherwise.

Data collection is frequently considered to be a time-consuming process and of   *Data Collection*
little interest to staff. Efforts should be made to utilize current documentation   *and Analysis*
and activities rather than develop new ones. In organizations fortunate enough
to have computerized information systems that can generate the appropriate
data from patient records, the collection process is streamlined. However, this is
usually not the case. When selecting criteria, thought needs to be given to how
the data will be obtained. If collection is from charts, the location in the record
must be identified. A trial run should be completed on two or three charts to see
if the criteria can be located. If not, another method such as direct observation
or patient interview may be required. If patient interviews are necessary, the data
should be obtained during routine patient rounds or during discharge preparation rather than a separate interview. Clerical staff on the unit should be able to
assist in data collection once indicators are selected and chart location determined. This, in fact, may be one of their responsibilities in the quality-
improvement process. Data collection by observation or patient interview can be
shared by all staff as long as the indicators are clearly identified.
    Once the data have been collected, the most important part of the quality-
improvement process begins. This is the analysis of the data. If no deficiencies
are identified after a reasonable sample of patients or activities have been reviewed, the indicator has been met and the staff can move on to the next priority
aspect of care. However, if the data show the thresholds have not been met, a
thorough analysis of the deficit areas is required. Staff involvement in this process is necessary in order to correctly identify which type of deficiency exists:
knowledge—behavior—or organization and system.
    A knowledge deficiency results when staff providing care do not know what
should be done or how to do it effectively. This is most often due to inexperi-
enced employees or to a new patient group or new procedure.
    Behavior deficiencies occur when staff know what should be done, but do not
do it. This is a time when there is frequently a tendency to blame rather than
constructively analyze the situation. Lack of time is frequently used to justify
behavior variations. This is especially true during these times of decreased
length of stay and personnel shortages. In-depth analysis is essential. Questions
to be asked include, Does this deficiency occur with all staff, on all shifts? If so, is
it related to the number or mix of staff on duty? Or is there an unreasonable
expectation that can no longer be met due to other changes? This has been

especially true in the area of patient education on the postpartum unit. Analysis may demonstrate that the indicator is no longer appropriate and must be revised. However, if staff believe the indicator is appropriate, behavior deficiencies need to be addressed in a different manner.

Deficiencies due to the organization or system frequently relate to unavailable supplies or equipment as well as to lack of support systems. Other organizational deficiencies may relate to lack of qualified staff, inadequate funds for orientation and staff education, or policies that inhibit quality care. An example of a policy deficiency may be rigid organization-wide visitation policies that are incompatible with family-centered maternity care philosophy.

Action Plan   Once analysis has been completed and there is agreement as to the root cause of the deficiency, an action plan is developed. Clearly, actions must be appropriate to the cause of the deficiency if quality improvement is to result. This is why analysis is so crucial to the quality-improvement process. Time and money are wasted if actions do not fit the need. Actions must be specific with dates for implementation and responsibilities specifically established. Vague action plans such as developing an educational program for nursing staff are inadequate. The program topic must be specific to the education need, with presentor named and time and place identified for the presentation. Even with knowledge deficiencies, education alone may not be sufficient. Assistance with utilization of the knowledge may be necessary through preceptors, peer support, or clinical care conferences.

Action plans for behavior deficiencies are usually more complex. System changes may be necessary to encourage behavior changes. If staff response to patient requests for pain medication is the deficiency, perhaps the staff can set a unit standard for response times. Clerical personnel who answer patient requests would need to be involved so that requests are routed appropriately. Individual staff behavior deficiencies may require the nurse manager to establish specific responsibility to meet these goals with a behavior change. Punitive action should only be a last resort when all other efforts have failed or the employee refuses to try to improve.

Organizational deficiencies always require multidisciplinary planning unless the deficiency is restricted to the specific nursing unit. Even then, if the nursing system deficiency is one that is present on all nursing units, joint planning with other unit staff should occur. A deficiency that relates to inadequate orientation of staff may require the overall nursing orientation plan to be revised in order to provide new employees prepared to deliver quality care. Deficiencies that cross department boundaries can be difficult to resolve if territoriality is part of the organizational culture. Ideally, these deficiencies should be resolved by those staff most closely involved in the situation. Realistically, it is usually the nurse manager or department director who must initiate the action to attempt to resolve the deficiency. It is important to focus on the lack of quality for the patient rather than inconvenience to staff if interdepartmental planning is to be accomplished.

Action plans must be implemented to be effective. Assignment of responsibility and specific time frames for actions to occur will provide the structure needed to put actions into place.

Once the corrective action has been taken, there needs to be sufficient time allowed for it to be assimilated into daily care activities. The length of time involved will depend on each situation. Follow-up evaluation should not take place until sufficient time has lapsed. For example, presenting an educational program on the fetal monitor strip interpretation will not improve practice the following day. The corrective action plan would include support and coaching for the staff as they work to improve their interpretation skills for a specific length of time. Once this has been completed, follow-up evaluation can be initiated. Sometimes the follow-up evaluation is confused with the support or implementation phase of the corrective action. Simply making a system or procedure change without actively working to put it into effect will rarely be successful. Nurse managers who understand change theory will be better prepared to fully implement change.

*Follow-up
Evaluation*

The nursing department plan should provide guidelines for the follow-up evaluation process. Usually, data collection and analysis are repeated but frequently not for as long a time as the original process. If the analysis shows improvement or correction, the staff need to determine if further monitoring and evaluation are required. Each situation is different, and those closest to the setting can usually make the best decision.

If the follow-up evaluation shows little or no improvement, analysis of both the deficiency and the corrective action will frequently show an incorrect diagnosis as to deficiency type. As in many problem-solving situations, there is a tendency to treat symptoms of the problem rather than the problem itself. It takes skill to get to the basic problem, and it will take staff time to develop this skill if they have little familiarity with the problem-solving process.

There are times when close scrutiny of unresolved behavior deficiencies shows that the issue is not considered by the staff or the nurse manager to truly be a factor in quality care and therefore not worth the effort to change. In these situations it is best to drop the topic and to select an aspect of care that all agree is a major issue. Monitoring and evaluating aspects of care that do not influence quality are a waste of time and resources and will not enlist staff support or participation. If the original effort spent in developing the important aspects of care is well guided, this should not happen.

Documentation of the quality-improvement process is essential as this communicates to the organization nursing's efforts to improve quality. There are usually department-wide nursing forms and documentation guidelines that should be brief and concise, yet document the process and the results obtained. The entire quality-improvement process must show continual improvement in the quality of care provided in the organization. The results of the unit-based quality-improvement efforts should be communicated to all appropriate groups. This includes the unit staff where the activity takes place and the nursing department quality-improvement coordinator where it is incorporated into the total nursing department report for communication throughout the organization.

JCAHO Clinical Indicators

For many years the primary quality-improvement activity in many hospitals was confined to review of mortality and morbidity data and infection rates. It was not until JCAHO began incorporating quality-improvement requirements into the accreditation process that organizational quality-improvement programs began to develop. The initial quality-improvement requirements focused on audits that basically involved lengthy chart reviews. Much of the criticism of JCAHO's quality-improvement process by professionals was that it focused on structure and documentation with little attention paid to patient outcome.

Agenda for Change

In 1987, JCAHO initiated its Agenda for Change—a major research and development project. An important aspect of this project is the survey and accreditation initiative intended to improve the JCAHO's capability to aid and stimulate health care organizations to provide high-quality care. It focuses on both clinical and organizational performance as both are considered essential components of quality. The commission does not propose to judge the quality of care or performance, but rather to evaluate the effectiveness of the organization in ensuring the provision of quality care and quality patient outcomes.

The initiative involved developing valid and reliable clinical, organizational, and management process and outcome indicators. These indicators are defined as measurable dimensions of quality care or appropriate performance. They are developed by task forces of experts chosen for their experience in evaluating quality care in their respective area of practice. The indicators are subjected to extensive testing by practitioners at various test hospitals as well as statistical analysis before they are accepted. The indicators themselves are not meant to be direct measures of quality, but rather to be used as screens to assist health care organizations in identifying possible substandard care requiring full peer review.

Obstetric Clinical Indicators

The first clinical area chosen for indicator development was obstetrics. The task force members and the twelve clinical indicators chosen for beta testing during 1990 are listed in Table 2-1. As the indicators were being refined and discussed throughout the country, there was concern expressed by nurses that there were no nursing indicators of care. This was a concern of nurse members of the task force initially, and much effort was spent in attempting to identify indicators relating to the family-centered maternity care concept, which is primarily a nursing concept. In order to be accepted as an obstetric clinical indicator, the indicator must be concise, measurable, and easily retrieved from the patient record, either through coding or from a portion of the chart that would be consistent nationally. Since there is no coding system in medical records for

TABLE 2-1
Obstetric Care Indicators Summary List

*1. Patients with primary cesarean section for failure to progress.

*2. Patients with attempted VBAC, subcategorized by success or failure.

*3. Patients with excessive maternal blood loss defined by either postdelivery red blood cell transfusion or a low postdelivery hematocrit or hemoglobin (Hct < 22%, Hg < 7 g) or a significant pre- to postdelivery decrease in hematocrit (decrease ≥ 11%) or hemoglobin (decrease ≥ 3.5 g) excluding patients with abruptio placentae or placenta previa.

*4. Patients with diagnosis of eclampsia.

*5. The delivery of infants weighing less than 2500 g, following either induction of labor or repeat cesarean section without medical indications.†

*6. Term infants admitted to a neonatal intensive care unit (NICU) within 24 hours of delivery and with NICU stay greater than 24 hours excluding admissions for major congenital anomalies.

*7. Neonates with Apgar score of 3 or less at 5 minutes and a birthweight greater than 1500 g.

*8. Neonates with a discharge diagnosis of meconium aspiration syndrome requiring either NICU oxygen therapy or admission for greater than 24 hours.

*9. Neonates with a discharge diagnosis of significant birth trauma.†

*10. Term infants with a diagnosis of hypoxic encephalitis or clinically apparent seizure prior to discharge from the hospital of birth.

*11. Deaths of infants or fetuses weighing 500 g or more subcategorized by intrahospital neonatal deaths, prepartum stillborns, and intrapartum stillborns.

*12. Intrahospital neonatal deaths of infants with a birthweight of 750 to 999 g born in a hospital with an NICU.

13. Maternal readmissions within 14 days of delivery.

14. Intrahospital maternal deaths occurring within 42 days postpartum.

15. Infants weighing less than 1800 g delivered in a hospital without an NICU.

16. Neonates transferred from a non-NICU hospital to a NICU hospital.

*The task force has recommended to JCAHO that indicators 1 through 12 be further tested for possible inclusion in the JCAHO performance monitoring system.

†In addition, the Obstetrical Care Task Force believes that all of the above indicators are of value and should be considered for use in individual hospital quality assurance progams.

nursing diagnoses, it was soon recognized that attempting to find nursing diagnoses or other nursing indicator data in patient charts would be impossible on a national level due to the vast differences in nursing records. Therefore, nursing diagnosis indicators are best identified on an individual organizational level. However, this does not mean the obstetric clinical indicators have no significance for nursing.

It is important to recognize that JCAHO's clinical indicators are clinical and are not related to one department or service. Nursing care impacts every patient and has the potential to influence all clinical indicators. This can best be demonstrated with an example. Indicator 3 relates to blood loss during labor, delivery, or postpartum from other than an abruptio placentae or placentae previa. If an organization's rate for excessive blood loss exceeds the threshold rate identified by JCAHO, the organization would conduct a thorough review of these cases. If it was found that the blood loss occurred during delivery, the primary focus would be on the performance of the physician or nurse midwife. However, if the blood loss occurred during the recovery phase, focus would include the nurse's performance including observations, care, and reporting activities. Review of blood loss during labor from any cause would also include scrutiny of the nurse's assessments and performance. Even an indicator such as indicator 2, which deals with vaginal births after cesarean (VBAC), can have significance for nurses. If the VBACs attempted are below the desired threshold and are found to be largely influenced by patient decisions, there may be an opportunity for nurses to develop VBAC education classes for potential patients. If the VBAC success rate is low, there may be a need for education of the labor and delivery nursing staff. Perhaps the staff are uncomfortable with the process, lack accurate information on risks, and are therefore unable to wholeheartedly support the patient during labor. Close review and analysis will show that most of the obstetric clinical indicators have a nursing component as well as a medical component and will frequently involve other departments such as the laboratory and anesthesia services.

Summary

Nurses in general have a major role in monitoring and evaluating the quality of care provided in today's complex health care organizations. Not only do they monitor and evaluate nursing care, but frequently identify potential quality concerns in other disciplines.

Obstetric, gynecologic, and neonatal nurses, with the opportunity to influence the health care of future generations, are particularly key to quality care. Mothers and infants are vulnerable to many risks, and obstetric, gynecologic, and neonatal nurses not only serve as their advocates but provide leadership in developing quality health care services to reduce these risks and promote a healthy, safe outcome. To accomplish these goals, the knowledge of and commitment to quality practice on an individual as well as universal level are mandatory.

References

1. Lang NM: Nurses are involved "closely and constantly" in quality of care. *HMQ* (First quarter), 1987.
2. Beyers M: Quality: The banner for the 1980's. *Nurs Clin N America* 23(3):619, 1988.
3. Pine M, et al.: Total quality management: Is your hospital ready? *AHA* 57(Oct), 1989.
4. Boggs JG: Intensive care unit use and collaboration between nurses and physicians. *Heart Lung* 18(4), 1989, 332–338.
5. Peters TJ, Waterman RH Jr: *In Search of Excellence.* New York, Harper & Row, 1982.
6. Naisbitt J, Aburdene P: *Re-inventing the Corporation.* New York, Warner, 1985.
7. Deming WE: *Quality, Productivity and Competitive Position.* Cambridge, Massachusetts Institute of Technology, 1982.
8. Schmele JA, Foss SJ: The quality management grid: A diagnostic method. *JONA* 19(9):29–34, 1989.

9. Crosby PB: *Quality Is Free.* New York, New American Library, 1979.

10. Smith-Marker CG: *Setting Standards for Professional Nursing: The Marker Model.* St. Louis, CV Mosby, 1988.

11. Joint Commission on Accreditation of Hospitals Organization: JCAHO, *Examples of Monitoring and Evaluation in Special Care Units—1988.* Chicago, JCAHO, 1988.

◆ 3 ◆

Risk Assessment

Joan Drukker Dauphinee

The challenge facing contemporary perinatal health care is to ensure that healthy mothers give birth to healthy infants, both capable of attaining maximum developmental potential. While this goal is mastered for most mother–fetus pairs, some patients experience poor perinatal outcomes—outcomes that might be prevented. Although technologies such as real-time ultrasound, Doppler, and other biochemical and biophysical assessments have enabled caregivers to better view the fetus, no perfect system for risk identification has surfaced. The role of risk assessment for intrapartum patients nevertheless remains vital to planning nursing care. The goal is to identify those mothers and fetuses at risk for developing antepartum, intrapartum, and postpartum or neonatal complications before appropriate intervention can take place. Risk assessment ideally begins prior to conception when preexisting medical and obstetric factors can be identified. At that time interventions can be designed to modify, reduce, or even nullify the risk. Most patients, however, come in for health care in the first trimester and thus may only benefit from assessment following conception.

The causal relationship between obstetric complications and perinatal outcome has long been recognized. In 1862, Little noted that abnormal labor and premature birth could be related to the child's later mental and physical conditions.[1] In 1951, Lilienfeld and Pasamanick showed that five factors—prematurity, multiple births, previous stillbirth, toxemia, and placental abnormalities—were related to cerebral palsy in infancy.[2] In 1958, Butler and Alberman coordinated the "British Perinatal Mortality Study," which reviewed all perinatal deaths over a three-month period.[3] The study identified women who might benefit from intensive prenatal care. Goodwin, Dunne, and Thomas, among others, have observed that multiple risk factors may occur in the same patient with cumulative adverse effects.[4-6] Other risk assessment studies have followed and have demonstrated a correlation between increasing risk and poor outcomes.[7,8]

Risk assessment tools typically evaluate demographic, psychosocial, obstetric, and medical factors, all of which have been identified as potential contributors to poor perinatal outcome. Specified factors are identified as either present or absent in a patient's history or current status, and a scoring system is applied. Some tools assign a number for each contributory factor and a total score is calculated, whereas others may designate that numbers for each factor identified be subtracted from a potentially perfect score. Once a final patient score is calculated, it is compared with a predetermined cutoff point, separating low-risk from high-risk patients. The term *at risk* is often used to differentiate those patients who are currently at high risk from those patients who are at risk for the development of a future problem. Thus, the patient who is currently in preterm labor may be high risk while her nonlaboring counterpart who has a history of previous preterm birth is at risk for preterm labor in the current pregnancy.

The effectiveness of a risk assessment tool lies in its ability to predict those patients who will develop poor perinatal outcomes (sensitivity) and those who will not (specificity). Those patients who are identified as low risk but who subsequently develop complications constitute false negatives, and those classified as at risk but who do not develop complications are false positives. Sensitivity should reach 80% in an effective risk assessment tool, while specificity is generally much higher.[9]

Although the number of factors assessed is variable among different tools, a tool that is highly complex may not be better than a simple and shorter form. Ease of administration is also a consideration, since each patient must be screened. The ideal tool is the shortest form that achieves the greatest sensitivity and specificity.

Dynamic Nature of Risk Assessment

Pregnancy is a dynamic state with a potential for change in risk status. A good risk assessment tool is a concise, legible, systematic method of collecting data that must also address the dynamic changes of pregnancy and the developing fetus (see Table 3-1). It is unclear whether risk assessment during the antepartum period adequately identifies the pregnancy at risk or if the combination of an antepartum assessment with an intrapartum component is a more reliable predictor. Some authors have purported that because of the many changes during labor, intrapartum assessment is the most predictive of outcome, since even antepartum patients at no apparent risk can become high risk in labor.[10-12]

There is no risk assessment method that correctly identifies all poor neonatal or maternal outcomes and even when identified not all problems may be averted. Current interventions may not be effective treatments for problems correctly identified, and thus some morbidity and mortality may simply not be preventable. Other pregnancies may be inappropriately identified as high risk but would never have bad outcomes.

TABLE 3-1
Requirements for a Good Risk Scoring System

Identify the patient at risk for poor perinatal outcome.
Anticipate health care needs of the woman and her fetus.
Predict potential perinatal complications.
Determine appropriate facility and resources for care.
Identify high-risk patients to access additional fees for more intensive care.
Identify candidates for alternative birthing options.
Reflect the dynamic changes of pregnancy.
Be easy to use yet comprehensive.
Facilitate communication among perinatal team members.
Be computer compatible to interpret and evaluate impact and outcome.
Be used for planning health care services.

Hobel developed a complex, comprehensive, specific, and objective perinatal scoring system.[10] The tool involved assessment of 51 prenatal factors and an additional 40 intrapartum and 35 neonatal factors. As well as being comprehensive, the scoring system accounted for changes in maternal and fetal condition over time. Assessment occurred at the initial prenatal visit, and developing problems were noted on subsequent prenatal visits, as were intrapartum and neonatal risk factors. All factors were assigned scores of 1, 5, or 10, and a cumulative antepartum or intrapartum score of 10 or more was considered high risk.

Nesbitt and Aubry devised a simple scoring method applied at the initial prenatal visit, during which only a limited number of factors were scored.[13-15] Of the clinic population, 30% were determined to be at risk as compared with 13% of the private population. Those identified as high risk accounted for almost one half of all poor neonatal outcomes and 60% of the maternal complications.

Numerous studies have demonstrated that, of those identified as high risk (about 25% of the total obstetric population), 25% (13.8% of the total obstetric population) account for only about one half of perinatal morbidity and mortality.[4,16-19] The other half come from the low-risk group (about 75% of the obstetric population).[20] In 1973, Hobel found that 23% of the population identified as low risk before labor subsequently were high risk during labor.[18] He also noted that low-risk antepartum patients met with greater morbidity and mortality than high-risk antepartum patients who did not become high risk during labor. Perhaps more intensive care is provided to patients labeled "high risk" than that given to those labeled "low risk."

Two studies demonstrated that approximately 20% of low-risk term patients screened for admission to a birthing center were subsequently transported to hospitals for additional care.[21,22] In 1989, Marshall compared Hobel's screening tool with the Maternity Center Association's tool.[23] Hobel's assessment achieved a sensitivity of only 33% and a specificity of 65%. The association's tool was more sensitive (88%) but far less specific (10%). Thus, predicting who will experience intrapartum problems is difficult.

To compensate for the dynamic changes of pregnancy, initial risk assessment should be completed as soon as the patient comes in for health care, with reassessment made later in pregnancy. A complete assessment must again be made when the patient is admitted to the labor and delivery unit. The frequency of ongoing evaluation depends on the assignment of antepartum and initial intrapartum risk.

The use of a systematic risk assessment program can result in the inappropriate assignment of risk and *undercalling* and *overcalling* of patient status. A well-known relationship exists between predicted risk and poor neonatal outcome; however, many high-risk patients have good neonatal outcomes. Oftentimes, identification of the high-risk patient results in assignment and implementation of intensive care and more frequent health care appointments. These factors may contribute to improved patient outcome, or perhaps the patient was inappropriately identified and the problem never existed. When overcalling occurs, patients may be subjected to increased testing, some of which may be unnecessary and stressful. When undercalling occurs, failure to identify the true high-risk patient results and, therefore, available intervention is withheld.

Regionalization

Properly identifying patients at risk is crucial to an effective program of regionalized care. The aim of regionalization is to concentrate resources and improve pregnancy outcome. Thus once patients are identified as high risk, appropriate care resources can be identified and patients can be assigned to the most suitable care provider and facility. This may result in consultation outside of the facility or referral to another service within the same facility. It may entail physical transfer of patients across town or across the state. Proper assessment may also identify those patients who require intrapartum transport. If time constraints prevent transport, risk assessment may reliably assist in predicting those patients who will require neonatal resuscitation, stabilization, and possibly transportation to another facility. A program of regionalized care should ensure that patients at highest risk be cared for in a center prepared to provide comprehensive health care services by a multidisciplinary perinatal team as well as a broad spectrum of specialists. Similarly, regionalized care and accurate risk assessment permit low-risk patients to remain in their community and have the safe choice of a hospital or alternative birthing experience.

Assessment Categories

Before nursing care of high-risk patients can be planned and implemented, assessment must be made, including risk assessment by the intrapartum nurse. Generally there are three categories of assessment: medical risk factors, obstetric risk factors, and psychosocial risk factors.

Medical factors include known medical complications that occurred prior to pregnancy or are diagnosed during the pregnancy. These include such disorders as diabetes mellitus, hypertension, sickle cell disease, and lupus. Prepregnancy counseling regarding the effects of these diseases on pregnancy should be offered to women in their childbearing years and should be specifically discussed before patients consider pregnancy. According to Gabbe, Niebyl, and Simpson, "A woman's health before conception influences her ability not only to conceive, but also to maintain pregnancy and to achieve a healthy outcome."[24] Ongoing assessments are then made during pregnancy regarding the effect of the disease on pregnancy and vice versa. Appropriate family members should always be included in these discussions, if the patient wishes.

Included in medical factors is a careful genetic personal and family history. Risks to the fetus are identified, and follow-up is provided as indicated. Nutritional and lifestyle factors should also be included as part of the medical assessment. Extremes in stature and alterations in nutrition may affect pregnancy outcome and are often amenable to nutritional therapy. Lifestyle issues such as smoking and substance abuse are assessed, and treatment offered as necessary.

Obstetric risk factors include issues regarding reproductive history such as previous preterm delivery, as well as conditions specific to the current pregnancy such as fetal size, pregnancy-induced hypertension, or placenta previa or placental abruption.

Psychosocial risk factors, assessed as socioeconomic and psychological status, may affect the pregnancy, treatment, and compliance to treatment. These include demographic data such as age, ethnicity, marital status, and level of education. This assessment should include fathers as well as mothers and at times siblings, grandparents, and other significant persons. Workplace exposure of the woman and her partner is also assessed. Adaptation to the tasks of pregnancy as well as attachment are important aspects of the psychological assessment. Psychological disorders should also be recognized.

Documentation

Good documentation, in the patient's record, and risk assessment must be concomitant and must continue throughout the antepartum, intrapartum, and postpartum periods. Long-hand SOAPE (subjective, objective, assessment, plan, and evaluation) notes and detailed paragraph notes are difficult to use when a patient's condition rapidly changes during the intrapartum period. Ongoing dynamic assessment can be most effectively accomplished with a flow sheet and labor curve. Optimally all the information must be contained on one or two pages—medical forms for oxytocin, magnesium sulfate, and vital signs should not be separate. Assessment wording is critical. If the fetal scalp pH is abnormal, the value should be reported and interpretations such as "fetal distress" avoided. According to ACOG and NAACOG, both nurses and physicians should comply with these recommendations.[25,26] Terminology must always be objective and accurate.

Once risk assessment is accomplished, a plan of care is developed by both the nurse and physician. If the patient is at no apparent risk, care is augmented with a standard care plan. Once risk is ascertained, the development of an individual plan of care is essential to provide the perinatal team with information for direction and continuity. Discussion concerning the patient's condition with the perinatal team will aid in continuing management. This is particularly true when a variety of caregivers are involved.

Studney et al. designed a computerized risk assessment system called COSTAR.[27] Although this system was designed for use by the entire hospital, each specialty had its own subsystem tailored to individual needs. The system provided consistent assessment and had also decreased previously duplicated paperwork. For example, the prenatal record was automatically included in the patient's hospital chart while a copy was sent to the nursery. Storing assessment results by computer facilitated collection of data, which were then readily retrieved and used for quality-assurance activities as well.

Starting a new risk assessment system is often difficult and met with resistance from both nurses and physicians. Preplanning with input from staff may encourage a smoother transition. In addition, all tools should be tested for appropriateness in the facility before other assessment systems are deleted. Ease of use and completeness of data are essential in gaining the support of the users. Studney and co-workers found unanimous and enthusiastic acceptance among staff concerning computer-generated assessments, even after 2½ years of use. The staff noted that continued availability of legible, concise data organized in standard format aided care management.[27]

Risk Assessment and the Caregiver

Good record keeping and history taking are essential in detecting patient risk; assessment forms may make caregivers aware of problems by requiring complete data collection. The use of forms, whether written or computer generated, provides a less-biased assessment than that obtained by practitioners based on clinical expertise and experience. Wall and Lesinski suggested that risk assessment systems are imprecise and may not be better than *good clinical judgment*.[12,28,29] Of course, not all practitioners have good clinical judgment. Some may never have learned it, and this is where a risk assessment system may help guide their judgment. Others such as nursing students, medical students, and residents may not have the skills to make assessments. A risk assessment tool, however, can often help students learn to collect complete data. Still others may have good skills to care for the normal patient, but are not able to manage the high-risk patient. Here a risk assessment system can help identify patients who should be referred or transferred to another delivery system. A systematic risk assessment tool may also help the practitioner keep up with ongoing changes in practice and technology.

In 1967, Drinkwater found that pilots made errors when their senses were overloaded.[30] Based on this work, McDonald demonstrated that medical errors were made because of the overwhelming amount of information that physicians had to continually process and not because of flaws in learning.[31] French then showed that the amount of data available per time unit is more than physicians can process without error.[32] Although risk assessments do not dictate management nor are they meant to replace practitioners, they do help to collect and store data that can then be used to identify those patients at risk. To decrease risk, the data cannot be ignored.

Nurses often perform the initial assessment when the patient comes to the labor and delivery area. Risk factors from the antepartum period should be clearly identified so they will not be missed as the intrapartum assessment is initiated. An intrapartum form designed to address risk assessment can guide the nurse and also be useful as findings are reported to the physician. The risk assessment form can be used as a checklist during verbal communication and also as space provided to document the content and time of physician verification.

Financial Aspects

Identifying high-risk patients may not be economically profitable. Many facilities providing high-risk care are finding current fee structures inadequate, because these patients are often charged the same rate as low-risk patients even though their care is more costly. As risk assessment facilitates identification of high-risk patients, intensive nursing care and additional equipment and resources can then be made available.

A well-defined classification system for labor and delivery patients has not yet been developed, although acuity systems are being used for patient assessment in other areas of the hospital. Part of the problem lies in the dynamic nature of pregnancy. DeJoseph, Petree, and Ross set up a simple system to identify high-risk patients and charge fees different than those charged for low-risk patients.[33] The cost difference of care for low- and high-risk patients was examined to assign the charge. Freitas and co-workers and Schwamb described classification systems for patients in labor that included acuity of the patients as well as length of time in the labor and delivery area.[34,35] Patient classification systems also help to assess and plan for staffing needs based on patient acuity. Used in conjunction with a call system, the hospital can maintain average staffing and call in additional nurses for peak times—the need identified either by acuity or numbers of patients. If a low census is noted, staffing can be decreased as necessary, decreasing costs and providing better patient coverage and, as a result, better patient care. Retention of nurses may also be improved because unscheduled overtime is decreased.

Risk assessment systems, although not perfect, can help caregivers identify high-risk patients who may need intensive care during their pregnancy and delivery. However, because of the dynamic state of pregnancy, it should never be taken for granted that patients will remain without risk or that the risk will not resolve. Careful ongoing systematic assessment helps to identify most high-risk patients in a timely manner during the antepartum and intrapartum periods. The risk assessment tool must be used by health care providers who are able to interpret the results and care for patients identified as high risk or, when appropriate, identify the need for patient transport. Only then will risk assessment be effective in the alteration of poor perinatal outcome.

References

1. Little WJ: On the influence of abnormal parturition, difficult labours, premature birth and asphyxia neonatorum on the mental and physical condition of the child, especially in relation to deformities. *Trans Obstet Soc London* 38:293, 1862.
2. Lilienfeld AM, Pasamanick B: The association of maternal and fetal factors with the development of cerebral palsy and epilepsy. *Am J Obstet Gynecol* 70:93, 1951.
3. Butler NR, Alberman ED: Perinatal problems. The Second Report of the 1958 British Perinatal Mortality Survey. Edinburgh and London, 1969.
4. Goodwin JW, Dunne JT, Thomas BW: Antepartum identification of the fetus at risk. *Canad Med Ass J* 101:57, 1969.
5. Halliday HL, Jones PK, Jones SL: Method of screening obstetric patients to prevent reproductive wastage. *Obstet Gynecol* 55:656, 1980.
6. Precht HRF: Neurological sequelae of prenatal and perinatal complications. *Brit Med J* 4:763, 1967.
7. Edwards LE, Barrada I, Tateau R, Hakanson EY: A simplified antepartum risk-scoring system. *Obstet Gynecol* 54(2):237, 1979.
8. Akhtar J, Sehgal N: Prognostic value of a prepartum and intrapartum risk-scoring method. *Southern Med J* 73:411, 1980.
9. Richards IDG, Roberts CJ: The "at risk" infant. *Lancet* 2:711–713, 1967.
10. Hobel CJ: Identification of the patient at risk, in Bolognese RJ, Schwarz RH (eds.): *Perinatal Medicine*, (2nd ed). Baltimore, Williams & Wilkins, 1977.
11. Sokol RJ, Rosen MG, Stojkov J, Chik L: Clinical application of high-risk scoring on an obstetric service. *Am J Obstet Gynecol* 128:652, 1977.
12. Wall EM: Assessing obstetric risk. A review of obstetric scoring systems. *J Fam Pract* 27:153, 1988.
13. Aubry RH: Identification of the high-risk perinatal patient, in Aladjem S, Brown AK (eds.): *Perinatal Intensive Care*. St Louis, C.V. Mosby, 1977.
14. Aubry RH, Pennington JC: Identification and evaluation of high-risk pregnancy: The perinatal concept. From the Department of Obstetrics and Gynecology, State University of New York, Upstate Medical Center, Syracuse, New York, 1973.
15. Nesbitt REL, Aubry RH: High-risk obstetrics; II: Value of semiobjective grading system in identifying the vulnerable group. *Am J Obstet Gynecol* 103:972, 1969.
16. Chez RA, Cefalo RC, Merkatz IR: Why it's important to help patients prepare for pregnancy. *Contemp Obstet Gynecol* 33:64, 1989.
17. Feldstein MS, Butler NR: Analysis of factors affecting perinatal mortality. *Br J Prev Soc Med* 19:128, 1965.
18. Hobel CJ, Hyvarinen MA, Okada DM, Oh W: Prenatal and intrapartum high-risk screening. *Am J Obstet Gynecol* 117:1, 1973.
19. Hobel CJ: Recognition of the high-risk pregnancy woman, in Spellacy WN (ed.): *Management of the High Risk Pregnancy*. Baltimore, University Park Press, 1975.
20. Wilson RW, Schifrin BS: Is any pregnancy low risk? *Obstet Gynecol* 55:653, 1980.
21. Dillon FT, Brenan BA, Dwyer J, et al: Midwifery, 1977. *Am J Obstet Gynecol* 130:917–926, 1978.

22. Faison JB, Pisani BJ, Douglas RG, et al: The Childbearing Center: An alternative birth setting. *Obstet Gynecol* 54:527–532, 1979.
23. Marshall VA: A comparison of two obstetric risk assessment tools. *J Nurse-Midwif* 34:1, 1989.
24. Gabbe SG, Niebyl JR, Simpson JL: *Obstetrics: Normal and Problem Pregnancies*. New York, Churchill Livingstone, 1986.
25. American College of Obstetrics and Gynecology and Nurses' Association of the American College of Obstetrics and Gynecology: Electronic fetal monitoring. Joint Statement, Washington, DC, ACOG/NAACOG, 1986.
26. NAACOG: Nursing responsibilities in implementing intrapartum fetal heart rate monitoring. Statement of the Organization for Obstetric, Gynecologic, and Neonatal Nurses. October, 1988.
27. Studney DR, Adams JB, Gorbach A, et al: A computerized prenatal record. *Obstet Gynecol* 50:82, 1977.
28. Wall EM, Sinclair AE, Nelson J, Toffler WL: The relationship between assessed obstetric risk and maternal-perinatal outcome. *J Fam Pract* 28:35, 1989.
29. Lesinski J: High-risk pregnancy: Unresolved problems of screening, management, and prognosis. *Obstet Gynecol* 48:599, 1975.
30. Drinkwater BL: Performance of civil aviation pilots under conditions of sensory overload. *Aerosp Med* 38:164–168, 1967.
31. McDonald CJ: Protocol-based computer reminders, the quality of care and the non-perfectibility of man. *N Engl J Med* 295:1351, 1976.
32. French N: Study suggests mental saturation causes MD oversights. *Comp World* June, 1977.
33. DeJoseph JF, Petree BJ, Ross W: Costing and charging: Pricing care in OB. *Nurs Manage* 15:36, 1984.
34. Freitas CA, Helmer T, Cousins N: The development and management uses of a patient classification system for a high-risk perinatal center. *JOGNN* Sept./Oct. 1987.
35. Schwamb J: A maternity patient classification system. *Nurs Manage* 20:66, 1989.

4
◆ ◆ ◆

Psychosocial Implications of High-Risk Intrapartum Care

Katharyn A. May

A significant minority of childbearing women and their families experience complications that require high-risk perinatal management. Conditions once regarded as beyond effective perinatal management are now more or less routinely managed in hospitals across the country. Advances in perinatal care have changed the appearance and function of conventional labor and delivery units, such that they now are specialized intensive care units with all of the attendant technological supports.

As a result, nursing responsibilities in the care of high-risk patients and their families during the intrapartum period have expanded dramatically. As is often the case, this rapid change in practice is reflected in an emphasis on technological aspects of care, both in the nursing literature and in continuing education efforts. While this focus is essential, it is insufficient alone. The psychosocial needs of families experiencing a high-risk labor and birth are urgent and complex and fall almost exclusively within the nurse's realm of responsibility.

The unique psychosocial needs of the high-risk intrapartum patient are universally acknowledged in the nursing literature. Truly expert clinicians are recognized as those who address these needs as an intrinsic part of their care. Clinicians use a kind of shorthand when describing care for such patients, "We know good support when we see it, and we know when it's needed." However, it is unclear how we come to know these things. Effective psychosocial support of high-risk intrapartum patients is still largely a product of the individual nurse's personal style and clinical trial-and-error.

Effective psychosocial care is difficult to teach, and even more difficult to measure or document, because it has been inadequately described and studied. Clinical and research literature in perinatal nursing remains relatively silent on the *specifics* of providing specialized psychosocial care to high-risk patients and their families during the critical intrapartum period. Statements such as "the nurse should provide sensitive and caring support" are far too general to provide clear direction. Many questions remain unanswered: What is effective support? What does it look like? When is such support needed? Under what conditions? How do we know it makes a difference?

Without more specificity, documentation of patient needs and necessary nursing resources, instruction on how to provide psychosocial care, and validation of the effectiveness of psychosocial care in the intrapartum period are hampered. Although psychosocial nursing care is not well described, and even less well understood from a research perspective, research indicates that psychological distress in the perinatal period can have lingering effects on individual and family well-being.[1,2] Further, it is clear that the dramatic and sometimes frightening intrapartum period can leave lasting impressions. It can enhance or inhibit the family's ability to integrate the birth experience into their lives and then make it difficult to move on to productive parenthood or to resolution of their perinatal loss, if that is the end result.[3,4]

This chapter will first review the growing research literature on psychosocial implications of at-risk childbearing, with a focus on causes and effects of distress in the perinatal period. Nursing responsibilities for psychosocial assessment and support during the intrapartum period will then be outlined, and expected outcomes for psychosocial nursing care will be proposed.

Given the lack of a well-developed body of research on the psychosocial aspects of high-risk labor and birth, these recommendations for specific assessment and intervention strategies should be seen only as guidelines against which to evaluate current practice. Much more focused attention by clinicians and researchers is needed before specific recommendations for psychosocial care of high-risk intrapartum patients and their families can be proposed with confidence.

Causes and Effects of Psychological Distress in the Perinatal Period

The transition to parenthood is a stress-producing process involving adaptation by both partners, even under the most favorable of circumstances.[5] Several studies have reported that families who have higher levels of potentially disruptive stress during pregnancy are also more likely to go on to develop perinatal complications.[6-8] The evidence is not sufficiently strong to suggest that high levels of preexisting psychosocial stress *cause* perinatal complications. However, nurses must be alert to the possibility that high-risk intrapartum patients and their families are not only dealing with the situational stressor of a high-risk condition, but also may be carrying a stress burden from preexisting stressors.

Preexisting Sources of Perinatal Stress

Information about a family's level of psychosocial adaptation during pregnancy may be available to the labor and delivery nurse only at the most general level, in anecdotal information on the prenatal record (*e.g.,* "pregnancy unplanned," "spousal conflict during pregnancy," "questionable social support available to mother," "maternal ambivalence about pregnancy." Admittedly, such factors are not within the scope of nursing management in the intrapartum period, even if there was sufficient documentation about the patient's psychosocial status. However, there is growing research evidence that preexisting distress and the effects of cumulative life stress can also directly affect individual and family well-being in the perinatal period.

ANXIETY, DEPRESSION, AND HIGH PERINATAL RISK

Anxiety and depression are emotional states that can be thought of as distress responses to stress. Some anxiety and depression are normal in both partners during the childbearing year, since this major life event demands changes in relationships and lifestyle. However, several studies link higher levels of emotional distress during pregnancy with poorer perinatal outcomes, as well as poorer family functioning in the childbearing year.[7-10] Mercer and others found levels of anxiety and depression were higher among parents experiencing a high-risk pregnancy than they were among those with a normal pregnancy, as would be expected; however, one half of high-risk women and almost one third of their mates demonstrated mood disturbance at levels suggestive of clinical depression.[1] Clearly, many families can be expected to enter the high-risk intrapartum experience with depleted emotional resources, especially if they have been coping with a high-risk pregnancy.

SELF-ESTEEM AND ADAPTATION TO AT-RISK CHILDBEARING

Several studies have focused on maternal self-esteem as a factor that may predict how a woman adapts to the reality of at-risk childbearing. In a study of women hospitalized for a high-risk pregnancy, low maternal self-esteem, high negative life stress, low social support, and an inadequate or absent mate relationship were predictive of high-obstetric risk.[11]

Self-esteem may not necessarily be of great importance in isolation, but may have more significance when taken into account with other aspects of a family's situation. For example, the results of a longitudinal study of women experiencing a high-risk pregnancy and birth showed that women with high self-esteem who experienced intimacy with spouse and·friends were likely to feel well-supported and as though they coped well with this stress.[12] Women with low self-esteem but adequate spousal support fared almost as well as women with high self-esteem. However, women with low self-esteem who had high intimacy with their own family of origin but not with spouse or friends reported they felt less well supported, experienced more significant levels of depression, and coped less well with an at-risk birth. Perhaps low self-esteem in a childbearing woman contributes to a certain isolation and a reluctance to distance herself from the family of origin. When an at-risk pregnancy results, the woman may perceive that she is getting insufficient support from those around her. This situation may characterize many young mothers who require high-risk perinatal care today.

HIGH-RISK PREGNANCY AS A PRELUDE TO HIGH-RISK LABOR AND DELIVERY

In a now classic work, Cohen identified four factors that contributed to maladaptation in pregnancy and the neonatal period: previous adverse experience in childbearing, conflicts or problems in support systems, inadequate preparation for childbearing or childrearing, and maternal health concerns.[13] Most, if not all, of these factors may have been present during pregnancy in a woman who now requires high-risk intrapartum care.

Further, if prescribed antepartum care has required the family to make major adjustments, such as loss of maternal employment, activity restriction, and multiple hospitalizations, the nurse can assume that the family will enter the intrapartum experience with a high level of preexisting stress. Support systems may be strained or depleted due to demands during pregnancy.[14] Assets the family usually uses to cope with stress, such as a satisfactory marital relationship, may not be optimal because of the challenge of coping with the high-risk pregnancy. Financial worries may be overwhelming, if there has been a loss of maternal employment during pregnancy and the family now faces the prospect of a high-risk delivery and neonatal course. These factors may be pushed into the background as the family copes with immediate events; however, the sum total of these stressors may result in a family system with barely adequate coping resources with which to deal with labor and birth.

EFFECT OF HIGH PERINATAL RISK ON PARENT–FETAL/INFANT ATTACHMENT

An issue frequently raised about the impact of high-risk childbearing is the possible effect on the process of parent–fetal/newborn attachment. The construct of maternal–fetal attachment, addressed in the research literature first by Cranley, suggests that feelings of connection to and protectiveness about the unborn arise for both parents prior to delivery, and factors such as self-esteem, emotional balance, and satisfaction in primary relationships (most often the mate relationship) are thought to enhance this emotional bond.[15]

Kemp and Page examined the relationship between at-risk pregnancy and maternal–fetal attachment in 54 low-risk and 32 high-risk pregnant women.[16] Women who experienced a high-risk pregnancy demonstrated lower self-esteem than their low-risk counterparts, but no differences were found in maternal–fetal attachment. A subsequent study of over 500 high- and low-risk pregnant women and their partners found, as expected, that levels of prenatal attachment are consistently higher in women than they are in their partners.[17] However, similar to Kemp and Page, these investigators found that a high-risk pregnancy requiring hospitalization had no effect on prenatal attachment. Further, this study also showed that factors such as self-esteem, anxiety, depression, or marital satisfaction did not contribute substantially to prenatal attachment in low-risk women and their partners or in high-risk women.

In addition, the relationship between prenatal and postpartum attachment is still not clear. Mercer et al. found that levels of prenatal attachment were not predictive of postpartum attachment in high-risk women or their partners.[1] Factors that appear to contribute to postpartum attachment in parents with a high-risk pregnancy include negative life events stress during pregnancy, self-esteem and sense of parental competence, low levels of depression, and higher perceived social support.

Thus, the consequences of a high-risk pregnancy and birth on the process of prenatal and postpartum attachment are as yet poorly understood, and clearly more research is needed before specific interventions can be recommended. At this point in the development of perinatal nursing practice and research, it may be productive to direct nursing time and energy toward control of environmental stressors, assisting parents in reframing expectations and supporting positive family coping, since these factors may contribute to greater emotional balance and positive adaptation in the postpartum period.

In addition, while preexisting psychological stress may be associated with the development of perinatal complications, the more important issue for nursing is the recognition that high-risk intrapartum patients may already have depleted their coping resources during pregnancy and face the probability of an at-risk birth with this deficit. Even when the pregnancy has been relatively stress-free, the diagnosis of "at risk" in the intrapartum period creates a storm of frightening possibilities with which families must grapple. When complications arise, all members of the family should be considered to be at risk for psychological distress. One source of immediate distress for high-risk childbearing families is the loss of emotional security when their own expectations for a normal birth are not met. This is worsened when the professionals caring for them respond rapidly to an at-risk condition that is difficult for parents to see and comprehend.

Shifting Expectations in the Intrapartum Period: Parental and Professional Perspectives

One of the first consequences of an at-risk intrapartum situation is the loss of the expected and hoped-for normal birth. When long-held expectations for birth are not met and families find themselves in situations unlike any they have experienced before, a period of adaptation is required during which the family re-orients themselves to their changed circumstances. Clearly, the most appropriate psychosocial care can be rendered only if the nurse recognizes what parents' expectations were and how rapidly they may be able to adapt to the new situation.

For the well-prepared, highly educated couple experiencing a "premium pregnancy," expectations for birth may be quite specific and may have focused on "options" such as use of a birthing room, avoidance of analgesia, and the presence of family and other support people. For them, control of the experience, more particularly, the avoidance of medical intervention, may have been an important expectation, because the health of mother and baby was largely assumed.

The reality of an at-risk birth introduces a sense of being helpless and out of control and reduces the usefulness of their coping strategies, which had been focused on achieving a "normal" (*i.e.,* low-intervention) birth. Such parents may very quickly recognize when things are not normal, but they may not be able to "shift gears" to concentrate on new priorities as rapidly as their level of mastery and preparation might suggest.[3]

Other families who are not as well educated, or as well prepared for childbirth, will still respond to unmet expectations in the face of an at-risk birth, although perhaps in different ways. Interventions, such as a cesarean delivery, may be viewed positively in and of themselves.[18,19] However, an at-risk situation introduces new and complicated explanations from professionals, sudden separation from family, and frightening new experiences. In both cases, parents may resist the efforts of professionals to deal with the at-risk condition or may deny that an at-risk condition exists. This behavior may be interpreted as overly controlling, obstructionist, or uninformed. However, what is more likely to be occurring in both of these cases is that parents have not yet shifted to a new set of expectations, already held by professionals, which focuses on doing what is necessary to achieve a positive outcome in the face of increased risk.

Adjusting to Crisis Management: A Major Stress for Families

In the high-risk intrapartum situation, professionals and parents are often adapting at different speeds and responding to different crises. Under the best of circumstances, parents have a limited repertoire of knowledge and experiences with which to cope with childbirth. They adapt to the current situation with difficulty and are unable to anticipate *what may happen* because adapting to *what is* requires all of their available energy. Professionals, on the other hand, adapt more quickly to changed circumstances because of their broader knowledge and experience and move quickly to anticipate what may happen.

Unfortunately, the professional's ability to anticipate sometimes creates rather than diminishes the family's distress, because it widens the gap between what the professional is responding to and what the family is experiencing. As professionals project forward to prevent problems, even as they are dealing with existing ones, they sometimes forget that parents are adapting at a slower pace.

In addition, it is sometimes difficult to determine whether professionals are responding to an actual emergency in which seconds count or to the potential emergency that the professional knows may arise and that can be prevented. In an actual emergency, quick and efficient action is needed, and some aspects of sensitive care must be sacrificed for the sake of effective crisis management. However, when the situation has worsened but no crisis yet exists, professionals nevertheless may still shift into crisis management. This shift occurs rapidly and far outpaces the family's ability to take in and process what is happening to them. An overly brisk transition to crisis management on the part of professionals has been aptly called "treating provider anxiety" or more graphically "the stormtrooper approach to obstetrics."

The stormtrooper approach is characterized by a number of occurrences: rushed or absent explanation of the situation to the woman and her family; no allowance for private discussion before a family decision is required or for privacy of any sort; a pressured quality in interactions; arbitrary and often unnecessary separation of the father or support person from the mother without appropriate follow-up; and (perhaps more common in teaching hospitals) twice as many bodies in the patient's room than are required to manage the situation.

This brisk shift to crisis management may occur without conscious thought and is based on the best of intentions. However, it is not without significant negative consequences. Some of the more disturbing memories and sense impressions parents carry away from the experience of an at-risk birth are those created by unthinking application of stormtrooper obstetrics.[3] Women experiencing unexpected cesarean births report that things "suddenly started moving very fast," with "lots of people in the room, telling (me) what to do"; that moment was intensely frightening and long remembered. Could necessary tasks have been completed with fewer people in the room, with a few moments of quiet while one person gave instructions? How much of the "hurry" was necessary, and how much was a consequence of caregiver anxiety? Fathers routinely spent periods waiting alone during high-risk intrapartum care. Was separation really necessary? In all but the most acute emergencies (which in reality are relatively rare), a more deliberate approach to care and provision of sensitive support is possible and may save patient and family considerable emotional distress.

Saving the family unnecessary distress in the face of an at-risk birth is an important nursing concern. Thus, reducing the environmental stress on families by actively managing the pace at which families are forced to adapt to the professional's mode of crisis management is an appropriate nursing intervention. This is not merely a nicety, since with the emergence of an at-risk condition, the patient and family should be supported in redirecting their energy to coping with the potential for serious loss.

During a complicated pregnancy, fear of potential loss is clearly a stressor affecting women and their families.[1,14] It is reasonable to assume that this fear also operates in the context of high-risk intrapartum care. Perinatal complications create the potential for varying degrees of loss: loss of the normal desired labor and birth, loss through maternal or fetal/neonatal injury, and loss of life.

Fear of Intrapartum Loss

While professionals understand the gradations of risk and the margins of safety associated with complications, parents and family usually do not have sufficient knowledge to make those distinctions. Because they lack sufficient knowledge to interpret the situation accurately, sometimes parents become fearful about potential loss which, in fact, is unlikely. For example, parents may interpret signs of increasing concern about fetal well-being as indications of a life-threatening complication, even when the objective risk is low and the problem can be managed with relative safety.

The nurse should remember that each parent brings a different set of concerns and expectations to the high-risk labor and delivery experience. If her physiological condition is unimpaired, the laboring woman is usually primarily concerned about the unborn. The mother is often acutely aware of subtle changes in professional behavior and will sometimes conclude that her unborn is in significant jeopardy, when professionals are only mildly concerned. However, medications, labor sensations, or physiological changes may limit the mother's perceptual field and dampen the intensity of her response. The father's anxiety level is likely to be high enough to make him exquisitely sensitive to environmental cues. However, his primary concern is usually his partner's well-being. Thus, based on what he sees unfolding before him, a father may conclude that his partner's life is in serious danger even though it is the unborn who is primarily at risk. In a large study of families in which the woman was hospitalized for complications in late pregnancy, fathers expressed fear of "leaving the hospital alone" in situations where, objectively speaking, only the fetus was at significant risk.[1] The urgency of actions surrounding an at-risk birth communicated a diffuse sense of danger to these fathers, leading them to fear greatly for their partners' lives, even when the condition being treated was fetal distress or preterm labor, in which maternal risk is relatively low.

Unfortunately, limited research attention has been paid to families' experiences of high-risk labor and birth irrespective of actual loss or to levels of emotional distress families experience during the process of high-risk intrapartum care. This is probably the result of the pressures of high-intensity care, the necessary concentration of maternal–fetal/neonatal survival, and the tendency to focus on situations such as poor neonatal outcome or perinatal demise as the only situational model for high emotional distress.

However, there is evidence to suggest that the long-term consequences of situational distress, even when maternal–neonatal outcomes are good, may be detrimental to individual and family well-being. Pioneering studies, such as those by Tilden and Lipson and Cranley, Hedahl, and Pegg have already documented that women may require months for the process of resolving grief and loss from a cesarean delivery.[20,21] Even though outcomes may be excellent, for many women the emotional impact of an at-risk delivery is not reduced. The same may be true for an increasing number of men, as more men become actively involved in the process of labor and birth. May and Sollid found that fathers were sometimes plagued with lingering guilt about "failing their partners" when an unexpected cesarean delivery was required.[3] They worried that their relationships with their infants were damaged because they "didn't bond" with their newborns immediately after delivery.

Helping the family focus their concerns about the at-risk situation without allowing these concerns to become overwhelming is a nursing responsibility in the intrapartum period. The nurse usually has enough information about preexisting family stressors, objective maternal–fetal risk, and the immediate situational factors affecting the family to provide reassurance, modify environmental stressors, and help the family focus its energy on achieving the best possible outcome.

Psychosocial Assessment and Intervention with the High-Risk Patient

Assessment and intervention related to psychosocial needs of high-risk intrapartum patients and their families are indeed a challenge. The intrapartum nurse must rely on information gathered by others regarding levels of family stress and adaptation during pregnancy. In addition, the nurse must gather information about individual and family responses to the stresses of labor quickly and under rapidly changing conditions.

As noted earlier, patterns of association between the quality of the mate relationship, self-esteem, and anxiety and depression in high-risk pregnancies have been identified in numerous studies. These factors may substantially contribute to the eventual adaptation of the woman and her family after an at-risk birth. Therefore, it may be reasonable to use these indicators in clinical care, in an effort to identify families with the greatest need for psychosocial support during an at-risk birth. The following issues may guide the nurse in an initial assessment of patient and family needs.

The nurse should note whether the mate relationship seems well established and secure: Are partners able to read and anticipate each other's needs? Does the woman express appreciation for mate's support and concern about his situation? Does the partner express concern about his mate's situation and a willingness to do what he can to assist? If there is expression of mutual concern, a desire to remain together, and some ability on the part of the mate to meet the woman's emotional needs in this stressful situation, it is likely that the relationship is providing an important level of support. In this case, nursing interventions may focus on supporting that closeness, monitoring fatigue and worry in the mate, and substituting for that support when separation of the partners is necessary.

Stability of Mate Relationship and Satisfaction with Support

If the nurse senses the partners are not able to support each other emotionally during this crisis, it may be useful to examine these issues: Was the pregnancy planned or desired by both partners? If pregnancy was not desired initially, has there been some resolution of ambivalence or resistance by both partners? Have both partners been involved in preparing for birth and new parenthood? If there was disagreement or ongoing tension in these areas, the nurse can anticipate that the mate relationship and the level of spousal support may be less than optimal. In this situation, the nurse may need to assess whose presence (other than the father of the baby) is most supportive and reassuring to the laboring woman and arrange for that person to provide additional support.

Assessment of parental self-esteem within the focused experience of prospective and new parenthood may yield cues to their probable responses in the intrapartum period. While it is clearly not feasible to "measure" self-esteem in the intrapartum period, the nurse can rely on possible clues, such as statements suggesting self-blame in respect to the risk condition or how well a high-risk regimen was adhered to during pregnancy.

Self-Esteem

The nurse should observe how the woman and her mate respond to praise for their efforts and reassurance about their ability to cope. If response is positive (*i.e.,* such comments appear to calm them), this type of focused support may be valuable. The nurse should also note that a woman or couple who appear not to need much reassurance and praise and who have a clear understanding of goals to be achieved may be at risk for judging themselves against performance expectations too harshly, especially in the rapidly changing circumstances of an at-risk labor and birth. For this family, it may be useful to provide praise for appropriate coping, but also to help the couple identify the need to remain "flexible" and to reframe expectations within what is possible.

Anxiety and Depression

High levels of anxiety or depression may be hinted at in the prenatal record, in notes regarding lack of partner support or involvement, missed prenatal visits or unexplained delays in seeking care, difficulty in meeting typical demands of pregnancy, and extremes in vigilance (very high or very low) about physical signs or symptoms or about fetal well-being. Depression is not a factor likely to require nursing attention in the intrapartum period. However, if there was evidence that the mother was depressed in the antepartum record, the nurse may need to adjust dynamics in the couple relationship during the intrapartum period, such as distancing and expressions of helplessness from the mate, blaming the baby for disruption of the marriage, or withdrawing from active involvement in labor support.

Assessing and intervening with maternal anxiety during labor are essentially the same process in the context of an at-risk birth. However, the nurse should also recognize that the latent fears of loss and injury experienced by any laboring couple become real and ominous under circumstances of at-risk childbearing. The nurse should be careful to explain and reinforce information about the nature of emerging threats and how professionals plan to deal with them. It is unwise to assume that parents understand information previously explained; the nurse should look for ways to assess understanding, reinforce positive points, and correct misconceptions (*e.g.,* "You remember that your wife's condition is stable—what we are concerned about right now is that the baby's heart rate appears to be slowing").

Parent– Unborn/Newborn Attachment

Since there is little evidence that at-risk childbearing negatively influences the process of parent–fetal/newborn attachment and since the demands of labor and delivery care rarely provide time for in-depth assessment and intervention in this area, the nurse's attention is better spent on assessing the impact of emergent distress on the family, as outlined later. Nevertheless, the nurse should be alert to cues that parents are emotionally tied to the fetus. Positive responses to fetal movement or physical evidence of the fetus (*e.g.,* ultrasound images and fetal heart rate tracings), reference to the fetus by name, or positive verbalizations are evidence of an established bond.

However, absence of such cues is *not* compelling evidence of a poor bond, since such behavior will be profoundly influenced by previous obstetric events (especially a previous loss), personality traits, cultural factors, and the intense nature of the intrapartum experience. However, when there is a fetal/neonatal loss, assessing the strength of the bond between parents and unborn/newborn and supporting the family through the resulting grief response clearly become a nursing priority.

Perhaps the most important area for nursing action in the psychosocial care of the high-risk intrapartum patient is in the control of the environment and the stressors therein. The nurse must constantly be on the alert for stormtrooper obstetrics and be assertive in exerting control over the patient's environment. The number of personnel and the number of entrances and exits from the patient's room can be kept to a safe minimum. Care and procedures can be clustered to avoid constant interruptions.

Environmental and Emergent Stress

The nurse should be especially vigilant to help patient and family cope with the rapidity of change and the behavioral changes demonstrated in providers as they adapt to clinical needs. When conditions are changing rapidly, the nurse should periodically step back and see how the patient and family are responding, and then step back in to ask, "What can I do to help you right now?"

The nurse should avoid "flying into action" with equipment and procedures without preparing the patient with a brief explanation and should remind other care providers to do likewise. Giving patient and family a few moments in which to adjust before the action resumes may be a valuable key. Also, "nursing" the equipment rather than the patient and family is a constant threat and must be guarded against.

The physical environment should be viewed from the family's eyes as much as possible. The nurse can suggest that "security" items might be brought from home and placed where the patient and family can see or touch them. Even in an intensive care environment, there is usually room for the patient to make choices about sounds, lighting, and arrangement of bedside space. However, patient choice is only possible if someone asks about preferences and then intervenes to honor them.

Finally, the nurse must remember that, even within the context of high-risk intrapartum care, the focus of care is the family, not the complication. There are, in reality, three patients requiring nursing care, the woman, the unborn, and the significant others. Family-centered care is even more important for high-risk patients than it is for their low-risk counterparts. At every opportunity the nurse should ask, "What can I do to support family well-being right now?" Needed interventions may include flexibility with visitors within safe limits, assigning some temporary and intensive support for a father who is at his own emotional limits, avoiding unnecessary and arbitrary separation of mates (even if it means questioning hospital policy), and teaching family members how to help each other focus their energy appropriately.

Such work is difficult. The nurse should also be sensitive to the fact that others must assist at times and that others may have insights into what may help a particular patient at a particular time. Consultation on psychosocial care is as important as consultation on physical or technical aspects of care, yet nurses sometimes hesitate to ask for help in this arena. Nurses also may be hesitant to communicate their observations and their plans of psychosocial care to other providers, because it seems "not as important" as information about obstetric status. Excellence in physical care must not be compromised; however, excellence in psychosocial care ought not to be.

Expected Outcomes of Psychosocial Care

Evaluating outcomes of intrapartum care in the psychosocial arena is notoriously difficult, because of the absence of reliable ways to measure comfort and distress, the constant and sometimes rapid change in patient condition, and absence of well-defined protocols for nursing care for emotional distress. The challenge is made even more difficult by the overlay of an at-risk birth, with the attendant threats to life and well-being.

However, it is possible to specify outcomes against which care can be judged and toward which progress can be made.

- Assess evidence of preexisting cumulative stress and, if necessary, seek additional information from prenatal care providers on which to base psychosocial support interventions.
- Keep patient and family informed of changes in condition and encourage them to freely ask questions of staff.
- Verify that patient and family can state basic understanding of patient's condition and the significance of changes in that condition.
- Encourage patient to express emotional distress and provide additional patient–family support as needed.
- Assess patient–family responses to psychosocial interventions and modify care to minimize apparent distress.
- Limit environmental stressors in keeping with patient–family wishes and safe standards of care.

The challenge is great, but the results of nursing efforts to provide sensitive psychosocial care within the context of increased perinatal risk are also important to parents and families. The blending of the best of "high tech–high touch" is the essence of excellence in intrapartum nursing care, and it is with high-risk patients and their families that nursing can demonstrate the best it has to offer.

References

1. Mercer R, Ferketich S, May K, DeJoseph J: Antepartal stress: Effect on family health and functioning. National Institutes of Health, National Center for Nursing Research Grant 5 RO1 NR0106 4-03. 1987.
2. Grossman F: Strain in the transition to parenthood, in Palkowitz R, Sussman M (eds.): *Transitions to Parenthood.* New York, Haworth Press, 1988.
3. May K, Sollid D: Fathers' responses to unanticipated cesarean delivery. *Birth* 11:87–95, 1984.
4. Parke R, Beitel A: Disappointment: When things go wrong in the transition to parenthood, in Palkowitz R, Sussman M (eds.): *Transitions to Parenthood.* New York, Haworth Press, 1988.
5. Belsky J, Pensky E: Marital change across the transition to parenthood, in Palkowitz R. Sussman M (eds.): *Transitions to Parenthood.* New York, Haworth Press, 1988.
6. Norbeck J, Tilden V: Life stress, social support, and emotional disequilibrium in complications of pregnancy: A prospective multivariate study. *J Health Soc Behav* 24:30–46, 1983.
7. Lederman R: Maternal anxiety in pregnancy: Relationship to fetal and newborn health status. *Ann Rev Nurs Res* 4:3–19, 1986.
8. Barnett B, Parker G: Possible determinants, correlates and consequences of high levels of anxiety in primiparous mothers. *Psych Med* 16:177–185, 1986.

9. White M, Dawson C: The impact of the at-risk infant on family solidarity. *Birth Defects: Orig Art Ser* 17(6):253–284, 1981.
10. O'Hara M, Rehm L, Campbell S: Postpartum depression: A role for social network and life stress variables. *J Nervous Mental Dis* 171:336–341, 1983.
11. Curry M, and Snell B: Antenatal hospitalization: Maternal behavior and the family. Final report, DHHS, HRSA, Division of Nursing, Nursing Research Support Section Grant 1 RO1 NU 00939. 1985.
12. Hobfoll S, Nadler A, Leiberman J: Satisfaction with social support during crisis: Intimacy and self-esteem as critical determinants. *J Personal Soc Psych* 51(2):296–304, 1986.
13. Cohen, R: Maladaptation to pregnancy. *Seminars in Perinatology* 3:15–24, 1979.
14. May K: Impact of home-managed preterm labor on families. Unpublished paper. 1990.
15. Cranley M: Development of a tool for the measurement of maternal attachment during pregnancy. *Nurs Res* 30(6):281–284, 1981.
16. Kemp V, Page C: Maternal prenatal attachment in normal and high-risk pregnancies. *Obstet Gynecol Neonat Nurs* 16(3):179–184, 1987.
17. Mercer R, Ferketich S, May K, et al: Further exploration of maternal and fetal attachment. *Res Nurs Health* 11:83–95, 1988.
18. Cummins L, Scrimshaw S, Engle P: Views of cesarean birth among primiparous women of Mexican origin in Los Angeles. *Birth* 15(3):164–168, 1988.
19. Sandelowski M, Bustamante R: Cesarean birth outside of the natural childbirth culture. *Res Nurs Health* 9:81–88, 1986.
20. Tilden V, Lipson J: Cesarean childbirth: Variables affecting psychological impact. *Western J Nurs Res* 3:127–132, 1982.
21. Cranley M, Hedahl K, Pegg S: Women's perceptions of vaginal and cesarean deliveries. *Nurs Res* 32(1):10–16, 1983.

II
♦ ♦ ♦

THE HIGH-RISK PATIENT

.5.
◆ ◆ ◆

Preterm Labor and Preterm Premature Rupture of Membranes

A. Diann Neal
Victoria Cahill Bockman

Supportive Data

Incidence

Preterm labor is defined as labor occurring prior to the completion of 36 weeks gestation.[1] Preterm births represent 8% to 10% of all births in the United States; however, this complication of pregnancy is responsible for 60% of all perinatal morbidity and mortality.[1,2] *Premature rupture of membranes* (PROM) is defined as rupture of the amniotic membranes prior to the onset of labor and is a condition not dependent on gestational age.[3] Approximately 30% of all preterm births have associated PROM.[3] *Preterm premature rupture of the membranes* (PPROM) refers to premature rupture prior to term or prior to 36 completed weeks gestation.[3] It is the single most common diagnosis associated with preterm birth and is also the most common event leading to a preterm infant's admission to a neonatal intensive care unit.[3,4]

Significance

Prematurity is the major unsolved problem in obstetrics today, and costs to society range well over a billion dollars annually.[5] The President's Panel on Mental Retardation in 1962 began the focus on high mortality and morbidity of low birthweight infants. Mental retardation was originally targeted as the major risk associated with prematurity and low birthweight, but blindness and developmental problems were other concerns also addressed. Neonatology began to develop as a specialty shortly thereafter, and studies by health care providers turned to the preterm infant.

The introduction of new pharmacologic agents to treat preterm labor has given some initial cause for optimism. However, no documented change in the incidence of preterm birth has occurred either in this country or in Europe.[6]

This failure may be due in part to a lack of early recognition and diagnosis of preterm labor precluding effective treatment. Further, lack of complete understanding of the physiology of labor and its complications affects the efficiency of both diagnosis and treatment for this group of patients.[7]

Neonatal survival rates increase proportionally with gestational age; however, technological advances in the field of neonatology continue to reduce the gestational age of viability.[1,2,8] Locally available infant care resources play a major role in medical management planning. The location of birth and support services, gestational age and maturity of the fetus, and risks of morbidity and mortality of mother and fetus will all be considered when making clinical care decisions.[9] Consultation with a neonatal team is important because medical management is ultimately guided by survival expectations weighed against the risks posed to mother and fetus by attempting to prolong the pregnancy.

Significant morbidity encountered by the preterm neonate may include respiratory distress syndrome, intraventricular hemorrhage, and necrotizing enterocolitis.[1,8] Retrolental fibroplasia is increasingly prevented but neurosensory impairment remains a serious potential long-term sequela.

Other long-term complications of preterm birth and neonatal prematurity include bronchopulmonary dysplasia and neurological handicaps such as cerebral palsy, blindness, and deafness, as well as developmental delays. Infants at greatest risk for morbidity are less than 32 weeks gestation, and the most commonly encountered problem is lung immaturity. Thus, respiratory distress syndrome in the severely immature infant is often a primary focus of management. Providing adequate alveolocapillary exchange of gases while preventing other complications requires delicate and constant care and monitoring. Surfactant therapies administered at birth offer new optimism for bronchopulmonary management of the preterm infant. Adequate surfactant lining layer introduced into the bronchopulmonary tree at birth may lead to normal lung function.

Fetal morbidity associated with PPROM in addition to the sequelae associated with preterm delivery includes specific problems associated with resultant oligohydramnios.[10] It has long been recognized that chronic leaking of amniotic fluid causes compression of the fetus. Lung volume may be reduced mechanically as well as restriction of fetal breathing by prevention of entry of amniotic fluid into the lungs.[11] Limited lung expansion may cause pulmonary hypoplasia, particularly in the very premature fetus.[11] Oligohydramnios can also lead to umbilical cord compression or entrapment, which occurs more often in breech presentations. Limb and facial deformities can also occur because of loss of the amniotic fluid cushion.[10] To date, efforts to reseal the leak have not proved practical on any reasonable scale.

Chorioamnionitis, another major complication of PPROM, may lead to fetal/neonatal infection. Presence of infection also results in an increased maternal consumption of oxygen, decreasing oxygen supplies available to the fetus. Surprisingly, PPROM patients without clinical signs of infection prior to 28 weeks gestation may not be as at great a risk for serious sequelae from chorioamnionitis as are term infants.[11,12] Conservative management (bedrest) without intervention is often employed with PPROM to allow for increasing gestational age and improved survivability. Tocolytics may also be employed to prevent preterm labor and allow the fetus additional time *in utero*.

The exact mechanism or event that initiates spontaneous labor remains obscure. The process appears to involve a complex series of interactions between hormones, enzymes, and cells and between fetus and mother (Figure 5-1). The appearance of certain physiologic events have been identified as occurring before or during labor. An active ripening process occurs within the cervix which involves a breakdown of collagen by collagenase resulting in changes in cervical connective tissue.[13] Increased fibroblast activity similar to an inflammatory tissue response also occurs during this ripening process, and the cervix becomes softer and shorter.[7,13,14] In addition to cervical ripening, gap junctions and oxytocin receptors appear in the myometrium.[15,16]

Gap junctions are neural contacts between cells which allow the instantaneous communication necessary for rhythmic and coordinated uterine contractions.[16] The formation of gap junctions also appears to be necessary for oxytocin stimulation of uterine contractions.[15]

The increase in number of oxytocin receptors at the time of labor is indicative of the important role oxytocin plays during the process of childbirth, increasing responsiveness of the uterus to oxytocin stimuli.[14,15] Serum levels do not rise appreciably before labor, but peak during the second stage.[14,15] Oxytocin receptors also found in the decidua stimulate the production of prostaglandins.

The role of estrogen and progesterone in the initiation of labor remains unclear. In sheep, rising fetal cortisol levels at term activate enzymes that alter

Etiology

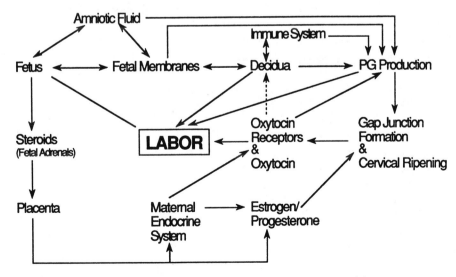

Figure 5-1. Factors associated with the initiation of spontaneous labor.

placental steroid production.[7,15] Estrogen is produced in greater quantities while progesterone secretion falls, resulting in increased prostaglandin synthesis. In humans, however, there is neither a demonstrable rise in fetal cortisol levels nor withdrawal of progesterone until after delivery of the placenta.[15] However, high levels of estrogen do have a stimulating effect on cervical ripening and gap junction formation while progesterone's effect is inhibitory.[15] It is possible that a change in the ratio of estrogen to progesterone may affect the initiation of labor in humans.[7,15]

Prostaglandins are the major hormones involved in the initiation of spontaneous labor. There is a dramatic rise in prostaglandin concentration in amniotic fluid during labor.[14] Arachidonic acid, the precursor of PGE_2 and $PGF_{2\alpha}$—the prostaglandins involved in parturition, is also found in increased concentration during labor. Prostaglandins not only affect cervical ripening, but also promote gap junction formation and stimulate uterine contractions.[7,15] The mechanism of prostaglandin action on uterine contractions appears to be mediated by the enhancement of calcium transport through the plasma membrane. Calcium is a vital component in the actin and myosin coupling process necessary for smooth muscle contraction.[7] Prostaglandins promote both the availability of intracellular calcium for uterine smooth muscle contraction, as well as the formation of myometrial gap junctions.[17] Together these two processes promote coordinated uterine contractions necessary for labor.

Prostaglandins are produced in the cervix, decidua, and myometrium. When infection or physical damage of the decidua, fetal membranes, or cervix occurs, increased prostaglandin synthesis is stimulated.[7] Because the decidua has many macrophage-like properties, decidual cells and macrophages both respond to infection by producing prostaglandins.[15] The tissue changes that occur during cervical ripening are in fact reminiscent of an inflammatory tissue response.[7,15] In addition, the amnion is apparently stimulated to increase production of prostaglandins through the influence of fetal urine. This effect is not noted until late in the gestation and is indicative of the possible communication occurring between mother and fetus, at least in part, via the amniotic fluid and fetal membranes.[18] The sequence of events that results in labor and parturition may be present but held in abeyance during pregnancy. It is speculated that when the fetal/placental unit somehow withdraws its support of the pregnancy, the initiation of parturition begins.[7,15]

The etiology of preterm labor is not readily apparent; however, numerous risk factors associated with preterm labor and birth have been identified (see Table 5-1). Risks associated with preterm labor are broadly categorized as medical and obstetric risks antedating pregnancy, current pregnancy-associated factors, and demographic and behavioral risks.[2,19]

Risk factors antedating the pregnancy include medical conditions associated with impaired renal function, hypertension, and decreased uterine perfusion. A history of a prior preterm delivery is a highly significant risk factor for preterm labor.[1,2,19] The risk decreases with each subsequent pregnancy carried to term and increases with each subsequent preterm birth.[19] One or more second tri-

TABLE 5-1
Risk Factors Associated with Preterm Labor and Birth

Medical or obstetric risks antedating pregnancy
    Prior preterm delivery
    Previous second-trimester abortion
    Cervical incompetence
    Uterine or cervical anomalies
    Renal disease
    Hypertension
Current pregnancy-associated risks
    Multiple gestation
    Placenta previa
    Placental abruption
    Fetal abnormality
    Hydramnios
    Abdominal surgery
    Maternal infection
    Maternal bleeding
    Cervical effacement or dilatation (more than 50% per 1 cm)
Demographic and behavioral risk factors
    Age (less than 19 or more than 40)
    Nonwhite
    Low socioeconomic status
    Single parent
    Smoking
    Substance abuse
    Prepregnancy weight less than 100 lb
    Poor weight gain
    Inadequate prenatal care
    Psychological stress

mester abortions are associated with increased risk for preterm labor in succeeding pregnancies.[18,19] Uterine anomalies, such as unicornate or bicornate uterus and uterine myomata, are also associated with greater risk for preterm labor.[19]

Cervical incompetence is a term used to describe the painless dilation of the cervix in the second or early-third trimester of pregnancy. It may be a result of diethylstilbestrol exposure *in utero,* cervical trauma during prior medical procedures, or oftentimes unknown causes.[12,18] Following dilation, prolapse of the membranes through the cervix occurs usually resulting in expulsion of a fetus who has not achieved viability.[12] This anatomic abnormality must be distinguished carefully from other recurrent causes of preterm pregnancy loss.[18] In select women, cervical cerclage may be beneficial in maintaining a pregnancy until fetal viability is attained.

Multiple gestation in the current pregnancy is the most significant risk factor predictive of preterm labor and/or birth.[1,19,20] Possible causes include uterine overdistention accompanied by stretching of the myometrial cells and possible decreased blood flow to the uterus. Increased pressure on the cervix may result in cervical dilation with increased exposure of the fetal membranes, predisposing to premature rupture. Similarly, hydramnios, related to fetal anomalies, maternal diabetes, or inhibition of fetal swallowing, is another potential cause of uterine overdistension and may subsequently lead to preterm labor.

Placental abruption associated with maternal hypertension and cocaine or crack use may lead to spontaneous preterm labor and subsequent preterm delivery. If bleeding is excessive and a threat to mother or fetus, prompt delivery may be required, resulting in a preterm birth.

There is also evidence linking infection to preterm labor and PPROM.[21,22] Bacterial infection and endotoxin production stimulate the biosynthesis of prostaglandin at the fetal membranes and decidua. Phospholipase A_2 is the liberating enzyme for arachidonic acid, the precursor for prostaglandin production. Bacterial action during the infection process releases phospholipase A_2 leading to prostaglandin prosynthesis. Prostaglandins E_2 and $F_{2\alpha}$ enhance uterine activity and dissolve and weaken collagen fibers.[23,24] Intrauterine infection most often occurs by an ascending route through the vagina, cervix, and maternal decidua. Bacteria invading the uterus are capable of crossing the fetal membranes to enter the intraamniotic space. The intervillous space and fetal vessels may be another possible route for infection, which when localized in the decidua and chorionic membrane can also lead to weakening of the membrane, resulting in membrane rupture. Focal weakening of the amniochorionic membranes is probably due to enzymatic bacterial action which may trigger the cascade of factors initiating labor. Changes in biochemical collagen metabolism occur in the amnion and chorion and lead to significant weakening of the membranes through collagenolysis.[25] Because of concentrations of bacteria, PPROM may be a variant of this normal process at an inappropriate time.

Systemic maternal infection, such as pyelonephritis, is also associated with preterm labor, suggesting the onset of labor in the presence of infection is a protective host response controlled by either mother and/or fetus.[21] Prostaglandin production, stimulated by the specific immunological response to infection, may initiate the birth process in response to a hostile maternal environment.

Certain sociological characteristics are associated with increased risk for preterm labor and delivery.[1] Single women, teenagers, and women over the age of 40 are at increased risk. Nonwhite women are statistically at greater risk for preterm labor than white women, and black women deliver babies prior to 37 weeks of gestation twice as often as do white women.[1,19] Low socioeconomic status and low educational attainment are reproducible demographic characteristics associated with an increased risk of preterm labor.[19] There is also an association between smoking and low birthweight.[2,19,45] Maternal smoking has been estimated to be a major contributing factor in 13% to 20% of preterm births in the United States.[19] Substance abuse is also associated with preterm labor (see Chapter 8). A prepregnancy weight of less than 100 lb and poor weight gain during pregnancy are associated risk factors for preterm labor.[2,27]

Physical work during pregnancy, which entails long hours, prolonged standing, and lifting, appears to increase the risk of preterm labor.[19,28] Compression of the pelvic vessels with decreased venous return and decreased uterine blood flow have been suggested as potential causes of preterm labor when pregnancy is accompanied by prolonged standing.[19] The physiologic effects of psychologic stress during pregnancy have not been fully elucidated, although the uterus can have a variable response to catecholamine release depending on the hormonal influences operating at the time. Whereas beta-adrenergic stimulation causes vasodilation in smooth muscle, alpha-adrenergic stimulation causes vasoconstriction and increased muscle tone.

It is not clear whether term parturition and the preterm birth process share similar mechanisms. The role of infection in the etiology of preterm labor is at this point in time the most clearly understood and perhaps correctable risk factor; however, infection is not responsible for or present in all cases of preterm labor. The complexity of identifiable risk factors strongly suggests multiple causes for preterm birth.

The etiology of PPROM is also poorly understood although associated factors are closely related to those of preterm labor: low socioeconomic status, smoking, poor diet, age, and single marital status.[3] In addition, history of sexually transmitted diseases has been linked to PPROM.[3] Contributing factors correlated with the occurrence of PPROM include incompetent cervix, infection or inflammatory weakening of the membranes, hydramnios, trauma, multiple gestations, maternal genital tract anomalies, and abruptio placentae.[3,29]

PRETERM LABOR

Framework for Accepted Therapy

There is much controversy across the country regarding the criteria for diagnosis of preterm labor. Although many believe a documented change in cervical dilation or effacement is necessary, uterine activity may prompt treatment in an effort to prevent cervical changes. Bedrest, hydration, and sedation are conservative measures that may halt preterm contractions in up to one half of patients. Bedrest in the lateral recumbent position and intravenous hydration promote increased intravascular volume, increased uterine blood flow, and decreased pressure on the cervix.[2,19] Failure of adequate maternal plasma volume expansion may be a possible cause of preterm contractions and may account in part for the therapeutic success of hydration and bedrest.[19] Additionally, a significant placebo effect may also be involved. Intravenous fluids should be limited to 400 to 500 ml and administered over 20 to 30 minutes as excessive hydration places the patient at increased risk for pulmonary edema should intravenous betamimetic or magnesium sulfate therapy become necessary.[30] Mild sedation may be appropriate for select patients who are very anxious.[31] Combined with reassurance, sedation may help decrease endogenous catecholamine production in a frightened woman.

Tocolysis refers to the pharmacological treatment of preterm contractions. Approximately one fourth to one half of women experiencing preterm contractions will not be in true preterm labor. Because success in postponing preterm birth is dependent on preventing significant cervical change, early intervention frequently precludes waiting to document cervical changes. Thus many women may be treated with tocolytic therapy unnecessarily. Unfortunately, advances in pharmacological treatments for preterm labor have not made a significant impact on the preterm birth rate. However, goals for tocolytic treatment of preterm labor are to inhibit uterine contractions, to prevent cervical change, and to prolong fetal time *in utero*.

The tocolytics most frequently used to halt uterine contractions are betamimetic agents, magnesium sulfate, prostaglandin inhibitors, and calcium channel blockers. The betamimetics used for the treatment of preterm labor include ritodrine hydrochloride and terbutaline sulfate. Isoxsuprine hydrochloride, because of its pronounced cardiovascular side effects, is rarely used today. Hexoprenaline is still in use in Europe, Africa, and at a few centers in the United States and Canada.[31,32] Hexoprenaline, like ritodrine and terbutaline, is considered to have a more direct effect on myometrial relaxation. Ritodrine is the only drug currently approved by the Food and Drug Administration for tocolytic use; however, no one drug has been proven superior to the others for intravenous use.[31,32,34,35]

Betamimetic agents work by stimulating beta-adrenergic receptors. Two types of beta receptors coexist throughout the body. Beta$_1$ receptors stimulate activity in heart, liver, pancreas, intestines, and adipose tissue. Beta$_2$ receptor stimulation causes smooth muscle relaxation in the uterus, bronchioles, and vasculature. The overlapping effects of beta$_1$ and beta$_2$ receptor activity are responsible for the adverse maternal and fetal side effects associated with these drugs. The tocolytic effect of betamimetic drugs occurs when beta receptor stimulation activates the enzyme adenyl cyclase; this then increases cyclic adenosine monophosphate (cAMP) within uterine smooth muscle cells. The effects of increased cAMP are a decrease in intracellular calcium, a necessary cofactor for muscle contraction, and decreased uterine smooth muscle activity. Betamimetic drugs are metabolized and inactivated by the liver and excreted in the urine.

The efficacy of betamimetic agents may be lost to desensitization or tachyphylaxis over time. After prolonged therapy, there is a decrease in the number of beta-adrenergic receptors resulting in a loss of efficacy. This phenomenon is known as down regulation, and when it occurs a tocolytic agent other than a betamimetic may be used.[36]

Conditions often cited as contraindications to tocolysis, or more specifically use of betamimetics, are numerous (Table 5-2). Presence of maternal cardiac disease, for example, may be readily identified as a contraindication to betamimetic therapy. However, it should be noted that previously undiagnosed cardiac disease as well as associated complications have been unmasked during tocolytic treatment with betamimetics.[37,38] Cerebral ischemia in patients prone to migraine headaches has been associated with the use of betamimetics.[37–39] A history of migraine headaches is particularly significant in the woman who is a candidate for tocolysis. Use of tocolytic agents in the presence of vaginal bleeding is dependent upon the reason for bleeding, maternal hemodynamic stability, fetal status, and goal of therapy.

TABLE 5-2
Relative and Absolute Contraindications to
Betamimetic Therapy

Maternal
　Cardiac disease
　Cardiac arrhythmias
　Uncontrolled diabetes
　Maternal infection
　Hyperthyroidism
　Pheochromocytoma
　Preeclampsia or eclampsia
　Uncontrolled chronic hypertension
　Active vaginal bleeding
　Hypovolemia
　History of migraine headaches
　Untreated urinary tract infection
　Chronic renal or hepatic disease
　Bronchial asthma already treated with betamimetics
　Advanced labor
　Fetal
　Fetal demise
　Fetal distress
　Intrauterine growth retardation
　Placental dysfunction
　Fetal anomalies incompatible with life

Ritodrine is administered orally or intravenously. Although clinical investigation suggests ritodrine can be given safely and effectively by intramuscular injection, this route is not approved by the Food and Drug Administration.[40] When using intravenous ritodrine, the initial infusion is begun at 50 to 100 μg/minute (0.05–0.1 ml/minute), and the maximum recommended dose is 350 μg/minute (0.35 mg/minute).[39]

Oral ritodrine is usually given 30 to 60 minutes before the intravenous infusion is stopped. The maximum recommended dose is 120 mg/day.[39] A higher dose (maximum of 360 mg/day) of ritodrine in a sustained-release formula is undergoing clinical investigation.[41] The benefit of this drug form is higher peak and trough plasma concentrations; however, the long-term effects of a sustained-release formula on the fetus must be considered.[30] Alternative protocols for administration, which include gradual reduction in infusion rate after effective tocolysis is achieved, have also been reported.[42]

Intravenous terbutaline is less costly than ritodrine, and its efficacy and safety appear to be comparable.[35,36] Intravenous regimes differ slightly from center to center. Terbutaline may be given by subcutaneous injection. The usual dosage is 0.25 mg terbutaline administered subcutaneously in the upper arm every 1 to 6 hours. The frequency of administration is determined by uterine activity and maternal pulse. Terbutaline has a rapid absorption rate and a half-life of 7 minutes.[43] Fewer and less severe side effects are seen with subcutaneous administration than with intravenous administration of any betamimetic drug.[43]

Betamimetics are potent drugs and require vigilant maternal and fetal assessment during intravenous use. Side effects and complications of betamimetic therapy are due to stimulation of beta-adrenergic receptors distributed throughout the body; adverse maternal effects may necessitate discontinuing the drug. The occurrence of side effects may be more frequent during increases in the infusion rate than during the maintenance infusion.[33,36] It should be remembered that oral therapy does not preclude development of significant side effects and complications. The most frequent side effect of betamimetic therapy is maternal tachycardia. Maternal heart rate increases 10 to 20 beats per minute as a partially compensatory response to vasodilation.[38] Discontinuing the infusion is recommended when maternal heart rate exceeds 140 beats per minute.[38] Cardiac arrhythmias have been reported in association with betamimetic therapy and may be asymptomatic. Associated myocardial ischemia may or may not occur.[37] Widening of the pulse pressure, an increased systolic and decreased diastolic pressure, is commonly seen without a significant reduction in mean arterial pressure. Hypotension occurs less frequently with $beta_2$ preferential drugs (*i.e.,* ritodrine), but it is still a potential side effect..

Shortness of breath and chest pain are the most common pulmonary side effects seen with betamimetic therapy.[38] Hyperventilation has also been reported.[38] Pulmonary edema is a serious and potentially fatal complication and, although the cause is not completely understood, it is most likely due to fluid overload and sodium retention.[37,38] Beta-adrenergic stimulation causes sodium and water retention, and excess fluid volume may result in spite of limiting intravenous fluid intake. Iatrogenic fluid overload may also lead to pulmonary edema. There remains disagreement about the safest type of intravenous solution to use.[37,38] Fluid intake should be carefully monitored and limited to 1 to 2 liters per day. Pulmonary edema may even occur after betamimetic infusion has been discontinued and during oral therapy. Risk factors for pulmonary edema include prolonged infusion (greater than 24 hours), subclinical chorioamnionitis, anemia, multiple gestation, persistent severe maternal tachycardia, and iatrogenic overload.[37] Glucocorticoid administration for fetal lung maturity has been implicated in the development of pulmonary edema, but its role remains controversial.[37,38] Delivery following betamimetic therapy also places the patient at increased risk for pulmonary edema. Close assessment of fluid balance and pulmonary status should continue for at least 12 hours following infusion therapy.

Beta-adrenergic stimulation causes glycogenolysis and hyperglycemia followed by hyperinsulinemia occurring within 4 hours of treatment.[36] Urine screening for glucose and ketones should occur at regular intervals. Ketoacidosis is a potential risk to patients with diabetes during betamimetic therapy, and a concomitant insulin infusion is often necessary. As a result of increased insulin secretion, potassium moves into the intracellular space during betamimetic administration causing decreased serum potassium.[38] There is no change, however, in the body's total potassium because potassium excretion is not increased and serum potassium levels usually return to normal within 24 hours.[37] Supplementation is rarely necessary unless serum potassium levels fall below 2.5 mg/100 ml.[37,38] Gastrointestinal side effects of betamimetic therapy include nausea, vomiting, ileus, and diarrhea. Anxiety, apprehension, and restlessness are also common effects of betamimetic therapy.

Fetal effects of betamimetic therapy are related to placental transfer of the drug and maternal metabolic alterations. Fetal tachycardia and arrhythmias have been reported.[38,44] Neonatal hypokalemia, hyperinsulinemia, and hypoglycemia may result if delivery occurs during a period of maternal metabolic changes due to betamimetic therapy.[42] Possible thickening of the intraventricular septum has been reported after prolonged exposure, but does not appear to be a permanent process and eventually normalizes.[42]

The tocolytic properties of magnesium sulfate ($MgSO_4$) are well accepted but not completely understood. Magnesium sulfate has fewer contraindications and less severe adverse effects than betamimetics and may be used in some conditions where betamimetics are contraindicated. Studies regarding the tocolytic efficacy of $MgSO_4$ have demonstrated success rates similar to that of betamimetic agents.[45–47]

The exact mechanism by which $MgSO_4$ interferes with uterine smooth muscle contraction is not clearly understood. On an intracellular level, magnesium affects cAMP concentration and interferes with the transport of calcium extracellularly. The net effect is less calcium available for the actin myosin coupling necessary for muscle contraction. Magnesium competes with calcium, which is necessary for the conduction of nerve impulses and affects nerve impulse transmission by decreasing the availability of the neurotransmitter acetylcholine and by reducing the sensitivity of the motor end plate to acetylcholine. Because $MgSO_4$ is cleared from the body via the kidneys, patients with impaired renal function are at risk for toxicity. Because of the effects of $MgSO_4$ on muscle contractility and nerve transmission, a history of myocardial infarction is a relative contraindication to the use of $MgSO_4$. The only absolute contraindication is maternal myasthenia gravis. The patient with this illness is already at high risk for serious respiratory compromise, and the effects of $MgSO_4$ on neurotransmission may result in respiratory arrest.

When $MgSO_4$ is used, a bolus of 4 to 6 g is usually given initially over 15 to 20 minutes followed by maintenance infusion administered at 2 to 3 g/hour by infusion pump. Therapeutic maternal serum levels of magnesium range between 4 and 8 mg/dl.[30] Magnesium sulfate has a slower rate of action than do the betamimetics, and contractions may persist for some time before diminishing completely. A single dose of subcutaneous terbutaline (0.25 mg) may be prescribed as an adjunct before sufficient serum levels of magnesium have been achieved.[48] Once contractions have stopped, oral betamimetic or other oral tocolytics are usually started and continued until 36 weeks gestation or until delivery. If contractions resume, reinstitution of intravenous $MgSO_4$ therapy may be required. One published report on long-term MgSO$_4$ tocolysis suggests that infusion therapy may continue for days or weeks without serious complications.[49]

The individual response to hypermagnesemia is varied. Side effects of MgSO$_4$ therapy are common, but rarely intolerable or life threatening and are dose related. Neuromuscular blockade of striated muscle is responsible for feelings of lethargy and weakness. Visual blurring and headache are also frequently experienced. Sensations of heat or burning at the intravenous site are common during the bolus infusion. Peripheral vasodilation frequently results in a generalized sensation of heat and complaints of nasal congestion. Transient hypotension may also occur. Gastrointestinal side effects including nausea and vomiting are common, and constipation may be troublesome.[49] Paralytic ileus is rare, but has been reported.[49] Pulmonary edema has been reported and is more likely to occur in women with an increased intravascular volume, such as those with multiple gestation or fluid overload.

If plasma concentration of magnesium exceeds 10 mg/dl, toxic effects may occur. Loss of deep tendon reflexes and respiratory depression accompany increasing neuromuscular depression. Alterations in myocardial conduction and function may result in cardiac arrest at levels above 12 mg/dl.[48] Calcium gluconate should be immediately available to reverse magnesium toxicity, should it occur.

Magnesium readily crosses the placenta resulting in fetal and neonatal hypermagnesemia. Reports on the fetal heart rate response to maternal MgSO$_4$ infusion have suggested either an increase or decrease in short-term variability.[50] Petrie suggested increased short-term variability may be due in part to increased placental perfusion with MgSO$_4$ therapy.[50] Loss of short-term variability should not be assumed to be a result of MgSO$_4$ therapy but should be further investigated. Neonatal hypermagnesemia may result in a lower Apgar score with points lost for muscle tone. The effects of hypermagnesemia on the preterm neonate have not been well studied to date.

Indomethacin functions as a prostaglandin inhibitor and has been used as a tocolytic. Prostaglandins, PGE$_2$ and PGF$_{2\alpha}$, play an important role in the pathogenesis of preterm labor.[51] These prostaglandins have proved to be potent uterotonic substances capable of inducing labor.[17] Prostaglandins E$_2$ and F$_{2\alpha}$ are highly unstable, localized hormones, produced and synthesized rapidly with a short half-life. They have conflicting and counteracting effects, often producing a cascade of events that may result in the body's natural induction of labor. Prostaglandins act on uterine smooth muscle by increasing gap junctions, which in turn improve the coordination of uterine contractions. Prostaglandin synthetase inhibitors retard this action by suppressing cyclo-oxygenase, which prevents the synthesis of prostaglandins from arachidonic acid.[52–54]

Indomethacin has been demonstrated to be significantly more effective than placebos in inhibiting preterm labor during a 24-hour course of therapy.[55] In one study, birth was delayed from 5 to 9 weeks and in some cases as long as 11 to 12 weeks.[54,56] Indomethacin can be given orally or rectally and is generally well tolerated by the mother. Intravenous tocolytic therapy may be discontinued during indomethacin administration.

The use of prostaglandin synthetase inhibitors is contraindicated in the presence of hypertensive disease of pregnancy, renal disease, peptic ulcers, aspirin sensitive allergy, and bleeding disorders.[52,57] Maternal side effects include epigastric pain with or without nausea, vomiting, and dyspepsia. As a result of platelet function interference, these inhibitors can cause gastrointestinal bleeding. Cervical and placental site bleeding may occur during labor and the postpartum period because of the relaxation of the uterine muscle as well as platelet aggregation dysfunction. Long-term administration may be associated with headaches, dizziness, depression, and psychosis.[18] Uteroplacental circulatory effects are contradictory as vasoconstriction and placental bed dilation both occur. No adverse neonatal effects have been demonstrated.[53,55,57]

Fetal physiologic effects of major concern include possible significant reduction in blood flow through the ductus arteriosus due to transient partial ductal narrowing. Doppler flow measurements have demonstrated a discernable reduction in blood flow through the ductus in about half the fetuses studied.[58] The reduction occurs 35 to 40 minutes after ingestion of indomethacin and is dose related. These cardiovascular effects appear to resolve within a day of treatment cessation.[54,58] The sensitivity of the ductus arteriosus to oxygen-mediated closure may increase with gestational age. The use of prostaglandin synthetase inhibitors is generally limited to gestations of less than 34 weeks to minimize this risk.[55]

Potential renal effects include reduced fetal urine output and a reduction in amniotic fluid production leading to oligohydramnios. Variable decelerations signaling umbilical cord compression may occur. When indomethacin use is discontinued, amniotic fluid volume quickly returns to normal, usually within 24 hours. No other significant adverse neonatal effects have been demonstrated to date.[53]

There are several other tocolytics currently under investigation, including calcium channel blockers and oxytocin analogues. Clinical trials have demonstrated that nifedipine, a calcium channel blocker, has a strong inhibitory effect on uterine activity. In one investigation, nifedipine was significantly more effective in halting preterm contractions than intravenous ritodrine.[59] Nifedipine has a selective inhibitory effect on "slow calcium channels." During a contraction, slow calcium channels are opened by depolarization, allowing calcium to diffuse into the cell through the membrane. In the presence of nifedipine these channels do not open, and the flow of the calcium is blocked, resulting in decreased uterine activity.[18] Nifedipine is given orally with an initial dose of 30 mg (three 10-mg capsules). Patients may be asked to crush or chew the capsules to speed absorption and the onset of effect. Following the initial dose 20 mg may be administered at 8- to 12-hour intervals for 3 days.

Adverse maternal reactions associated with use of nifedipine are related to inhibitory effects on smooth muscle contraction. Women receiving nifedipine experience transient flushing of the face, neck, and chest due to vasodilation.

While maternal heart rate increases, this effect is transitory. Read and Welby, however, noted a rise in fetal heart rates clinically similar to the effect of ritodrine.[59] Blood pressure decreases slightly in some patients, but no significant hypotensive episodes generally occur.[59,60] Animal research has suggested fetal acidosis and hypoxemia may occur during nifedipine administration, although these effects have not been demonstrated in the human fetus.[61,62] No fetal deaths or neonatal morbidity have been associated with nifedipine.[18]

Research continues to search for the safest and most effective tocolytic. Oxytocin analogues, aminophylline, and diazoxide are receiving some attention for their ability to suppress smooth muscle contractility. However, at this time both magnesium sulfate and the beta-adrenergic drugs are most widely used.

PRETERM PREMATURE RUPTURE OF MEMBRANES

During therapeutic management of PPROM, fetal risks and benefits of intra- versus extrauterine life are weighed. In the presence of chorioamnionitis, the fetus and the mother are generally at less risk if delivery is accomplished quickly. In the absence of infection, intrauterine management is usually attempted until fetal lung maturity is reached or another complication becomes of primary concern.

One study suggests the outcome of preterm pregnancies with PPROM can be improved, as well as an immature lecithin-to-sphingomyelin ratio, by the concurrent use of corticosteroids and antibiotics.[63] Patients in this study demonstrated a reduction in the incidence of respiratory distress syndrome and other infant morbidity while demonstrating no difference in the incidence of maternal or neonatal infection.

Oligohydramnios may lead to umbilical cord compression and variable decelerations and has also been linked to intrauterine growth retardation. It is unclear if physical compression of the cord is a cause of decreased fetal growth. Ultrasound and biophysical profile are major tools used for assessment of the fetal condition (Figure 5-2). Ultrasound scans for fluid pockets, compromised intrauterine growth, and fetal breathing may be done serially. The absence of fetal breathing is associated with risk for infection.[10,11,64,65] Amniocentesis may be done for serial assessment of fetal lung maturity and presence of bacteria. Once lung maturity is established, delivery is indicated to avoid the risks of expectant management: maternal and/or fetal infection, oligohydramnios, abruptio placentae, or fetal distress from cord entrapment or compression.[66] Antibiotic therapy is indicated when chorioamnionitis is diagnosed because of the risk for septicemia. Antibiotic therapy is necessary in the treatment of (*a*) beta-hemolytic streptococci, (*b*) *Neisseria gonorrhoeae*, and (*c*) *Chlamydia trachomatis*.[1,64] Data regarding the use of prophylactic antibiotic therapy are inconclusive to date.[1]

The stress of PPROM is believed by some to enhance fetal lung maturity by stimulating the production of glucocorticoids by the fetal adrenals. This action in turn stimulates production of lecithin, a lung surfactant, by the fetal lungs.[67] The use of glucocorticoid therapy has been suggested to enhance fetal lung maturity

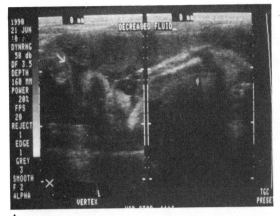

A

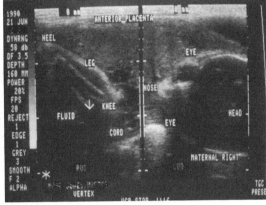

B

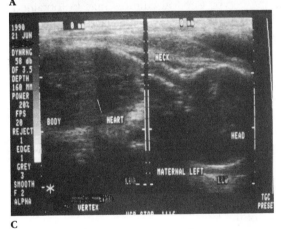

C

Figure 5-2. Ultrasound assessment of a patient at 35 weeks gestation with PPROM. A. The fetal body is in direct contact with the placenta and the uterus. The arrow points to a single pocket of fluid. B. Two small pockets of fluid are shown by the fetal knee and nose. C. Fetus is in direct contact with the placenta and uterus. No fluid is seen.

when preterm delivery is probable. Administration of corticosteroid therapy prior to delivery may accelerate lung maturation and create a "window" of time during which birth may occur with a reduced incidence of respiratory distress syndrome. This window occurs between 24 hours and 7 days after therapy completion.[8,68,69] Therapy may be repeated weekly until delivery.[12] The mechanism of action of glucocorticoid therapy is not understood but appears to stimulate at least transient fetal surfactant production.

There are potential adverse maternal effects from glucocorticoid therapy. Pulmonary edema has been reported in some women receiving simultaneous betamimetic therapy and glucocorticoids.[70] Other potential adverse effects on the mother receiving glucocorticoids include destabilization of the patient with diabetes, accelerated deterioration of pregnancy-induced hypertension, impaired wound healing, and increased risk of infection.[12] Fetal deterioration may be a potential consequence. Risks and benefits must be weighed prior to initiation of treatment.

Assessment

Preterm labor is a significant complication and thus nursing assessment of the mother and fetus begins as quickly as possible and continues throughout hospitalization. Upon admission, maternal vital signs and fetal status are evaluated concurrently with assessment of uterine activity and vaginal discharge. A careful history is taken to identify gestational age, prenatal care, and risk factors such as multiple gestation, hydramnios, history of previous preterm deliveries, uterine anomalies, and history of precipitating events.

Uterine activity and irritability are best assessed by a tocodynamometer and palpation. If the membranes are intact, cervical dilation, effacement, consistency, and position may be evaluated by gentle digital exam. If ruptured membranes are suspected, a sterile speculum exam is done to document the presence of amniotic fluid and to visualize the cervix. Cervical cultures may be obtained.

During assessment, the patient is usually placed in the lateral recumbent position to increase blood flow to the uterus, and bedrest is prescribed. The patient is hydrated with intravenous fluids to increase blood flow to the uterus. Systematic and serial assessment continues throughout treatment and is best accomplished by continuity of care providers so as to identify subtle changes in patient status from day to day. Serial cervical assessment by speculum or gentle digital exam tracks cervical changes. Changes in cervical tissue consistency, cervical position, and station of the presenting part may indicate advancing labor. The patient is monitored for associated symptoms which include the following:

1. Passage of cervical mucus, often slightly blood-tinged
2. Low backache
3. Pelvic pressure due to descent of the fetus
4. Menstrual-like cramps
5. Intestinal cramping with or without diarrhea[71]

Uterine activity is closely monitored and although cessation of uterine contractions is a treatment goal, progressive cervical change is the true indication of labor.[12] Evidence suggests that patterns of daily uterine contractility observed in patients after an episode of preterm labor can identify those at greater risk for a preterm delivery as uterine activity appears to be significantly higher in this group.[72]

Diagnosis of preterm labor is generally accepted and confirmed when progressive cervical dilation reaches 2 cm, and cervical effacement reaches 80%.[18,73] Advancement of cervical dilation beyond 4 cm is usually an indication that tocolytic therapy and other attempts to halt labor may be unsuccessful.[74] Digital cervical examinations are limited to avoid the possibility of stimulating labor. In the presence of PPROM, digital exams increase the risk of infection by carrying organisms through the vagina to the endocervical canal; these are therefore avoided during management of PPROM until delivery is imminent.

TABLE 5-3
Initial Management of Preterm Premature Rupture of Membranes[a]

The confirmation of rupture of the amniotic membranes
Determination of pathologic bacterial infection at the time of rupture
Documentation of gestational age
Determination of fetal pulmonary maturity
Early detection of developing maternal and/or fetal infections
Early detection of fetal compromise

[a]From Crenshaw[76].

Amniotic fluid examination for the lecithin-to-sphingomyelin ratio and presence or absence of phosphatidylglycerol concentration assists in the evaluation of fetal pulmonary maturity. If the specimen is retrieved through amniocentesis rather than by vaginal collection, it may also be examined for bacteria. Tests may include Gram's stain, cultures, and C-reactive protein studies as indicators of the presence of infection.

The *p*H of amniotic fluid is essentially neutral (6.5–7.5), while cervical mucus is usually slightly acidic (5.0–6.0). Urine may normally vary in *p*H from 4.5 to 8.0. Maternal blood near the cervix may also be near neutral (7.4).[66] The overlap of these values makes nitrazine testing of a vaginal fluid specimen ineffective for the diagnosis of PROM. Examination of vaginal fluid for ferning after drying the specimen on a glass slide has proved to be a more sensitive test to confirm the presence of amniotic fluid in the vaginal vault.[75] Alone, none of these tests are completely reliable, but an analysis of physical findings and history is necessary for diagnosis (see Table 5-3).

Fetal heart rate and uterine activity are monitored closely, so that any deterioration in fetal status which might require a change in the management plan of care can be recognized. Monitoring may be intermittent, continuous, or involve daily nonstress tests depending on the patient's clinical status.

Serial ultrasound for examination of the amount of amniotic fluid, fetal size, presentation, lower uterine segment funneling, presence of fetal breathing, and placental location and status all aid in improved assessment of maternal–fetal condition.

Formulation of Nursing Diagnoses

Nursing diagnoses are derived by reviewing the actual and potential problems of the woman experiencing preterm labor. The diagnosis formulates a starting point on which the nursing plan of care is based. The more specific the nursing diagnosis, the more readily interventions can be planned. Nursing interventions are much more easily evaluated and revised throughout the woman's hospitalization when nursing diagnoses are specific and measurable.

The patient in preterm labor faces the potential for delivering a premature infant at risk for morbidity related to prematurity. The anxiety the woman may experience in the face of her own hospitalization, loss of control of her body, and potential injury to her baby are assessed. Significant stress may be a deleterious factor in prolongation of the pregnancy.

Nursing diagnoses during tocolytic therapy also address prevention of severe maternal and fetal complications related to the specific drug used. For example, the potential for alteration in tissue perfusion during ritodrine infusion is related to severe maternal tachycardia, hypotension, myocardial ischemia, and an altered intravascular volume. Nursing interventions are directed toward resolving the individual's specific and immediate problems identified by the nursing diagnoses.

- Potential fetal injury related to prematurity
- Potential fetal injury related to PPROM or oligohydramnios
- Infection, potential for, related to PPROM
- Potential maternal–fetal injury related to infection
- Anxiety related to preterm labor and possible preterm delivery
- Fluid volume alteration: excess related to betamimetic tocolysis
- Potential alteration in tissue perfusion: cardiopulmonary, related to betamimetic tocolysis as evidenced by severe maternal tachycardia, chest pain, or tightness
- Potential metabolic alterations related to betamimetic tocolysis, hyperglycemia, and hypokalemia
- Potential for ineffective breathing patterns related to $MgSO_4$ tocolysis
- Alteration in comfort related to tocolytic side effects and preterm labor
- Alterations in maternal–family coping related to hospitalization during preterm labor or PPROM

Theoretical Basis for the Plan of Nursing Care and Intervention

A patient admitted to the hospital for preterm labor is placed in the lateral recumbent position, and strict bedrest is prescribed. Initial assessment and interventions are carried out concurrently. During the initial observation period, intravenous hydration may be appropriate if contractions persist. Intake and output are monitored and documented immediately in the event tocolytic therapy is started.

It is possible that uterine activity can be stimulated by high levels of endogenous catecholemines produced during states of anxiety and fear.[31,64] The anxious, frightened patient should be provided with a calm environment and frequent reassurance. It may be appropriate, at some point during the patient's hospitalization, to provide the patient with support from a psychologist or social worker. Historically, nurses have been aware that providing continuity of care promotes rapport and trust between patient and caregiver, thus alleviating anxiety. Explanations concerning the plan of care, treatment, surveillance techniques, and expected outcome of the baby may need to be repeated once the patient's level of anxiety diminishes.

Nursing care of the patient in preterm labor includes an ongoing assessment of uterine activity by palpation and/or electronic monitoring. Fetal well-being is assessed with continuous fetal heart rate monitoring or frequent auscultation.

During tocolytic therapy, nursing actions are directed toward monitoring and documenting the effects of tocolysis on uterine activity. If contractions continue despite tocolytic therapy, cervical changes and the station of the presenting part must be assessed and documented. Effective tocolysis is achieved when contractions become milder and less frequent. Six or more contractions in an hour should prompt physician notification and reevaluation of the method of tocolysis. In general, the frequency of digital cervical exams is determined by the clinical status of the mother. It is beneficial to limit such exams as much as possible as cervical manipulation can potentially stimulate prostaglandin production and uterine activity. In the presence of ruptured membranes, vaginal exams are limited because of the potential for infection. If possible, vaginal exams should be performed by the same examiner in order to detect any subtle changes in the cervix. Nursing management during tocolytic therapy includes prevention and recognition of serious adverse effects. Nursing management also includes minimization of the uncomfortable side effects related to drug administration.

Betamimetic agents are potent drugs requiring vigilant nursing management during intravenous infusion. Vital signs are taken at least hourly during the maintenance infusion. More frequent monitoring is warranted during infusion increases and in any patient with risk factors. Baseline tests prior to infusion therapy may include a maternal electrocardiogram, complete blood count, electrolyte level status, and urinalysis. Monitoring of the fetal heart rate and uterine activity should continue throughout the infusion.

The maternal fluid volume status is followed closely during betamimetic therapy. The patient must have nothing orally during the tocolytic infusion with strict intake and output records maintained. If a urinary catheter is in place, intake and output can be assessed hourly, otherwise at least every 4 hours. The betamimetic solution is added, mixed in a separate infusion bag, and piggybacked into a mainline. The use of an infusion pump is mandatory for precise dosage administration. It is prudent to control the mainline by infusion pump to maintain accurate intake and to avoid fluid overload. Daily weights and serial hemograms also aid in assessing fluid status.

Cardiopulmonary complications of betamimetic therapy can be life threatening; close monitoring of cardiopulmonary status is essential. Lung fields are auscultated for the presence of adventitious sounds. Continuous cardiac monitoring is recommended when maternal heart rate is greater than 120 beats per minute and whenever symptoms suggesting arrhythmias are present, such as an irregular heart rate. A maternal heart rate greater than 120, a systolic pressure less than 90 mmHg or a diastolic pressure less than 40 mmHg require immediate physician notification. The betamimetic infusion is decreased or discontinued. Complaints of chest pain, shortness of breath, or any other abnormal reactions to the drug also require immediate physician notification and evaluation. The patient must be monitored for cardiopulmonary complications for 12 to 24 hours after the infusion has been discontinued. Monitoring includes strict intake and output assessment, auscultation of lung fields, and monitoring of vital signs. The patient receiving betamimetic tocolysis is usually restless and apprehensive, and nursing management should include comfort measures and provisions for periods of rest.

Prior to $MgSO_4$ tocolysis, a baseline assessment includes vital signs and deep tendon reflexes. These important clinical parameters are assessed during the maintenance infusion as hypotension may occur particularly during the bolus infusion. Positioning the patient on her side and assessing blood pressure levels frequently minimize the risks to mother and fetus. Care providers are alerted to early signs of magnesium toxicity through assessments of the respiratory rate and deep tendon reflexes. A respiratory rate less than 12 per minute or absent deep tendon reflexes require immediate physician notification. A magnesium serum level is drawn and the infusion discontinued if magnesium toxicity is suspected. To reverse magnesium toxicity, calcium gluconate should be readily available. The recommended dose is 1 g of calcium gluconate (10 ml of 10% solution) administered intravenously over a 5- to 10-minute period. A physician should be present during calcium gluconate administration.

Fluid restriction is necessary to minimize the risks of pulmonary edema. A total hourly or daily intake should be clarified with the physician. The use of an infusion pump is mandatory to maintain precise control of the dosage administration and to control the mainline rate. Lung fields are auscultated for the presence of adventitious sounds. A urinary catheter is usually not necessary unless urinary retention is a problem or urinary output falls, but output must be assessed and documented. The frequency, quality, duration, and patient perception of uterine contractions are monitored closely. Mild, infrequent contractions usually do not result in cervical change.[48] The fetus should be monitored closely as well.

As with any tocolytic therapy, the patient receiving indomethacin requires careful monitoring for effectiveness of the therapy. Indomethacin is usually well tolerated by patients. Gastrointestinal side effects can be minimized by administering oral medication with food. Antacids may also help to relieve gastrointestinal discomfort. Fetal heart rate monitoring is specifically concerned with identifying variable decelerations, which may indicate cord compression due to reduction in amniotic fluid.

Once the fetal membranes have ruptured, nursing management includes the continuing assessment of the patient for signs of infection. Fetal tachycardia is often the first sign of infection, but other clinical signs or symptoms include maternal tachycardia, rising temperature, fever, chills, uterine tenderness, foul-smelling vaginal discharge, and purulent vaginal or cervical discharge. Patients with ruptured membranes must be educated about the need for careful perineal hygiene.

Expected Outcomes

The optimal outcome for a woman in preterm labor is to effectively prolong the pregnancy until 37 weeks gestation or fetal lung maturity is achieved. Unfortunately this is not always a realistic expectation. While mothers experiencing preterm labor require reassurance from the health care team, they should never be offered false hopes if a preterm birth is inevitable.

The expected outcome for both mother and baby depends on the clinical status of the patient and estimated gestational age. The outcome for a woman in advanced labor with ruptured membranes and chorioamnionitis at 33 to 34 weeks gestation will be different than that for a woman at the same gestational age with intact membranes and a closed cervix. The expected outcome for the woman with ruptured membranes and chorioamnionitis might be vaginal delivery before significant maternal and fetal compromise occur. The goal of nursing care is to protect both mother and fetus from further harm through continuous maternal–fetal assessment and communication with the physician and other health care team members.

The ultimate goal in the treatment of preterm labor in the intrapartum setting is to prevent significant maternal and neonatal morbidity and mortality. The optimal outcome for the fetus/neonate is delaying birth until term or until lung maturity is attained. If cervical change continues, delaying the delivery until steroids are administered may be a more realistic goal than prevention of a preterm birth. Optimal maternal outcomes include protection from potential complications of tocolytic therapy, avoiding significant infection especially following rupture of membranes, and a thorough understanding by the woman of the treatment and care she is receiving.

PRETERM LABOR WITH TOCOLYSIS
The patient will

1. Continue the pregnancy until 37 completed weeks or until fetal lung maturity has been achieved.
2. Maintain effective breathing patterns as evidenced by normal maternal respiratory rate and volume.
3. Maintain normal tissue perfusion as evidenced by the absence of chest pain, a maternal heart rate of less than 120 beats per minute, and a reassuring fetal heart rate tracing.
4. Maintain a normovolemic state as evidenced by an adequate urine output, normal breath sounds, and a systolic blood pressure greater than 90 mm Hg (or normal blood pressure).

5. Be free of significant side effects of tocolytic treatment as evidenced by the presence of deep tendon reflexes, absence of electrocardiogram changes, and subjective complaints of shortness of breath or chest pain.

PRETERM PREMATURE RUPTURE OF MEMBRANES
The patient will

1. Remain free from infection as evidenced by absence of foul-smelling or purulent amniotic fluid and/or temperature elevation.

PSYCHOSOCIAL WELL-BEING
The patient will

1. Verbalize decreased fear and increased understanding of the risks of prematurity to the baby.
2. Verbalize understanding of the need for and potential side effects of tocolytic therapy.
3. Verbalize understanding of the process of monitoring for uterine activity and fetal heart rate patterns.
4. Verbalize her perception of support from family and significant others.

FETAL WELL-BEING
The fetus will

1. Maintain a baseline heart rate between 110 and 160 beats per minute.
2. Maintain a reassuring fetal heart rate pattern as evidenced by (*a*) heart rate accelerations (as appropriate for gestational age), (*b*) absence of periodic patterns, and (*c*) absence of variable decelerations after rupture of membranes.
3. Maintain usual activity, as perceived by mother.

References

1. American College of Obstetricians and Gynecologists: Preterm labor. *ACOG Technical Bulletin* No. 133, Washington, DC, ACOG, Oct. 1989.
2. Bennett NJ, Botti JJ: New strategies for preterm labor. *Nurse Pract* 14(4):27–38, 1989.
3. American College of Obstetricians and Gynecologists: Premature rupture of membranes. *ACOG Technical Bulletin* No. 115, Washington, DC, ACOG, Apr. 1988.
4. Kalterider DF, Kohl S: Epidemiology of preterm delivery. *Clin Obstet Gynecol* 23:17–31, 1980.
5. DeCaria D: Preterm labor: New approaches to an old problem. *Baby Care Forum* Fall, 1989.
6. Hemminke E, Starfield B: Prevention and treatment of premature labor by drugs. *Brit Obstet Gynecol* 85:411, 1978.
7. Liggins GC: Initiation of spontaneous labor. *Clin Obstet Gynecol* 26(1):47–55, 1983.
8. Harris J: Premature labor: Who is at risk, who can be helped, and how. *Consultant* 24:256–260, 1984.

9. Bowes WA: Clinical management of preterm delivery. *Clin Obstet Gynecol* 32(3):652–661, 1988.
10. Blott M, Greenough A: Neonatal outcome after prolonged rupture of the membranes starting in the second trimester. *Arch Dis Child* 63:1147, 1988.
11. Kilbride H, Yeast J, Thibeault D: Intrapartum and delivery room management of premature rupture of membranes complicated by oligohydramnios. *Clin Perinatol* 16(4):863–888, 1989.
12. Cunningham FG, MacDonald PC, Gant NF: *Williams' Obstetrics* (18th ed.). Norwalk, CT, Appleton and Lange, 1989.
13. Uldbjerg N, Ulmsten U, Ekman G: The ripening of the human uterine cervix in terms of connective tissue biochemistry. *Clin Obstet Gynecol* 26(1):14–25, 1983.
14. Brindley BA, Sokol RJ: Induction and augmentation of labor: Basis and methods for current practice. *Obstet Gynecol Surv* 43(12):730–743, 1988.
15. Casey ML, MacDonald P: Biomolecular processes in the initiation of parturition: Decidual activation. *Clin Obstet Gynecol* 31(3):533–552, 1988.
16. Garfield RE, Hayashi RH: Appearance of gap junctions in the myometrium of women during labor. *Am J Obstet Gynecol* 140(3):254–259, 1981.
17. Ulmsten U: Prostaglandins in high risk obstetrics, in Brody S, Ueland K (eds.): *Endocrine Disorders in Pregnancy.* Englewood Cliffs, NJ, Appleton Lange, 1989.
18. Creasy R, Resnick R: *Maternal-Fetal Medicine: Principles and Practice* (2nd ed.). Philadelphia, W.B. Saunders, 1989.
19. Main D: The epidemiology of preterm birth. *Clin Obstet Gynecol* 31(3):521–531, 1988.
20. Hunter L: Twin gestation: Antepartum management. *J Perinatal Neonatal Nurs* 3(1):1–13, 1989.
21. Romero R, Mazor M: Infection and preterm labor. *Clin Obstet Gynecol* 31(3):533–582, 1988.
22. Toth M, Witkins S, Ledger W, Thaler H: The role of infection in the etiology of preterm birth. *Obstet Gynecol* 71(5):723–726, 1988.
23. Bejar R, Curbelo V, Davis D: Premature labor. II: Bacterial sources of phospholipase. *Obstet Gynecol* 57(4):479–486, 1981.
24. Rayburn, W: Prostaglandin E_2 gel for cervical ripening and induction of labor: A critical analysis. *Am J Obstet Gynecol* 160:529–534, Mar. 1989.
25. Vadillo-Ortega F, Gonzalez-Avial G, Karchmer S, et al: Collagen metabolism in premature rupture of amniotic membranes. *Obstet Gynecol* 75(1):84–88, 1990.
26. Aaronson L, Macnee C: Tobacco, alcohol, and caffeine use during pregnancy. *JOGNN* 18(4): 279–287, 1989.
27. Jacobson H: Prevention of prematurity: The role of diet in health care. *P-N* 17–22, Apr. 1983.
28. McDonald A, McDonald J, Armstrong B, et al: Prematurity and work in pregnancy. *Brit J Indust Med* 45:56–62, 1988.
29. Olds S, London M, Ladewig P: *Maternal Newborn Nursing: A Family Centered Approach* (3rd ed.). Addison-Wesley, Reading, MA, 1988.
30. Givens S: Update on tocolytic therapy in the management of preterm labor. *J Perinat Neonat Nurs* 2(1):21–23, 1988.
31. Niebyl JR, Caritis S, Lipshitz J, Petrie R: Tocolytics: When and how to use them. *Contemp Obstet Gynecol* 27:146–162, June, 1986.
32. Lipshitz J, Baillie P, Davey DA: A comparison of the uterine beta$_2$-adrenoreceptor selectivity of fenoterol, hexoprenaline, ritodrine and Salbutamol. *S Am Med J* 50:1969–1972, 1976.
33. Caritis SN, Toig G, Heddinger L, Ashmead G: A double blind study comparing ritodrine and terbutaline in the treatment of preterm labor. *Am J Obstet Gynecol* 150(1):7–14, 1984.
34. Merkatz I, Peter J, Barden T: Ritodrine hydrochloride: A betamimetic agent for use in preterm labor. *Obstet Gynecol* 56(1):7–12, 1980.
35. Moore B, Briggs G, Freeman R: Terbutaline for tocolysis: Do advantages outweigh risks? *Contemp Obstet Gynecol* 32(3):53–65, September, 1988.
36. Caritis S, Lin L, Toig G, Wong LK: Pharmaco-dynamics of ritodrine in pregnant women during preterm labor. *Am J Obstet Gynecol* 147(7):752–759, 1983.
37. Benedetti TJ: Maternal complications of parenteral β-sympathomimetic therapy for premature labor. *Am J Obstet Gynecol* 145(1):1–6, 1983.

38. Graber E: Dilemmas in the pharmacological management of preterm labor. *Obstet Gynecol Surv* 44(7):512–517, 1989.

39. Bardon TP, Peter JB, Merkatz I: Ritodrine hydrochloride: A betamimetic agent for use in preterm labor. I: Pharmacology, clinical history, administration, side effects and safety. *Am J Obstet Gynecol* 56(1):1–6, 1980.

40. Gonik B, Benedetti TJ, Creasy RK, Lee AF: Intramuscular versus intravenous ritodrine hydrochloride for preterm labor management. *Am J Obstet Gynecol* 159(2):323–328, 1988.

41. Witter FR, Benedetti TJ, Petty BG, et al: Pharmacodynamics and tolerance of oral sustained release ritodrine. *Am J Obstet Gynecol* 159(3):690–695, 1988.

42. Caritis S, Darby M, Chan L: Pharmacologic treatment of preterm labor. *Clin Obstet Gynecol* 31(3):635–651, 1988.

43. Stubblefield P, Heyl P: Treatment of preterm labor with subcutaneous terbutaline. *Obstet Gynecol* 59(4):457–462, 1982.

44. Aarimaa T, Ekbald U, Erbkola R, et al: Effect of antepartum ritodrine on the cardiorespiratory status of the newborn after elective cesarean section. *Gynecol Obstet Invest* 23:160–166, 1987.

45. Hollander D, Nagey D, Pupkin M: Magnesium sulfate and ritodrine hydrochloride: A randomized comparison. *Obstet Gynecol* 156(3):631–637, 1987.

46. Miller J, Keane M, Horger R: A comparison of magnesium sulfate and terbutaline for the arrest of premature labor: A preliminary report. *J Reprod Med* 27(6):348–351, 1982.

47. Thiagarajah S, Harbert G, Bourgeois FJ: Magnesium sulfate and ritodrine hydrochloride: Systemic and uterine hemodynamic effects. *Am J Obstet Gynecol* 153(6):666–674, 1985.

48. Elliott J: Magnesium sulfate as a tocolytic agent. *Contemp Obstet Gynecol* 25:49–61, June 1985.

49. Dudley D, Gagnon D, Varner MW: Long-term tocolysis with magnesium sulfate. *Obstet Gynecol* 73:373, 1989.

50. Petrie RH: Tocolysis using magnesium sulfate. *Sem Perinatol* 5(3):266–273, 1981.

51. Zuckerman H, Reiss U, and Rubenstein I: Inhibition of human premature labor by indomethacin. *Obstet Gynecol* 44:787–792, 1974.

52. Few B: Indomethacin for treatment of premature labor. *MCN* 13:93, 1988.

53. Morales WJ, Smith S, Angel JL, et al: Efficacy and safety of indomethacin versus ritodrine in the management of preterm labor: A randomized study. *Obstet Gynecol* 74(4):567–572, 1989.

54. Zuckerman H, Shalev E, Gilad G, Katzuni E: Further study of the inhibition of premature labor by indomethacin. *J Perinat Med* 12:19–23, 1984.

55. Niebyl JR, Witter FR: Neonatal outcome after indomethacin treatment for preterm labor. *Am J Obstet Gynecol* 55:747–749, 1986.

56. Niebyl JR, Blake DA, White RD, et al: The inhibition of premature labor with indomethacin. *Am J Obstet Gynecol* 136:1014–1019, 1980.

57. Abdella T: A decision analytic approach to delivery of the very low birth-weight infant. Presentation to The Society of Perinatal Obstetricians, Sixth Annual Meeting, San Antonio, Texas. Jan. 30–Feb. 1, 1986.

58. Moise K, Jr, Huhta J, Troffater K, Sharif D: Low dose aspirin therapy in the treatment of lupus anticoagulant: Effects on the human ductus arteriosus. *Soc Perinat Obstet Ann Meeting* 123, 1988.

59. Read WD, Welby DE: The use of a calcium antagonist (nifedipine) to suppress labor. *Brit J Obstet Gynecol* 93:933–937, 1986.

60. Ulmsten U, Andersson KE, Wingerup L: Treatment of premature labor with the calcium antagonist nifedipine. *Arch Gynecol* 229:1–5, 1980.

61. Duscay CA, Thompson JS, Wu AT, Novy MJ: Effects of calcium entry blocker (nicardipine) tocolysis in rhesus macaques: Fetal plasma concentrations and cardiorespiratory changes. *Am J Obstet Gynecol* 157(6):1482–1486, 1987.

62. Mari G, Kirshon B, Moise KJ, et al: Doppler assessment of the fetal and uteroplacental circulation during nifedipine therapy for preterm labor. *Am J Obstet Gynecol* 161(6, part 1):1514–1518, 1989.

63. Morales WJ, Angel JL, O'Brien WF, Knuppel RA: Use of ampicillin and corticosteroids in premature rupture of membranes: A randomized study. *Obstet Gynecol* 73(5):721, 1989.

64. Sachs B, Ringer S: Intrapartum and delivery room management of the very low birthweight infant. *Clin Perinatol* 16(4):809–823, 1989.

65. Vintzileos AM, Campbell WA, Nochimson PJ, Weinbaum PJ: Fetal breathing as a predictor of infection in premature rupture of the membranes. *S Am Obstet Gynecol* 6:813–817, 1986.

66. Nagey DA, Saller DN: An analysis of the decisions in the management of premature rupture of the membranes. *Clin Obstet Gynecol* 29:826–834, 1986.

67. Weitzel H, Lorenz I, Kipper B: Clinical aspects of antenatal glucocorticoid treatment for prevention of neonatal respiratory distress syndrome. *J Perinatol Med* 15:441–444, 1987.

68. Felton G, Martin B: The high cost of preterm labor. *RN* 48:47–51, 1985.

69. Gazaway P, Mullins C: Prevention of preterm labor and premature rupture of the membranes. *Clin Obstet Gynecol* 29(4):835–849, 1986.

70. Jacobs M, Knight A, Arias F: Maternal pulmonary edema resulting from betamimetic and glucocorticoid therapy. *Obstet Gynecol* 56(1):56–59, 1980.

71. Herron MA, Katy M, Creasy RK: Evaluation of a preterm birth prevention program: Preliminary report. *Obstet Gynecol* 59:452, 1982.

72. Bustman LE, Langer O, Damus K, et al: Uterine contractility patterns after an episode of preterm labor. *Obstet Gynecol* 75(3):346, 1990.

73. Leveno KJ, Cunningham FG: Dilemmas in the management of preterm birth, in Pritchard JA, McDonald PC, Gant NF (eds.): *Supplement to Williams' Obstetrics,* 17th ed., vol. 12. Norwalk, CT, Appleton and Lange, 1987.

74. Liu DTY, Fairweather DIV: The management of preterm labor, in Elder MG, Hendricks CH (eds.): *Obstetrics and Gynecology. I: Preterm Labor.* London, Butterworth, 1981.

75. Reese EA, Chervenak FA, Maya FR, Hobbins JC: Amniotic fluid arborization: Effect of blood, meconium, and pH alterations. *Obstet Gynecol* 64:248, 1984.

76. Crenshaw C: Preterm premature rupture of the membranes (Foreword). *Clin Obstet Gynecol* 29(4):735–738, 1986.

6

❖ ❖ ❖

Prolonged Pregnancy

Marian F. Lake

Supportive Data

Incidence

Pregnancy is defined as *prolonged* when it exceeds 42 weeks or 294 days from the first day of a woman's last menstrual period (LMP). Prolonged gestation occurs in approximately 10% of all pregnancies, with 5% extending beyond 43 weeks of gestation.[1,2]

Accurate calculation of prolonged pregnancy depends upon an accurate assessment of the fetal gestational age. Assessment of gestational age traditionally relies on the establishment of an estimated date of confinement based on the first day of the woman's last menstrual period. Unfortunately, a woman may not be able to recall her last menstrual period, may have experienced irregular periods, or may have had delayed ovulation, all of which potentially contribute to an unreliable estimated date of confinement.

Other means of assessment that increase the accuracy of gestational dating include documentation of the following:

- A positive urine pregnancy test within 6 weeks after the last menstrual period or serum pregnancy test within 2 weeks of it.
- First documentation of audible fetal heart tones by unamplified auscultation using a DeLee fetal stethoscope usually between 17 and 19 weeks gestation.
- Maternal perception of first fetal movement usually noted between 16 and 20 weeks.
- Serial measurement of fundal height between 22 and 30 weeks.
- Ultrasound measurement of fetal size prior to 26 weeks with crown rump length, femur length, or biparietal diameter.

Early access to prenatal care clearly enhances the accuracy of these measurements. Without knowledge of pregnancy duration, the risk of inaccurate gestational age assessment increases. As a result, it has been suggested that perhaps more than 50% of pregnancies classified as prolonged are actually of normal length.[2,3]

Significance

Prolonged pregnancy is associated with an increased risk for both the fetus and mother. Fetal risks are for the most part associated with progressive, degenerative placental changes, whereas maternal risks heighten during labor, delivery, and the immediate postpartum period.

Placental function reaches a peak by 36 weeks. Thereafter functional efficiency begins to diminish. As the placenta ages, intervillous infarcts may develop resulting in placental infarcts.[2] This phenomenon, though not exclusive to prolonged pregnancy, can progress and worsen as gestation advances beyond term.

Analyses of pregnancy outcome in the 1960s and 1970s demonstrated that as gestation progressed beyond 42 weeks, the risk of stillbirth increased.[2] In the normal population, perinatal death occurs in 1% to 2% of term pregnancies. In 1963, McClure-Brown showed that the death rate doubled at 43 weeks and quadrupled at 44 weeks.[4] However, more recent analyses have not revealed the same risk for stillbirth in this group of patients.[5,6,7] Technologic advances used in determining gestational age along with improved maternal and fetal surveillance may account for this trend. Notwithstanding, sizeable fetal and neonatal risks remain.

One of those risks is the neonatal syndrome of postmaturity. Postmaturity is a condition seen in approximately 20% to 30% of neonates whose mothers were assessed as being past the due date originally set.[7-9] Postmaturity syndrome may only be diagnosed after examination of the infant and is therefore a neonatal rather than an obstetric condition. The characteristics of a postmature neonate are the result of advanced fetal development, prolonged exposure to amniotic fluid, and exposure to placental insufficiency. The baby typically exhibits meconium staining (Figure 6-1); long nails; wrinkled, peeling skin (Figure 6-2); increased alertness; decreased subcutaneous fat; and long hair (Figure 6-3). The fetus who remains *in utero* beyond 42 weeks gestation and who does not exhibit this syndrome as a neonate nevertheless remains at risk before delivery.

Even though placental function slows after 36 weeks, placental and fetal growth continue until delivery. Macrosomia may result and occurs in 20% to 25% of prolonged pregnancies.[5,10,11] When the fetus is macrosomic, shoulder dystocia and trauma at delivery may occur. Fractured humerus or clavicle, brachial plexus, facial nerve palsy, asphyxia, and death have all been associated with shoulder dystocia at delivery.[12,13]

The maximum amount of amniotic fluid volume in a normal pregnancy is 1000 to 1200 cc, and this volume is reached at approximately 38 weeks gestation, after which time the volume gradually decreases. By 42 weeks, the volume has decreased to approximately 300 cc and continues to decrease at 43 and 44 weeks.[2] Amniotic fluid acts as a cushion for the umbilical cord, helping to protect it from deleterious compression. Abnormally small volumes of fluid (*i.e.,*

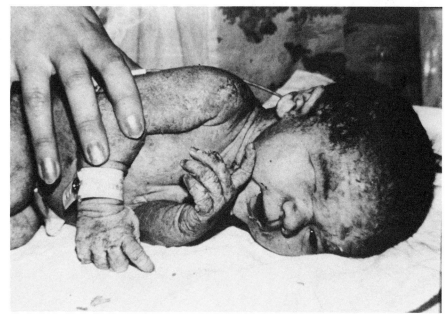

Figure 6-1.
Postmature infant
with meconium
staining, imme-
diately after birth.

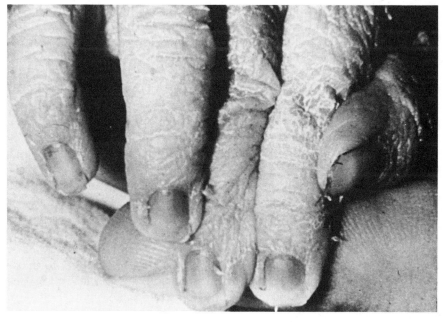

Figure 6-2.
Postmature infant
with characteristic
long nails and peel-
ing, wrinkled skin.

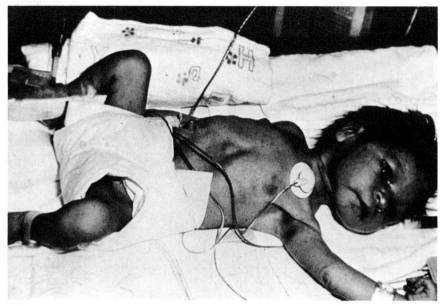

Figure 6-3.
Postmature infant in Figure 6-1 at two days of age showing increased alertness, decreased subcutaneous fat, and long hair.

oligohydramnios) have been associated with fetal cord compression in labor[14,15] and postmaturity syndrome in the neonate.[8]

Meconium-stained amniotic fluid, a condition also associated with prolonged gestation, poses increased fetal risk. The proposed mechanism for intrauterine meconium passage is stimulation of smooth muscle in the fetal colon, which is caused by hypoxia and results in defecation. Whether meconium passage is stimulated by hypoxia from placental insufficiency or cord compression is unclear. However, the incidence of meconium in prolonged pregnancy increases if oligohydramnios is also present.[15] The presence of meconium and, in particular, thick meconium is associated with an increased risk of fetal distress during labor and acidosis at birth.[7,16-18] Meconium aspiration syndrome—a neonatal complication that can result in mechanical airway obstruction, chemical pneumonitis, pneumothorax, and eventual death—has been reported to occur eight times more frequently in prolonged pregnancy than in normal length gestation.[19]

Prolonged pregnancy also increases the risk of maternal complications. Of the women with this diagnosis 15% to 30% will have cesarean sections.[7,19,20] Fetal macrosomia, fetal compromise, and prolonged labor contribute to this increased risk.

Induction of labor with the intravenous administration of oxytocin, whether for maternal or fetal indications, is often employed in these cases. Oxytocin use is associated with maternal uterine hyperstimulation; this can lead to uterine rupture and antidiuresis, which results in water intoxication.[21]

When fetal macrosomia is present, the incidence of cephalopelvic dispropor- tion, uterine dysfunction, and prolonged labor are increased and the risks of maternal exhaustion and intrapartum infection rise.[21] In addition, fetal mac- rosomia with uterine overdistention, operative delivery, traumatic vaginal deliv- ery resulting in vaginal or cervical lacerations, and administration of oxytocin during labor increase the maternal risk of postpartum hemorrhage.

Finally, often overlooked but nonetheless important complications for the woman with a prolonged pregnancy are frustration and emotional turmoil from anxiety and fear.[22] When these emotions are not acknowledged, the woman may become angry and resentful toward her health care providers. Overwhelming anxiety may interfere with the woman's ability to understand and facilitate her therapy.

The significance of prolonged pregnancy rests in its association with fetal death, fetal compromise, neonatal illness, and maternal complications during labor, delivery, and the immediate postpartum period. The intrapartum period appears to be the time at which the risks of prolonged pregnancy are at their peak.

Etiology

The cause of prolonged pregnancy is unknown. There are, however, certain fetal and maternal conditions that seem to increase the risk of occurrence. Several factors that may cause decreased estrogen levels in pregnancy have been associ- ated with prolonged pregnancy. Fetal pituitary or adrenal gland insufficiency, as seen in anencephaly, are two such conditions.[2,23] Insufficient amounts of the precursor hormone dehydroisoandrosterone sulfate, which maintains appropri- ate levels of estradiol and estriol, also may cause prolonged gestation.[21] Another factor linked with this condition is placental sulfatase deficiency, an uncommon genetic disorder that also leads to decreased estriol levels. Other fetal anomalies include hydrocephaly and osteogenesis imperfecta.[24]

Prolonged pregnancy occurs more often in certain groups of women than it does in others. For example, primigravid women 15 to 20 years of age are more likely to have a postterm pregnancy than are multigravid women of the same age. Multigravid women over 35 years of age are more likely than primigravid women.[2] Women who have had one prolonged pregnancy have a 50% risk of recurrence.[25] Although no consistent cause for prolonged pregnancy has been found, identifying the woman or fetus in whom it is more likely to occur should heighten the health care provider's awareness of potential maternal or fetal jeopardy.

Framework for Accepted Therapy

Accepted antepartum therapy during prolonged pregnancy focuses on evalua- tion of the fetal–placental unit. Deteriorating placental function places the fetus at risk for inadequate nutrition and oxygenation. Uteroplacental function and the intrauterine environment are evaluated to assess fetal well-being and identify potential jeopardy during this high-risk period.

A variety of protocols using some or all of the antepartum assessment meth- ods outlined in Table 6-1 may be used. The most common tests are the nonstress

TABLE 6-1
Antepartum Fetal Surveillance in Prolonged Pregnancy

Clinical Finding/Test	Result		
	Normal	*Suspicious*	*Abnormal*
Uterine measurement	Increasing	No change	Decreasing
Maternal weight	Increasing	Decreasing	——
Maternal perception of fetal activity	Unchanged	Decreasing	Cessation
Biophysical profile	≥8	5–7	≤4
Nonstress test	Reactive	Reactive with variable decelerations	Nonreactive, variable, or late decelerations
Fetal movement	Normal	Diminished	None
Fetal tone	Normal	Diminished	Flaccid
Fetal breathing	Normal	Diminished	None or gasping
Amniotic fluid volume	Normal	Diminished	Oligohydramnios
Fetal growth by ultrasound	Continued growth	Unchanged	Growth retardation
Contraction stress test	Negative	Equivocal	Positive

Source: Adapted from Campbell WA, Nochimson DJ, Vintzileos AM: Prolonged pregnancy, in Knuppel RA, Drukker JE (eds.): *High Risk Pregnancy: A Team Approach*. Philadelphia, WB Saunders, 1986.

test, the contraction stress test, and the biophysical profile, which includes the assessment of amniotic fluid volume.

The nonstress test (NST) is based on the assumption that a fetus with an intact central nervous system and in whom there is adequate oxygenation will exhibit transient fetal heart rate (FHR) accelerations in response to fetal movement. The presence of two accelerations of 15-beats-per-minute amplitude that last at least 15 seconds within a 10- to 20-minute time period is considered a reactive, or normal, reassuring test. Occasionally, acoustic stimulation with a device similar to an artificial larynx is applied to the maternal abdomen in an attempt to awaken or stimulate the fetus during the NST. In prolonged pregnancy, placental dysfunction and potential disruption in fetal oxygenation may result in a nonreactive test. A nonreactive test, despite attempts to arouse the fetus, indicates the need for further fetal evaluation.

Spontaneous variable decelerations during a nonstress test may occur in as many as 33% of the patients tested. This finding suggests cord compression and oligohydramnios and is associated with meconium passage, fetal distress in labor, and low 1-minute Apgar scores.[26,27] Assessment of amniotic fluid volume is generally made when variable decelerations are observed.

The contraction stress test (CST) may be the primary means of fetal assessment in prolonged pregnancy, or it may be used in conjunction with the NST. The CST is based on the premise that the fetus with uteroplacental insufficiency will exhibit signs of hypoxia with late decelerations in response to spontaneous or induced contractions. When the late decelerations occur with 50% or more of the contractions, the CST is classified as "positive."[28] In prolonged pregnancy, degenerative placental changes are most likely responsible for the uteroplacental insufficiency. Variable decelerations (*i.e.,* evidence of cord compression and oligohydramnios) may also occur during a CST.

The biophysical profile is a means of antepartum assessment that incorporates evaluation of the NST, fetal movement, fetal breathing movements, fetal tone, and amniotic fluid volume. A score is assigned to the assessment based on findings. Each parameter is given a score of 0 to 2, with 2 assigned if evaluation is normal. A score of 8 to 10 with adequate fluid volume is considered normal. It has been shown that the biophysical profile allows identification of the fetus in jeopardy and thereby improves outcome.[29,30,31]

The risks of placental dysfunction, oligohydramnios, and potential fetal compromise indicate the need for continual FHR monitoring during labor. The potential for uteroplacental insufficiency and cord compression is increased, and both complications produce recognizable periodic and baseline changes in the FHR.

When uteroplacental insufficiency is present, fetal chemoreceptors are stimulated by decreasing fetal Po_2 and the parasympathetic nervous system is stimulated, causing the FHR to slow in a characteristic, uniform pattern of late decelerations. During cord compression fetal hypertension and subsequent hypotension stimulate baroreceptors, while chemoreceptors, stimulated by the acute fall in Po_2 during cord compression, also exert an influence on FHR control. The result is parasympathetic stimulation, which produces the pattern of variable decelerations. As the fetal condition worsens and the insult becomes chronic, sympathetic nervous system response may produce tachycardia.

When the normal interplay between the parasympathetic and sympathetic nervous system is dampened by hypoxia, variability decreases. If hypoxia continues and becomes chronic, the fetus uses all metabolic reserves and evidence of severe fetal distress develops including loss of variability with late decelerations, severe variable decelerations, or bradycardia.

Accurate assessment of all parameters of fetal status necessitates precise reception of FHR and fetal heart beat intervals. Auscultation or external electronic fetal monitoring may limit reception of this information and therefore impede the interpretation of these parameters, especially if the woman is frequently changing positions or is obese. Applying an internal fetal electrode will allow for more precise interpretation of the FHR.

Evaluation of fetal acid–base status may become necessary during labor. If fetal hypoxia persists and anaerobic metabolism occurs, fetal acidosis may develop. Assessment of fetal acid–base status can be achieved through the technique of scalp blood sampling. A confirmed fetal capillary blood *p*H of 7.20 or lower is associated with serious fetal jeopardy.[17,32]

Intrapartum risk to the postterm fetus can be substantial. Astute observation of FHR and periodic acid–base evaluation give the practitioner a means of assessing fetal well-being and identifying potential jeopardy.

The uteroplacental insufficiency that produces hypoxia and subsequent late decelerations may have one or more causes. Degenerative placental changes may impede the supply of blood to the fetus, decreasing fetal P_{O_2} and leading to hypoxia.[2] When cord compression occurs, the mechanical force impedes oxygen flow to the fetus. Excess uterine activity may severely limit intervillous gas exchange as intraspiral vessels are occluded by myometrial muscular contraction. Maternal hypotension resulting from vena caval compression by the gravid uterus or regional anesthesia may result in an inadequate supply of oxygen to the uterus and placenta.

Regardless of cause, therapy is directed toward facilitating or improving oxygen transfer to the fetus. Such measures include the following:

- Lateral positioning to facilitate venous return and increase cardiac output while relieving hypotension.
- Repositioning in an attempt to relieve mechanical compression of the umbilical cord
- Maternal oxygen administration to raise maternal–fetal oxygen concentration gradient
- Discontinuing oxytocin infusion if uterine hyperstimulation is evident

The technique of amnioinfusion has been described as a method of relieving umbilical cord compression in the presence of oligohydramnios.[33] Warmed or room-temperature normal saline is infused into the uterine cavity through an intrauterine pressure catheter (IUPC). Variable decelerations have been relieved in more than 50% of patients. It is also associated with a significant reduction in cesarean sections due to fetal distress.[34,35]

Labor may be induced in prolonged pregnancy to avoid or check fetal risk. The condition of the cervix may influence this decision and the course of induced labor. Induction success rate is increased, length of labor shortened, and the potential for cesarean section decreased if the cervix is "favorable" for induction (*i.e.,* it has begun to dilate, efface, soften, and move to an anterior position and the fetus has begun to descend into the pelvis).[19,36] However, less than 10% of women who are postterm have a cervix favorable for induction.[10]

Inducing labor under any circumstance carries maternal and fetal risk. Overstimulation of uterine activity and subsequent uteroplacental insufficiency are perhaps the most significant. Assessment of uterine activity during induction is essential, and the placement of an IUPC may be required for evaluation of the frequency, intensity, and duration of contractions and the degree of uterine relaxation between contractions. The IUPC may be placed by the physician or, with appropriate institutional policies and procedures, by the registered nurse.[37] Observation of quantified uterine activity made possible by use of the IUPC aids in the detection of uterine dysfunction and overstimulation from oxytocin.

The woman with prolonged pregnancy is at risk for dysfunctional labor. Careful assessment of the frequency and intensity of contractions allows accurate diagnosis. If labor is assessed as inefficient and no contraindications exist, augmentation of labor may be undertaken. Although frequency and relative duration of uterine activity can be evaluated by palpation or with an externally applied tocodynamometer, an IUPC will provide more precise information about these two parameters.

Preparing for delivery with personnel skilled in pediatric resuscitative techniques can reduce neonatal morbidity and mortality. If fetal distress from uteroplacental insufficiency or cord compression has been evident in labor, personnel in attendance at delivery must be prepared to resuscitate the depressed infant. When cord compression has occurred in the late stages of labor, the neonate may exhibit respiratory acidosis. If fetal distress has been chronic and exemplified by late decelerations and loss of variability, metabolic acidosis may be present.[32]

The presence of meconium also requires preparation and intervention at the time of delivery. Neonatal complications can be reduced with suctioning of the infant's mouth and nostrils before delivery of the shoulders from the vagina or uterine incision. Further suctioning of the trachea must be accomplished immediately after delivery under direct visualization by laryngoscopy and intubation. Fetal acidosis occurs more frequently when meconium passage has occurred *in utero,* and vigorous resuscitation may be necessary.

Assessment

Nursing assessment is determined by the stage of labor at the time of admission (see Table 6-2). When admission occurs for elective induction or early labor, thorough, orderly assessment is possible. Intrapartum evaluation begins with a review of the prenatal record if available and expands to include continual assessment of fetal and maternal factors. Maternal and fetal jeopardy may not occur until delivery, and assessment must therefore continue.

When a prolonged FHR deceleration or severe variable decelerations occur immediately prior to delivery, preparations are made for neonatal resuscitation. These patterns may be missed if lack of continuous FHR monitoring or astute auscultation immediately before delivery occurs. Thus FHR monitoring in the delivery room is essential.

The need for resuscitation is often determined at the time of delivery. If oligohydramnios is present and the color of the amniotic fluid has not been determined, *in utero* meconium passage may not be evident until after birth. Shoulder dystocia is generally not predicted until after the fetal head is delivered. If the shoulders become trapped, delayed delivery may result in a depressed infant.

Maternal assessment in the immediate postpartum period focuses on the risk of postpartum hemorrhage. Assessment of vital signs, blood loss at delivery, trauma at delivery, uterine tone, and amount of lochia and urinary output are crucial.

TABLE 6-2
Nursing Assessment of the Patient with Prolonged Pregnancy

Assessment of Prenatal Information

I. Reliability of gestational age (GA)
   A. Date of pregnancy documentation
   B. GA at time of first prenatal visit
   C. Ultrasound results
   D. First documentation of FHR with fetoscope
   E. Practitioner's assessment of GA reliability
II. Maternal and fetal risk factors
   A. History of prolonged pregnancy
   B. Fetal anomalies
III. Antepartum surveillance
   A. Trends in fundal height
   B. Maternal perception of recent fetal movement
   C. NST/CST
   D. Biophysical profile
   E. Amniotic fluid volume

Intrapartum Assessment

Maternal Factors	Fetal Factors

I. Status of cervix on admission
II. Uterine activity
  A. Frequency
  B. Intensity
  C. Duration
  D. Resting tone
III. Knowledge and understanding
  of procedures and status
IV. Status during delivery
  A. Lacerations
  B. Blood loss
	I. FHR
	  A. Baseline characteristics
	    1. Rate
	      a. Tachycardia
	      b. Bradycardia
	    2. Variability
	  B. Periodic changes
	    1. Late decelerations
	    2. Variable decelerations
	II. Amniotic fluid
	  A. Volume
	  B. Color and consistency
	III. Acid–base status
	IV. Status during delivery
	  A. Undetected meconium
	  B. Delivery of shoulders

Formulation of Nursing Diagnoses

The physiologic aberrations that can occur in the placental fetal unit during prolonged pregnancy are the basis for the development of nursing diagnoses and care. Those diagnoses are the following:

- Potential for impaired placental function and fetal compromise
- Potential for a difficult labor (dystocia)

- Potential for fetal or maternal injury
- Anxiety and fear about maternal and fetal well-being
- Potential for impaired neonatal tissue perfusion

Theoretical Basis for the Plan of Nursing Care

Shortly after admission to the labor and delivery unit, the nurse's documentation of the progress of labor begins with assessment of three factors:

1. Documentation of onset of regular uterine activity
2. The status of the cervix
3. The quality of contractions

Application of the tocodynamometer on an external fetal monitor can assist in evaluating frequency and duration of contractions. The maternal abdomen must be palpated to determine intensity of uterine contractions and to assess uterine resting tone.

Fetal well-being during the intrapartum period is dependent on adequate oxygenation. A fetus whose gestation has progressed beyond 294 days is at risk for inadequate or interrupted oxygenation during labor.

Evaluation of fetal status may be most efficiently and consistently achieved in this high-risk situation with continuous electronic fetal monitoring. With the application of the monitor, the nurse maintains an interpretable tracing. Application of the spiral electrode provides a means of accurately assessing all characteristics of the FHR. It is therefore appropriate for the registered nurse, under the guidance of state nurse practice acts and supportive hospital policies, to use this method when indicated. Current guidelines for FHR assessment by auscultation in high-risk pregnancies recommend auscultation every 30 minutes during the latent phase of labor, every 15 minutes in the active phase, and every 5 minutes in the second stage.[38] Baseline heart rate and decelerations not related to contractions (nonperiodic changes) are best detected between contractions while the uterus is relaxed. To detect periodic changes, auscultation must be performed during and for 30 seconds immediately following a contraction.[39] To assess FHR variability, time intervals between successive heart beats must be compared. Because auscultation precludes measurement of this time interval, however, assessment of FHR variability is prevented. Nevertheless, the nurse's care must include regular observation of and comment on baseline and periodic characteristics of FHR from admission through delivery.

Nonreassuring patterns require intervention. Late decelerations are the result of uteroplacental insufficiency from maternal hypotension, placental dysfunction, or excess uterine activity. Nursing intervention in response to this pattern should include the following:

- Repositioning the patient on her side
- Correcting maternal hypotension if evident

- Discontinuing oxytocin infusion if hyperstimulation is present
- Administering oxygen
- Notifying the physician of the nonreassuring pattern and corrective actions taken

Though there are several potential causes of decreased variability during labor, hypoxia must be considered a cause. If it is observed, appropriate nursing interventions must promote fetal oxygenation by positioning the woman on her side and administering oxygen. Implementation of these and all interventions must be followed by comprehensive documentation and observation of fetal response to the actions.

If a pattern of variable decelerations develops, nursing care is directed toward relieving cord compression by repositioning the patient and administering oxygen. If the decelerations are mild and variability is reassuring, no further intervention may be indicated. If they are severe and variability is nonreassuring, intervention includes oxygen administration and discontinuation of oxytocin. A vaginal examination is indicated to rule out a prolapsed cord. If cord compression is severe and prolonged and not relieved by these conventional means, amnioinfusion may be employed. Normal saline is gradually instilled as artificial amniotic fluid in an attempt to cushion the cord against further compression. Although this procedure has been described as a nursing function, the nurse may also assist the physician with the procedure.[33] Approximately 500 cc of normal saline is infused into the uterus through an IUPC over 30 minutes. Repeat infusions are determined by fetal status. Nursing interventions should include a thorough explanation to the patient, support during the procedure, careful calibration and recalibration of the IUPC after the infusion, and documentation of the procedure and fetal response.

Fetal acid-base assessment by fetal scalp sampling may be undertaken if signs of fetal hypoxia persist. Nursing intervention will include preparing the patient by explaining the procedure and supporting her during its performance, preparing the equipment and supplies, and positioning of the patient in the lithotomy position. Care must be taken to detect possible maternal supine hypotension during the procedure and to document the time and results of sampling on the FHR tracing and in the patient's chart.

The nursing care of the woman with a prolonged pregnancy who is being induced must center around deliberate, continuous observation of uterine activity and FHR response. The reader is referred to the earlier section describing the procedure for administering oxytocin. Placement and calibration of an IUPC once membranes have ruptured will allow the nurse to precisely evaluate all aspects of uterine activity. Applying a fetal scalp electrode provides the nurse with precise information concerning the FHR. Prior to beginning induction, the nurse must evaluate fetal status. The fetus of the postterm pregnancy faces labor at appreciable risk for uteroplacental insufficiency, and documentation of a reassuring tracing prior to oxytocin administration is imperative. When administered in amounts of 20 mU or more, oxytocin can produce a potent antidiuretic effect (see Chapter 7).[21]

Uterine dysfunction may produce prolonged labor. In the case of prolonged pregnancy, the uterine dysfunction may be caused by uterine overdistention. The definition of prolonged latent or active phase of labor relies on fairly precise documentation of cervical dilation over time.[40] It is the intrapartum nurses' responsibility to carefully document this as well as the quality and quantity of uterine activity. Plotting this information on a partogram often facilitates detection of abnormal patterns of progress in labor.[41,42]

Quantification of uterine activity in millimeters of mercury (mmHg) can only be achieved with an appropriately calibrated IUPC. Though the catheter can be placed only after spontaneous rupture of membranes or artificial rupture by the physician, placement and calibration are recognized as functions of the registered nurse. Thus nursing intervention includes the appropriately timed placement of an IUPC, particularly in the case of labor induction or augmentation with oxytocin infusion.

Prolonged labor leading to maternal exhaustion or intrauterine infection, fetal macrosomia resulting in shoulder dystocia, the risk of operative delivery, and the risk of postpartum hemorrhage may lead to fetal or maternal injury. Maternal exhaustion and intrauterine infection are well-recognized risks associated with prolonged labor. Nursing intervention is formulated to control these risks and reduce their intensity. The nurse must diligently work to maintain a tranquil atmosphere for the patient and her coach by providing information, explanations, reassurance, and encouragement in a calm, clear manner. Breathing and comfort techniques should be taught or reinforced for both the patient and her coach. Adequate hydration must be maintained. Signs of infection such as maternal fever, maternal or fetal tachycardia, or foul-smelling or purulent vaginal discharge must be recorded and reported promptly.

Fetal macrosomia occurs in up to 25% of prolonged pregnancies. For that reason prudent nursing care includes preparing for this possibility in all patients with prolonged pregnancy. Knowledge of the availability of anesthesia personnel will be necessary. Cooperation of the patient and her coach at the time of delivery is essential and will be enhanced by nursing care that includes maintaining support through eye contact and clear, calm direction. The nurse may be called on to facilitate delivery by applying suprapubic pressure under the direction of the physician while he or she performs downward traction on the fetal head or by repositioning the woman's legs into a sharply flexed position on her abdomen in an attempt to free the trapped shoulder. Nursing intervention includes the presence of a second member of the labor unit staff at delivery if at all possible.

Postpartum hemorrhage is also a risk of prolonged pregnancy. Fetal macrosomia may be a contributing factor. Delivery of a large infant may be complicated by vaginal or cervical lacerations. In this instance, the uterine muscles are more likely to be "overstretched" and become hypotonic after delivery. Hypotonia prevents the postpartum uterus from contracting down and constricting vessels at the placental implantation site. Thus, uterine atonia and hemorrhage may result. In addition, both prolonged labor and oxytocin administration are risk factors associated with postpartum hemorrhage.[43]

Nursing care is facilitated by early recognition and prompt treatment of postpartum hemorrhage. Recognizing the risk factors and maintaining a heightened awareness of the possibility of excessive blood loss are important. Further nursing care will include maintaining a patent intravenous line, administering dilute oxytocin solution when ordered, performing routine uterine massage with assessment of uterine tone, assessing blood loss at delivery and immediately afterward, avoiding bladder distention, assessing and documenting vital signs, and preparing for possible administration of ergonovine (Ergotrate) or methylergonovine (Methergine) if bleeding is excessive. Both of these agents may cause serious hypertension and must be administered with caution. A derivative of prostaglandin $F_{2\alpha}$ (Prostin 15M) has been shown to be effective in controlling hemorrhage secondary to uterine atonia when given intramuscularly.[44]

As the woman progresses past her due date, both she and her family members may begin to experience and express concern for the baby's well-being. A lack of clear information about the indication for and results of antepartum surveillance may heighten those fears. She may feel a lack of control over her body and her pregnancy. These factors, combined with added fatigue, may result in feelings of frustration, anger, and anxiety.[22] The intrapartum nurse's plan of care must address these feelings.

The nurse can direct care by providing clear, concise explanations of all interventions and by allowing the woman and her coach the opportunity to express their concerns. During labor, explanations should be given repeatedly. The level of activity and the woman's anxiety may prevent her from hearing them completely the first time. A few simple phrases such as, "Tell me what has been on your mind these last few weeks" or "What's been the most difficult part of these last few days" will give the patient and her coach the opportunity to talk about their fears. Encouraging her to ask questions will also help to allay fears. It is helpful for the nurse to offer encouragement and support about those aspects that are normal, such as reactive NSTs, adequate amniotic fluid volume, and a reassuring intrapartum tracing. However, it is also important to review available prenatal records which may reveal the discovery of fetal anomalies such as anencephaly. In this case, the need for emotional support during labor and delivery intensifies. Through these actions, the nurse will assist in helping the woman control what may seen like overwhelming fear and anxiety.

Impaired uteroplacental function or excessive uterine activity places the fetus at risk for hypoxia, acidosis, and asphyxia. Resulting fetal compromise is associated with low Apgar scores and neonatal depression at birth. Meconium-stained fluid particularly in the presence of oligohydramnios increases this risk. Delayed delivery subsequent to shoulder dystocia in the macrosomic infant may result in neonatal trauma and severe asphyxia. The postmaturity syndrome, seen in 20% to 30% of prolonged pregnancies, develops as the result of chronic placental dysfunction, and asphyxia and acidosis at birth are not uncommon in these neonates.

The intrapartum nurse must be skilled in immediate neonatal assessment and resuscitation. If available, pediatric personnel should be in the delivery room at the time of birth. Nursing care also involves ensuring the availability and preparation of resuscitative equipment including the laryngoscope, endotracheal tubes, suction equipment, appropriately sized anesthesia bags and face masks, and an adequate oxygen supply. Documentation of all resuscitation efforts should be accomplished.

Expected Outcomes

In caring for the patient with a prolonged pregnancy, the intrapartum nurse gathers information during assessment. From this compilation of information, nursing diagnoses are formulated and a plan of care developed and implemented.

The outcomes that are expected from this intervention serve as goals toward which nursing care is directed. The expected outcomes for prolonged pregnancy are the following:

1. The patient will experience normal progress in labor and an atraumatic delivery.
2. The fetus and neonate will maintain adequate oxygenation and tissue perfusion.
3. The fetus will be delivered without trauma.
4. The patient will maintain normal circulating postpartum blood volume.
5. The patient and her coach will express concern appropriate for her condition and will avoid excessive anxiety.

Prolonged pregnancy can result in significant fetal and maternal risk. That risk intensifies during the intrapartum period. Knowledge of why these risks exist allows the intrapartum nurse to develop a plan of care in which intervention is applied to reduce or eliminate them. The implementation of nursing diagnoses upon which care is planned will promote a healthy outcome for the mother and child.

References

1. Beischer NA, Evans JH, Townsend L: Studies in prolonged pregnancy. I: The incidence of prolonged pregnancy. *Am J Obstet Gynecol* 123:67, 1975.
2. Vorherr H: Placental insufficiency in relation to postterm pregnancy and fetal postmaturity. *Am J Obstet Gynecol* 123:67, 1975.
3. Boyd ME, Usher RH, McLean FH, Kramer MS: Obstetric consequences of postmaturity. *Am J Obstet Gynecol* 158:334, 1988.

4. McClure-Brown JC: Post maturity. *Am J Obstet Gynecol* 85:573, 1963.

5. Eden RD, Seifert LS, Winegar A, Spellacy WN: Perinatal characteristics of uncomplicated postdate pregnancies. *Obstet Gynecol* 69:296, 1987.

6. Sachs BP, Friedman EA: Results of epidemiologic study of postdate pregnancy. *J Reprod Med* 31:162, 1986.

7. Schneider JM, Olson RW, Curet LB: Screening for fetal and neonatal risk in the postdate pregnancy. *Am J Obstet Gynecol* 131:473, 1978.

8. Rayburn WF, Molley ME, Stempel LF, Gendreau RH: Antepartum prediction of the postmature infant. *Obstet Gynecol* 60:148, 1982.

9. Cucco C, Osborne MA, Cibils LA: Maternal–fetal outcomes in prolonged pregnancy. *Am J Obstet Gynecol* 161:916, 1989.

10. Harris BA, Huddleston JF, Sutliff G, Perlis W: The unfavorable cervix in prolonged pregnancy. *Obstet Gynecol* 62:171, 1983.

11. Hauth JC, Goodman MT, Gilstrap LC, Gilstrap JE: Post-term pregnancy. I. *Obstet Gynecol* 56:467, 1980.

12. Benedetti TJ, Gabbe SG: Shoulder dystocia: A complication of fetal macrosomia and prolonged second stage of labor with mid-plane delivery. *Obstet Gynecol* 52:526, 1978.

13. McCall JO: Shoulder dystocia: A study of after effects. *Am J Obstet Gynecol* 83:1486, 1962.

14. Leveno KJ, Quirk JG, Cunningham FG, et al: Prolonged pregnancy. I: Observations concerning the causes of fetal distress. *Am J Obstet Gynecol* 150:465, 1984.

15. Phelan JP, Platt LD, Yeh S, et al: The role of ultrasound assessment of amniotic fluid volume in the management of the postdate pregnancy. *Am J Obstet Gynecol* 151:304, 1985.

16. Miller FC, Read JA: Intrapartum assessment of the postdate fetus. *Am J Obstet Gynecol* 141:516, 1981.

17. Shaw K, Clark SL: Reliability of intrapartum fetal heart rate monitoring in the postterm fetus with meconium passage. *Obstet Gynecol* 72:886, 1988.

18. Zolar RW, Quilligan EJ: The influence of scalp sampling on the cesarean section rate for fetal distress. *Am J Obstet Gynecol* 135:239, 1979.

19. Usher RH, Boyd ME, McLean FH, Kramer MS: Assessment of fetal risk in postdate pregnancies. *Am J Obstet Gynecol* 158:259, 1988.

20. Fleisher A, Schulman H, Farmakedes G, et al: Antepartum nonstress test and the postmature pregnancy. *Obstet Gynecol* 66:80, 1985.

21. Cunningham FG, MacDonald PC, Gant NF: *Williams' Obstetrics* (18th ed.). Norwalk, CT, Appleton & Lange, 1989.

22. Affonso DD, Harris TR: Postterm pregnancy. *J Obstet Gynecol Neonat Nurs* 9:139, 1980.

23. Naeye RL: Causes of perinatal mortality excess in prolonged gestations. *Am J Epidemiol* 108:429, 1978.

24. Clifford SH: Postmaturity. *Adv Pediatr* 9:13, 1957.

25. Campbell WA, Nochimson DJ, Vintzileos AM: Prolonged pregnancy, in Knuppel RA, Drukker JE (eds.): *High Risk Pregnancy: A Team Approach*. Philadelphia, WB Saunders, 1986.

26. Benedetti TJ, Easterling T: Antepartum testing in postterm pregnancy. *J Reprod Med* 33:252, 1988.

27. Phelan JP, Platt LD, Yeh S, et al: Continuing role of the nonstress test in the management of postdate pregnancy. *Obstet Gynecol* 64:624, 1984.

28. American College of Obstetricians and Gynecologists: Antepartum fetal surveillance. ACOG Technical Bulletin No. 107, Washington, DC, ACOG, 1987.

29. Eden RD, Gergely RZ, Schifrin BS, Wade ME: Comparison of antepartum testing schemes for the management of the postdate pregnancy. *Am J Obstet Gynecol* 144:683, 1982.

30. Johnson JM, Harman CR, Lange IR, Manning FR: Biophysical profile scoring in the management of the post term pregnancy. *Am J Obstet Gynecol* 154:269, 1986.

31. Manning FA, Basket TF, Morrison I, Lang I: Fetal biophysical profile scoring: A prospective study in 1184 high risk patients. *Am J Obstet Gynecol* 140:289, 1981.

32. Parer JT: *Handbook of Fetal Heart Rate Monitoring*. Philadelphia, WB Saunders, 1983.

33. Galvan BJ, VanMullem C, Broekhuizen FF: Using amnioinfusion for the relief of repetitive variable decelerations during labor. *J Obstet Gynecol Neonat Nurs* 18:222, 1989.

34. Miyazaki FS, Taylor NA: Saline amnioinfusion for relief of variable or prolonged decelerations. *Am J Obstet Gynecol* 146:670, 1985.

35. Nageotte MP, Freeman RK, Garite TJ, Dorchester W: Prophylactic intrapartum amnioinfusion in patients with preterm rupture of membranes. *Am J Obstet Gynecol* 153:557, 1985.

36. Bishop EH: Pelvic scoring for elective induction. *Obstet Gynecol* 24:266, 1964.

37. Nurses' Association of the American College of Obstetrics and Gynecology: *Standards for Obstetric, Gynecologic, and Neonatal Nursing.* (3rd ed.). Washington, DC, NAACOG, 1986.

38. American Academy of Pediatrics and American College of Obstetricians and Gynecologists. *Guidelines for Perinatal Care* (2nd ed.). Washington, DC, AAP/ACOG, 1988.

39. American College of Obstetricians and Gynecologists: Intrapartum fetal heart rate monitoring, ACOG Technical Bulletin No. 132, Washington DC, ACOG, 1989.

40. Cohen W, Friedman EA: *Management of Labor.* Baltimore, University Park Press, 1983.

41. Studd JW: A visual method of charting labor: The partogram. *Contemp Obstet Gynecol* 18:25, 1981.

42. Earn AA: The partographic labor board: An alternative for earlier decisions regarding management during labor. *Am J Obstet Gynecol* 144:858, 1982.

43. Benedetti TJ: Obstetric hemorrhage, in Gabbe SG, Niebyl JR, Simpson JL (eds.): *Obstetrics: Normal and Problem Pregnancies.* New York: Churchill Livingstone, 1986.

44. Hayashi RH, Castillo MS, Noah ML: Management of severe postpartum hemorrhage with a prostaglandin F_2 alpha analogue. *Obstet Gynecol* 63:806, 1984.

.7.

◆ ◆ ◆

Induction and Augmentation of Labor

Susan Pozaic

Supportive Data

Incidence

Pregnancy, in the majority, is a self-limiting event, although some gestations require assistance in bringing about parturition. Modern obstetrics employs a number of pharmacologic and mechanical methods to initiate or enhance the labor process. According to the 1980 National Natality Survey, artificial methods to initiate or stimulate labor were used in 43% of all hospital births.[0] Therefore, a common and specialized part of obstetric nursing practice is direct care of these patients. This entails responsibility for and regulation of the pharmacologic means of stimulation of labor—specifically, the prostaglandins and oxytocin. The use of these two methods will be the focus of this chapter.

Augmentation is defined as artificial stimulation of labor that began spontaneously but has progressed abnormally. Additional uterine activity is stimulated, usually by pharmacologic means, in order to bring about more progressive cervical dilation and effacement and descent of the fetus. *Induction* is the initiation of labor by artificial means prior to its spontaneous onset. Uterine activity is initiated in order to produce uterine contractions of sufficient quality to progressively efface and dilate the cervix and bring about the descent of the fetus. Induction of labor is carried out when there is a medical indication to end the gestation.

Significance

Pharmacologic methods to enhance labor have significantly contributed to decreasing maternal and fetal/neonatal mortality rates over the past 3 decades.[1] Unfortunately, however, induction and augmentation of labor, whether by pharmacologic or nonpharmacologic means, carry some degree of morbidity for the mother and newborn.

The most frequently used method of nonpharmacologic stimulation of labor is amniotomy. According to the 1980 National Natality Survey, 7.75% of hospital births were the result of labors stimulated by amniotomy alone.[0] Associated potential hazards include maternal–fetal infection, umbilical cord prolapse— which is rare when the vertex is engaged—and umbilical cord compression.[2] Stripping the membranes to induce labor is associated with premature rupture of the fetal membranes, risk of infection, as well as the danger of disrupting a low-lying placenta.

Pharmacologic agents to stimulate labor include oxytocin and prostaglandins. Nearly one quarter of all hospital births in 1980 were induced or augmented by oxytocin alone.[2] The widespread use of this drug makes understanding the associated complications essential to the care of women undergoing this procedure. Hyperstimulation of the uterus may occur either as a result of high dosage or increased patient sensitivity to oxytocin. Tetanic contractions produce excessive and extreme tension within the uterine musculature, thereby increasing the risk of uterine rupture, cervical lacerations, amniotic fluid embolus, and decreased uteroplacental perfusion with subsequent insufficiency of oxygen transfer to the fetus. Uteroplacental insufficiency causes fetal heart rate changes including late decelerations, bradycardia, tachycardia, premature ventricular contractions, and possibly death secondary to asphyxia. Another important property of oxytocin is its antidiuretic effect. When oxytocin infusions are prolonged and the infusion rate approaches 40 mU/minute, there is a dramatic drop in urinary output and potential exists for water intoxication.[3] Rapid intravenous infusion of oxytocin has been noted to cause severe maternal hypotension, increased heart rate, venous return, cardiac output, and electrocardiographic changes that are indicative of cardiac ischemia.[4] These cardiovascular effects may be especially hazardous to women who are hemorrhaging, those receiving regional anesthesia, or those with valvular heart disease. However, these effects should not occur when oxytocin is properly diluted and administered by infusion pump.

Women who receive oxytocin intrapartally are thought to be at higher risk for postpartum hemorrhage secondary to uterine atony. Hemorrhage may be related to oxytocin-induced thrombocytopenia, afibrinogenemia, and hypoprothrombinemia.[4] By carefully controlling delivery and by continuing the oxytocin infusion postpartally, this complication may be prevented.

Allergic reactions including anaphylaxis can occur and may be fatal. Injudicious use of oxytocin has resulted in maternal deaths due to hypertensive episodes and subarachnoid hemorrhage.[4]

Neonates who are delivered following oxytocin-induced labor are 1.6 times more likely to develop hyperbilirubinemia than are neonates who were not exposed to oxytocin induction or augmentation.[4] Hyperbilirubinemia is also more likely with very high doses of oxytocin.[5] The principal fetal hazard is iatrogenic prematurity and related respiratory distress syndrome. Iatrogenic prematurity and increased cesarean sections are major problems associated with elective induction of labor. For these reasons, elective induction or termination of pregnancy strictly for patient or physician convenience is not recommended by the Food and Drug Administration.[6]

Prostaglandin gel preparations are frequently used intravaginally or intracervically for the purpose of cervical preparation prior to induction. However, such use has not been approved by the Food and Drug Administration and, therefore, should be used only with clear indication and informed patient consent. Since this preparation is not commercially available in the United States, the potential for variability of drug concentrations exists. Inconsistent effects may result. Prostaglandins are associated with nausea, vomiting, diarrhea, pyrexia, shivering, and uterine hyperstimulation.

Etiology

Despite the risks associated with pharmacologic and nonpharmacologic methods of induction and augmentation, the needs of the mother and fetus may necessitate their use. The physician must therefore consider whether labor manipulation would more likely harm or benefit both mother and fetus. Labor manipulation is indicated when the mother and/or her fetus would benefit physiologically from delivery. Indications for delivery are usually relative and dynamic in the sense that they change as modern obstetrical practice changes. Maternal factors may include pregnancy-induced or chronic hypertension; diabetes mellitus; antepartal bleeding including partial placenta previa or mild abruptio placentae; premature rupture of the membranes in a term pregnancy; chorioamnionitis; history of recurrent fetal death; and renal, cardiac, hepatic, pulmonary, or malignant diseases.[3,7] Fetal indications include isoimmunization, intrauterine growth retardation, intrauterine fetal death, prolonged gestation, major anomalies, and fetal distress evidenced by biochemical or biophysical indicators.[7,8]

In general, any contraindication to spontaneous vaginal delivery is a contraindication to induction of labor. Maternal contraindications to labor induction include complete placenta previa, vasa previa, classical uterine incision, pelvic structural deformities, active genital herpes infection, invasive cervical carcinoma, hypertonic uterine activity, and maternal exhaustion.[3,7] Relative contraindications include grand multiparity and uterine overdistention, as a result of hydramnios or multiple gestation.[8] Fetal contraindications to labor induction include abnormal presentation (*e.g.,* transverse lie), funic presentation, presenting part above the pelvic inlet, and fetal distress.[3,7]

Labor induction is initiated in the anticipation of a favorable outcome— spontaneous vaginal delivery. The likelihood of this occurring is increased when the cervix demonstrates readiness to progressively efface and dilate. Bishop developed a method by which the cervix can be clinically evaluated and scored to assist in predicting the likelihood of successful induction.[9] Position of the cervix as it relates to the vagina; cervical consistency, dilation, and effacement;

TABLE 7-1
Bishop's Pelvic Scoring

	0	1	2	3
Dilation (cm)	0	1–2	3–4	5–6
Effacement (%)	0–30	40–50	60–70	80
Station	−3	−2	−1 to 0	+1, +2
Consistency	Firm	Medium	Soft	—
Position	Posterior	Midposition	Anterior	—

and station of the fetal presenting part are evaluated and given a numerical value (see Table 7-1). The range of scores is 0 to 13, with low numbers indicating an unfavorable cervix and high numbers indicating a favorable cervix.

In a study conducted in 1966 by Friedman and co-workers, a cervical score of 1 to 4 was associated with an induction failure rate of 19.5%; a score of 5 to 8 with a 4.8% failure rate; and a score of 9 to 12 with no failures.[10] Since cervical condition plays such an important role in the induction of labor—the latent phase in particular—a variety of methods to prepare the cervix for labor have been tried. These include relaxin, laminaria, catheters, breast stimulation, oxytocin, estrogen, and prostaglandin E and prostaglandin F.

Augmentation of labor is indicated when there is a lack of labor progress (*i.e.,* cervical effacement and dilation) or when the fetus fails to descend with inadequate quantities of uterine contractions. A lack of labor progress can be identified only after the woman has been in active labor, since hypotonic uterine dysfunction occurs most frequently when the cervix is dilated to 4 cm or more. One of the most common errors is the treatment of uterine dysfunction or hypotonus when the woman is not yet in active labor.[11]

An understanding of the normal labor curve developed by Friedman helps to illustrate the normal labor progress of cervical dilation and fetal descent.[12] Labor disorders that may be treated with oxytocin include hypotonic uterine dysfunction, protraction disorders, and arrest disorders. Uterine dysfunction is frequently caused by pelvic contractures, fetal malposition, and uterine overdistention. Cervical rigidity is an uncommon cause.[11] In hypotonic uterine dysfunction, basal tonus is normal and there is only a slight rise in pressure during a contraction that is insufficient to dilate the cervix. If, indeed, the patient had been in active labor, as evidenced by rhythmic, uncomfortable uterine activity that has produced cervical effacement and dilation of at least 4 cm, and cephalopelvic disproportion is not present, augmentation is considered.

Protraction disorders include the following:

1. Protracted active phase dilation in which cervical dilation is less than 1.2 cm/hour in the nulliparous patient and less than 1.5 cm/hour in the multiparous patient
2. Protracted descent in which the maximum slope of descent of the fetal presenting part is less than 1 cm/hour in the nulliparous patient and less than 2 cm/hour in the multiparous patient.

One third of these cases are due to cephalopelvic disproportion of varying degrees.[11] In this case, cesarean section is the preferred treatment. If cephalopelvic disproportion is not present, treatment is controversial but may include augmentation.

Arrest disorders include prolonged deceleration phase, secondary arrest of dilation, arrest of descent, and failure of descent. A prolonged deceleration phase occurs when the termination of transition exceeds 3 hours in the nulliparous patient and 1 hour in the multiparous patient. Secondary arrest of dilation exists when there is no further cervical dilation for greater than 2 hours in the active phase. Arrest of descent is present when there is no further descent of the fetus for greater than 1 hour. Failure of descent exists when there is no descent either during the deceleration phase of the first stage of labor or during the second stage of labor. If cephalopelvic disproportion is not present, augmentation of labor may be attempted.

In order to understand the mechanisms of methods used to prepare or "ripen" the cervix and induce or augment labor, uterine physiology as it relates to the initiation of labor must be reviewed. The exact mechanism responsible for the initiation of labor has not been determined; however, a number of physiologic events are known to occur prior to or during labor. The onset of labor requires the myometrial inhibiting effect of progesterone to be diminished. Progesterone, along with estrogen, facilitates increased prostaglandin synthesis. These substances play a role in the cascade of labor events—cervical ripening, gap junction formation, the increase in oxytocin receptors, and increased responsiveness of the uterus to substances that produce contractions.[13] (For a detailed description of the underlying physiology involved in initiation of parturition, refer to Chapter 5, pages 59–60.)

Framework for Accepted Therapy

CERVICAL RIPENING

Cervical ripening refers to softening and effacement and is thought to represent the maturation of the reproductive system in terms of labor-induction readiness. The mechanism is not well understood, but it is thought to be stimulated by estrogen and prostaglandins.[14] This maturational process involves biochemical changes in the cervical components: smooth muscle, connective tissue, and collagen.[15]

Cervical changes can be produced using mechanical or chemical means. Devices used to mechanically dilate the cervix are laminaria and catheters. The mechanism of action is simple expansion, which then promotes prostaglandin production, which in turn changes the collagen matrix of the cervix.[16] Mechanical dilators may be indicated when pharmacologic means to ripen the cervix are contraindicated or are not feasible.

Chemical agents used to enhance cervical maturation include relaxin, oxytocin, estrogen, and prostaglandin E and F. The hormone relaxin has been shown to be effective in ripening the cervix.[17,18] In many species, though not human, serum relaxin rises 24 hours prior to labor. Elevated levels of relaxin produce softening, effacement, and dilation of the cervix. Relaxin probably facilitates connective tissue restructuring, which causes ripening effects without producing uterine contractions.[17] Purified porcine relaxin in gel form is administered vaginally or intracervically in doses ranging from 1 to 4 mg.[17,18]

Oxytocin, used by many to induce labor, may be used in various ways to induce cervical ripening. It is likely that oxytocin works to enhance cervical ripening by inducing uterine contractions that produce biophysical and biochemical changes similar to those that occur naturally during the early latent phase of labor.[19] Oxytocin is administered by slow intravenous infusion for up to 20 hours or serially over a period of days to produce cervical change.[19,20] Use of the body's natural physiologic functioning in the form of breast stimulation to cause endogenous release of oxytocin has been shown to be effective in priming the cervix.[21,22] The method of breast stimulation should be carefully evaluated for incidence of uterine hyperstimulation.[23] Gentle unilateral stimulation produces less hypertonus.[21]

Various estrogens have been used to induce cervical ripening. An increased estrogen–progesterone ratio is thought to enhance collagen breakdown in the cervix without producing prominent uterine contractions. It is also believed that estrogen promotes sensitivity of the cervix to prostaglandins.[24]

Prostaglandins are hormones produced by most organs, especially the endometrium in the female. Prostaglandin E_2 (PGE_2) is the primary prostaglandin produced by the cervix and trophoblast.[13] Precursors of prostaglandins are stored as phospholipids in the cell membrane. Prostaglandins are formed just prior to their release, since they are rapidly metabolized by the lungs, kidneys, and liver.[25] The most important prostaglandins involved in reproduction are prostaglandin E_2 (PGE_2) and $F_{2\alpha}$ ($PGF_{2\alpha}$) formed from arachidonic acid. Exogenous sources of PGE_2 produce the same biochemical changes that occur naturally in the ripening cervix, without increasing uterine activity.[13,14] Prostaglandin E_2 may also alter the myometrium by changing membrane excitability, which thereby prepares the uterus for parturition.[26] It is administered locally (*i.e.*, intracervically or vaginally in dosages ranging from 0.5 to 5 mg).[13]

Prostaglandins used to induce labor may be given systemically. This should be accomplished cautiously because of the side effects and risk of hyperstimulation resulting from variable effective dose, narrow therapeutic range, and longer myometrial effects than those expected from the rapid degradation of prostaglandins systemically.[14] Prostaglandins are not approved by the Food and Drug Administration for either cervical ripening or induction of labor.

LABOR INDUCTION AND AUGMENTATION

The methods described to artificially ripen the cervix may also induce labor in certain patients. Nonpharmacologic methods to induce labor will be briefly described and more detailed information will be presented regarding the pharmacologic methods of labor induction since the nurse is responsible for patient assessment and nursing management.

Nonpharmacologic methods to induce or augment labor include stripping of the membranes and amniotomy. Stripping of the membranes is the manual separation of the chorioamniotic membranes from the lower uterine segment. Cervical stretching is often accomplished simultaneously. This procedure may initiate labor by stimulating an autonomic neural reflex, releasing endogenous oxytocin from the maternal pituitary, and by locally releasing prostaglandins.[27] Disadvantages of this procedure are as previously mentioned, and variable results make its usefulness questionable and beyond the scope of nursing practice.

Amniotomy is thought to stimulate labor by the release of arachidonic acid and subsequent formation of the prostaglandins. These prostaglandins are thought to potentiate the action of oxytocin so that myometrial activity is initiated or maintained.[28] In a study of the fetal membranes, it was determined that the fetal head alone exerts more force against the cervix than does the head covered with the membranes. However, before the head is directly applied to the cervix, the membranes play an important role as dilator.[29] After thorough consideration of the risks involved, the physician or nurse midwife may elect to rupture the membranes in order to augment the labor process once the presenting part is well applied to the cervix. Very often, amniotomy is used concurrently with a pharmacologic agent to further augment the labor process.

Oxytocin increases uterine contractility by increasing free intracellular calcium. This is accomplished by increased calcium influx, mobilization of calcium stores, and inhibition of the calcium extrusion pump. Calcium is vital for the activation of smooth muscle. Sensitivity of the uterus to oxytocin depends on the concentration of myometrial oxytocin receptors. Oxytocin receptors increase throughout pregnancy with a sharp rise during parturition as a result of the increased estrogen–progesterone ratio and prostaglandin synthesis. As the oxytocin receptors increase through gestation, myometrial sensitivity to oxytocin increases and the amount of oxytocin necessary to produce uterine contractions decreases. Oxytocin probably also enhances prostaglandin production in the decidua which, in turn, stimulates uterine contractions.[30]

Gap junctions in the myometrium allow rapid communication between large numbers of cells which then are capable of producing the expulsive forces necessary for delivery. Commercially available oxytocin is a synthetic form of the hormone secreted by the hypothalamus and stored in the neurohypophysis. The only route currently approved by the Food and Drug Administration for the induction or augmentation of labor is by continuous intravenous infusion. Oxytocin is removed from plasma by the kidneys and liver and is inactivated by placental oxytocinase in the blood. Initial uterine response to intravenous oxytocin may occur almost immediately and the effect may persist for up to 1 hour.[4] The pharmacokinetic half-life of oxytocin is generally 3 to 5 minutes. The time to reach steady-state drug concentrations in the blood is three to five times the half-life. Earlier oxytocin induction and augmentation protocols were based on this information and provided for an upward adjustment in dosage every 15 to 20 minutes. However, more recent data suggest that the pharmacokinetic half-life of oxytocin is not consistent with the time to reach maximum pharmacologic effect.

In vivo studies conducted by Seitchik and others demonstrated that the interval to reach the maximum pharmacologic effect of oxytocin is 40 minutes.[31,32] Indeed, other studies have demonstrated benefits in extending the dosing interval. These benefits include less uterine hyperstimulation, less abnormal fetal heart rate tracings, and lower maximal dose.[33,34] Seitchik and Castillo demonstrated that 45% of patients with augmented labor will require less than 2.5 mU/minute; 45% will require 2.5 to 5 mU/minute, and 10% will require greater than 5 mU/minute.[35] Stated differently, 90% of patients will require less than 6 mU/minute.[7] Since small doses will produce adequate uterine activity and cervical dilation, the initial and incremental doses should be small, 0.5 mU to 1 mU/minute initially and 1 to 2 mU/minute incrementally.

Assessment

The decision of whether to induce or augment labor is based on physical benefit to the mother and/or fetus as addressed earlier. Also, contraindications to induction or augmentation should not be present. A physician who is qualified to perform cesarean deliveries should evaluate the patient in terms of indications versus contraindications to induction and augmentation and should be readily available to manage any complications. The patient should be examined by the physician prior to labor induction to determine fetal presentation, station of presenting part, and adequacy of pelvic size. Additionally, obstetric personnel who understand oxytocin effects and who are able to identify maternal and/or fetal complications should be present.[36] Proper equipment such as an infusion pump and fetal monitor must be present and available. A written protocol for the preparation and administration of oxytocin, as well as nursing responsibilities, should be established by the obstetrics department in each institution. The patient should be informed of the clinical indication and procedure to be implemented and be emotionally prepared. Many patients have been informed by peers that induced labor is more painful than spontaneous labor. Oxytocin protocols that advocate low initial dosage and gradual dosage increases more closely approximate spontaneous labor with gradual onset of painful contractions as the woman adjusts to the labor process.

Immediately prior to beginning induction, the physician or nurse must perform a vaginal exam to determine cervical status.[36] Leopold's maneuvers should also be employed to verify fetal position. Baseline laboratory values including complete blood count, serum electrolyte levels, and blood type and hold should be obtained.

Baseline maternal vital signs, uterine activity, and fetal heart rate should be evaluated prior to initiation of the labor induction procedure. Findings of the initial assessment including maternal emotional assessment and coping should be documented in the clinical record.

Nursing Diagnoses

Nursing diagnosis is an essential component of the nursing process. Formulating a nursing diagnosis is the link between gathering information and developing a plan of care. It demands astute, holistic clinical judgment based on a sound knowledge base. The following are nursing diagnoses that are appropriate for patients undergoing induction or augmentation of labor.

MATERNAL STABILITY
- Alterations in cardiac output: decreased related to side effects of prostaglandins and oxytocin
- Potential fluid volume overload related to oxytocin infusion
- Potential for injury: uterine hyperstimulation
- Impaired physical mobility related to continuous monitoring

PSYCHOSOCIAL WELL-BEING
- Alterations in comfort: pain related to intense uterine activity
- Ineffective individual coping related to intense uterine activity
- Fear related to unknown methods: induction and augmentation techniques
- Fear related to self and fetal well-being
- Knowledge deficit related to unknown methods: induction and augmentation techniques
- Disturbance of self-concept: role performance related to altered birth plan

FETAL WELL-BEING
- Potential for injury: fetal compromise related to decreased oxygenation
- Potential for injury: fetal compromise related to infectious process

Theoretical Basis for the Plan of Nursing Care and Intervention

The nurses' role prior to initiating any procedure is to prepare the patient emotionally as well as physically. An assessment of the patient's knowledge of the procedure including the reason for its use, possible side effects and how they will be managed, how the procedure is performed, and her anxiety related to the procedure is conducted. If the physician elects to use prostaglandins for the purpose of cervical ripening, the nursing role is one of support. This includes preparing the equipment, initiating maternal–fetal monitoring, positioning the patient in the lithotomy or dorsal position, and providing emotional support. The patient may be encouraged to use relaxation techniques. Following the procedure, fetal surveillance continues, vital signs are reassessed, and the patient rests. Documentation includes cervical examination results, drug dosage, route, side effects, and patient reaction.[25]

Prostaglandin gel may be followed by oxytocin for labor stimulation. Oxytocin is approved by the Food and Drug Administration for induction or augmentation of labor by the intravenous route. It must be diluted since rapid infusion can cause maternal hypotension, cardiac ischemia, and uterine tetany. Oxytocin is commercially available as 10 U/1 ml and is added to a balanced salt solution such as lactated Ringer's or 0.9% sodium chloride. A balanced salt solution will not exacerbate the water-retentive properties of oxytocin. The concentration should be standardized according to institutional policy. Oxytocin dosage is measured in milliunits per minute. A common dilution is 10 U of oxytocin per 1000 ml intravenous fluid. This yields a concentration of 10 mU/1 ml. An alternative dilution is 15 U of oxytocin per 250 ml intravenous solution, yielding a concentration of 60 mU/1 ml. This dilution is convenient for dosage administration since milliliters per hour are equivalent to milliunits per minute. The following formulas may be useful in calculating oxytocin dosages for administration.

1. **Determine milliunits of oxytocin per milliliters as follows:**

$$\frac{\text{Units of oxytocin}}{\text{milliliters of intravenous fluid}} \times 1000 = (\text{mU/ml})$$

2. **Determine milliunits of oxytocin per minute as follows:**

$$\frac{\text{mU/ml}}{1} \times \frac{\text{ml}}{60 \text{ minutes}} = (\text{mU/minute})$$

Example: **15 U oxytocin mixed in 250 ml intravenous fluid with infusion pump set to deliver 1 ml/hour**

1. $\dfrac{15 \text{ U}}{250 \text{ ml}} \times 1000 = 60 \text{ mU/ml}$

2. $\dfrac{60 \text{ mU/ml}}{1} \times \dfrac{1 \text{ ml administered}}{60 \text{ minutes}} = 1 \text{ mU/minute}$

Table 7-2 lists oxytocin conversions for the previously discussed dilutions. The medication sticker on the oxytocin solution should note the concentration. In order to administer precise dosages, an infusion pump must be utilized. At the most proximal port, the diluted solution is then piggybacked into a primary intravenous line containing electrolyte solution. A primary intravenous solution is used to keep the line open should the medication need to be discontinued and/or should an intravenous fluid bolus be necessary.

Prior to initiating the infusion, baseline vital signs (*i.e.,* temperature, pulse, respirations, and blood pressure) and fetal and uterine status should be assessed. Use of continuous electronic fetal monitoring permits more thorough assessment of fetal heart rate responses and uterine activity. Internal or direct

TABLE 7-2
Oxytocin Conversions

Rate (mU/minute)	Solution Concentration	
	10 U Oxytocin/1000 ml (10 mU/ml)	15 U Oxytocin/250 ml (60 mU/ml)
	ml/hour	ml/hour
0.5	3	0.5
1	6	1
2	12	2
3	18	3
4	24	4
5	30	5
6	36	6
7	42	7
8	48	8
9	54	9
10	60	10
11	66	11
12	72	12
13	78	13
14	84	14
15	90	15
16	96	16
17	102	17
18	108	18
19	114	19
20	120	20

electronic monitoring methods permit the most accurate evaluation of fetal heart rate variability and strength of uterine activity and require cervical dilation and rupture of the membranes. As these occur, a fetal spiral electrode and intrauterine pressure catheter may be considered.

The infusion should be initiated with a low dose since the effective dose varies greatly among women. It is increased by small, set increments after steady state has been achieved with the previous dosage adjustment. This should produce a gradual onset of labor equivalent to the early latent phase of labor. It should also decrease the total dose of oxytocin and the incidence of hyperstimulation of the uterus. Three factors are continually assessed in order to determine a patient's therapeutic oxytocin dose: uterine activity, fetal response, and cervical effacement and dilation. Uterine activity goals consist of uterine contractions with a frequency of 2 to 3 minutes, duration of 40 to 90 seconds, and intensity of 40 to 90 mm Hg by intrauterine monitoring.[37] The resting tone must be less than 20 mm Hg by intrauterine monitoring. If intrauterine pressure monitoring is not used, contractions should be moderate to firm to palpation and resting tone should be adequate as identified by lack of sensation of intrauterine pressure on the examiner's hand. Should hyperstimulation occur, the infusion is decreased or discontinued. The fetal response to uterine activity must then be assessed. If nonreassuring signs become evident, the oxytocin infusion should be decreased or discontinued.

The definitive measurement of adequate oxytocin dosage is cervical dilation. Dilation should progress by at least 1 cm/hour. The need to assess cervical change is balanced with the potential risk of infection in performing vaginal examination.

Water intoxication, a complication of prolonged high-dose oxytocin administration, is prevented by using balanced salt intravenous solutions, decreasing the total dose of oxytocin, monitoring intake and output, and observing at-risk patients for signs and symptoms (*i.e.,* weakness, restlessness, nausea, vomiting, diarrhea, polyuria or oliguria, and seizures).

In summary, ongoing assessment of the patient undergoing induction or augmentation of labor consists of maternal vital signs, uterine activity, fetal response, cervical dilation, and observation for conscientious fluid management. As labor progresses to the active phase, the dose of oxytocin may need to be gradually decreased as the concentration of oxytocin receptors increases through labor, making lower doses more effective. Oxytocin is often continued in the immediate postpartum period to prevent postpartum hemorrhage.

Expected Outcomes

MATERNAL STABILITY

The patient will do the following:

1. Maintain vital signs within normal ranges.
2. Maintain adequate output.
3. Avoid vena caval compression and hypotension by maintaining a lateral position.
4. Achieve adequate uterine activity.
5. Avoid uterine hyperstimulation and subsequent injury.

PSYCHOSOCIAL WELL-BEING

The patient will do the following:

1. Verbalize understanding of procedures including risks.
2. Verbalize understanding of the monitoring process.
3. Verbalize decreased fear of procedure and unknown.
4. Demonstrate ability to relax during uterine activity.
5. Verbalize feelings related to role performance.
6. Demonstrate normal maternal–infant bonding.

FETAL WELL-BEING

The fetus will do the following:

1. Maintain fetal heart rate between 110 to 160 beats per minute.
2. Maintain a reassuring fetal heart rate pattern on the electronic fetal heart rate monitor as evidenced by: (*a*) minimal or greater fetal heart rate variability; (*b*) presence of long-term variability; (*c*) absence of fetal heart rate decelerations; (*d*) presence of accelerations.
3. Exhibit intrauterine activity.

References

0. Hutchins V, Kessel SS, Placek PJ: Trends in maternal and infant health factors associated with low infant birth weight, United States, 1972 and 1980. *Public Health Reports* 99(2):162–172, March–April 1984.
1. Blakemore KJ, Petrie RH: Oxytocin for the induction of labor. *Obstet Gynecol Clin N America* 15(2):339–353, 1988.
2. Niswander KR: Induction of labor, in Sciarra JJ. (ed.): *Gynecology and Obstetrics,* vol. 2. pp. 1–7. Lippincott Harper Medical, 1986.
3. Musacchio MJ: *Oxytocins for Augmentation and Induction of Labor.* New York, March of Dimes, 1990.
4. American Society of Hospital Pharmacists: *AHFS Drug Information 1990.* Bethesda, MD, ASHP, 1990.
5. Beazley JM, Alderman B: Neonatal hyperbilirubinemia following the use of oxytocin in labor. *Brit J Obstet Gynecol* 82:265–271, 1975.
6. Food and Drug Administration: New restrictions on oxytocin use. Washington, DC, *FDA Drug Bulletin* 8(5):30, 1978.
7. ACOG: Induction and augmentation of labor. *ACOG Tech Bull* 157, 1991.
8. O'Brien WF, Cefalo RC: Labor and delivery, in Gabbe SG, Niebyl JR, Simpson JL (eds.): *Obstetrics: Normal and Problem Pregnancies.* New York, Churchill Livingstone, 1986.
9. Bishop EH: Pelvic scoring for elective induction. *Obstet Gynecol* 24(2):266–268, 1964.
10. Friedman EA, Niswander KR, Bayonet-Rivera NP, Sachtleben MR: Relation of prelabor evaluation to inducibility and the course of labor. *Obstet Gynecol* 28(4):495–501, 1966.
11. Cunningham FG, MacDonald PC, Gant NF: *Williams' Obstetrics* (18th ed.). East Norwalk, CT, Appleton & Lange, 1989.
12. Friedman EA: The graphic analysis of labor. *Am J Obstet Gynecol* 68(6):1568–1575, 1954.
13. Schulman H, Farmakides G: Role of the unfavorable cervix in the induction of labor. *Clin Obstet Gynecol* 30(1):50–55, 1987.
14. Andersson KE, Forman A, Ulmsten U: Pharmacology of labor. *Clin Obstet Gynecol* 26(1):56–77, 1983.
15. Danforth DN: The morphology of the human cervix. *Clin Obstet Gynecol* 26(1):7–13, 1983.
16. Newton ER: Using mechanical dilators for cervical ripening. *Contemp Obstet Gynecol* 30:47–64, 1987.
17. MacLennan AH, Green RC, Grant P, Nicolson R: Ripening of the human cervix and induction of labor with purified porcine relaxin. *Obstet Gynecol* 68(5):598–601, 1986.
18. Evans MI, Dougan MB, Noawad AH, et al: Ripening of the human cervix with porcine ovarian relaxin. *Am J Obstet Gynecol* 147(4):410–414, 1983.
19. Chez RA, Barton DM, Miller FC, Petrie RH: When and how to induce labor. *Contemp Obstet Gynecol* 32:145–153, 1988.
20. Merrill PA, Freeman RK: Serial induction of labor. *Contemp Obstet Gynecol* 27:51–54, 1986.
21. Salmon YM, Kee WH, Tan SL, Jen SW: Cervical ripening by breast stimulation. *Obstet Gynecol* 67(1):21–24, 1986.

22. Elliott JP, Flaherty JF: The use of breast stimulation to prevent postdate pregnancy. *Am J Obstet Gynecol* 149(6):628–632, 1984.

23. Curtis P, Evens S, Resnick J, et al: Uterine responses to three techniques of breast stimulation. *Obstet Gynecol* 67(1):25–28, 1986.

24. Uldbjerg N, Ulmsten U, Ekman G: The ripening of the human cervix in terms of connective biochemistry. *Clin Obstet Gynecol* 26(1):14–26, 1983.

25. Glazer G, Hulme MA: Prostaglandin gel for cervical ripening. *MCN* 12(1):28–31, 1987.

26. Schulman H: Prostaglandins, in Fuchs F, Klopper A. (eds.): *Endocrinology of Pregnancy*, 3rd ed. New York, Harper & Row, 1983.

27. McKay S, Mahan CS: How worthwhile are membrane stripping and amniotomy? *Contemp Obstet Gynecol* 184:173–181, 1983.

28. Husslein P, Kofler E, Rasmussen AB, et al: Oxytocin and the initiation of human parturition. IV: Plasma concentrations of oxytocin and 13,14-dihydro-15-ketoprostaglandin $F_{2\alpha}$ during induction of labor by artificial rupture of the membranes. *Am J Obstet Gynecol* 147(5):503–507, 1983.

29. Manabe Y, Sagawa N, Mori T: Experimental evidence for the progress of labor with the increase in the force of cervical dilatation after rupture of the membranes. *Am J Obstet Gynecol* 152(6):696–704, 1985.

30. Fuchs AR, Fuchs F: Physiology of parturition, in Gabbe SG, Niebyl JR, Simpson JL (eds.): *Obstetrics: Normal and Problem Pregnancies*. New York, Churchill Livingstone, 1986.

31. Seitchik J, Castillo M: Oxytocin augmentation of dysfunctional labor. I: Clinical data. *Am J Obstet Gynecol* 144(8):899–905, 1982.

32. Seitchik J, Amico J, Robinson AG, Castillo M: Oxytocin augmentation of labor. IV: Oxytocin pharmacokinetics. *Am J Obstet Gynecol* 150(3):225–228, 1984.

33. Blakemore KJ, Qin NG, Petrie RH, Paine LL: A prospective comparison of hourly and quarter-hourly oxytocin dose increase intervals for the induction of labor at term. *Obstet Gynecol* 75(5):757–761, 1990.

34. Foster TCS, Jacobson JD, Valenzuela GJ: Oxytocin augmentation of labor: A comparison of 15- and 30-minute dose increment intervals. *Obstet Gynecol* 71(2):147–149, 1988.

35. Seitchik J, Castillo M: Oxytocin augmentation of dysfunctional labor. III: Multiparous patients. *Am J Obstet Gynecol* 145(7):777–780, 1983.

36. American Academy of Pediatrics and the American College of Obstetricians and Gynecologists: *Guidelines for Perinatal Care* (2nd ed.). Elk Grove Village, IL, AAP/ACOG, 1988.

37. Petrie RH, Williams AM: Induction of labor, in Knuppel RA, Drukker JE (eds.): *High Risk Pregnancy: A Team Approach*. Philadelphia, Saunders, 1986.

8
◆ ◆ ◆

The Chemically Dependent Pregnant Woman

Karen L. Starr
Gay M. Chisum

Supportive Data

Incidence

Chemical dependence among women of childbearing age is a growing problem and has brought new challenges to health care professionals. The National Institute of Alcohol Abuse and Alcoholism indicated that 2.25 million women in the United States are problem drinkers.[1] In 1986, a survey of the National Institute of Drug Abuse revealed that 1 in 10 women of childbearing age had used cocaine the previous year.[2]

The incidence of chemical dependence during pregnancy was reviewed in a 36-hospital survey conducted by the National Association of Perinatal Addiction Research and Education. It revealed an 11% incidence of illicit "substance abuse" during pregnancy.[3] Reported hospital rates of chemical dependence during pregnancy varied from 0.4% to 27% and were directly related to the thoroughness of the substance use assessment. In 1988, an estimated 375,000 babies had been prenatally exposed to illegal substances, although current figures do not account for exposure to alcohol, cigarettes, over-the-counter drugs, and prescribed medications.[3]

In this country, chemical dependence among pregnant women is probably underestimated because of society's biases and stereotypes of the alcohol and drug user. The media have focused on minority women and women of low socioeconomic status, although no specific patient profile exists because the illness affects women of all ages, races, and ethnic and socioeconomic statuses. Lack of formal training in perinatal chemical dependence for health care providers also impedes the identification process. Without a working knowledge of the addictive process and its effects and good assessment skills, health care professionals may lack the tools for proper identification of chemically dependent pregnant women. When all these factors are taken into account, the number of pregnant women who use alcohol and other drugs is probably greater than estimated.

Significance

Pregnant women who *continue* to use alcohol and other drugs during pregnancy are chemically dependent; therefore, terms such as "substance abuser" or "substance abuse" should be avoided. Health care professionals have long used the term "abuse" when discussing these women. Terminology such as this implies deliberate behavior or control over actions and frequently reflects individual value systems. An effort should be made to avoid these negative terms when discussing chemical dependence and pregnancy.

Maternal chemical dependence has been associated with numerous medical and obstetric complications. Alcohol and other drugs used during pregnancy have adverse effects on the mother, fetus, and neonate. The severity of complications is associated with the specific type of drugs used during the pregnancy. Other issues regarding maternal substance use, which contribute to adverse pregnancy outcomes, include polydrug use, nutritional deficits, medical complications, trauma, poor health practices, risk for human immunodeficiency virus exposure, hepatitis B, and low socioeconomic status.

Maternal morbidity and mortality have been directly related to the type of drug used, timing of drug use, and the route of administration. Early research focused on opiate use during pregnancy, and maternal morbidity and mortality arising from intravenous heroin dependence associated with infections and lack of prenatal care. The most frequently occurring complications noted in these early studies were endocarditis, hepatitis, cellulitis, urinary tract infections, and venereal diseases. In 1982, Rosner and Chasnoff found that pregnant opiate-dependent women who had been closely supervised in a methadone program and then later in an intensive prenatal clinic had no drug-related maternal complications.[4] Rarely today do pregnant patients use only one substance. The drugs most frequently used by pregnant women are alcohol, cigarettes, marijuana, and cocaine across all socioeconomic strata.

Women (and men with chronic alcoholism) have less alcohol dehydrogenase activity in the gastric mucosa than men without alcoholism. This enzyme detoxifies alcohol, thus deficiency results in higher bioavailability of alcohol. Women, therefore, suffer the effects of alcohol intake at much lower doses in a shorter time span and are generally sicker than men.[5]

Alcohol is a mood elevating, central nervous system depressant that affects every organ system in the body, but it has its most profound effect on the central nervous system. The areas of the brain associated with the most highly integrated functions are depressed—first, producing loss of control, disorganized thought processes, and decreased coordination. Alcohol is a respiratory depressant and also affects temperature-regulating mechanisms in the body. Polyneuropathy, Wernicke's disease, and Korsakoff's psychosis with memory loss are potential long-term complications of alcoholism. Wernicke's syndrome consists of neurologic problems such as ataxia, nystagmus, and paralysis of certain ocular muscles. Korsakoff's syndrome consists of psychological symptoms such as severe recent memory loss, confusion, and confabulation (made-up stories to fill in gaps in memory loss).

Alcohol alters normal systemic hormonal balance and carbohydrate metabolism, sometimes resulting in glucose intolerance. It also interferes with adrenocortical, adrenomedullary, thyroid, gonadal, and pituitary functioning. Megaloblastic anemia resulting from granulocytopenia due to direct toxic effects of ethanol on bone marrow and severe folate deficiency, or sequestration of white cells in the spleen and thrombocytopenia related to alcohol intake are a few hematologic abnormalities observed. In addition, alcoholics are especially vulnerable to contracting infectious diseases and have difficulty combating them.

Cardiomyopathy in patients with long-standing alcohol intake also occurs. Its characteristics include breathlessness, easy fatigability, palpitations, anorexia, and dependent edema. Hypertension is prevalent in the alcoholic population, as are coronary artery disease and cardiac dysrhythmias.

There is an increased incidence of esophageal cancer, cancer of the mouth, pharynx, larynx, and liver, as well as esophageal and gastric varices, peptic ulcer disease, duodenitis, esophagitis, pancreatitis, and other pancreatic conditions.[6,7] Malabsorption and alteration in intestinal motility, structural changes in the upper gastrointestinal tract, and impaired transport of glucose, amino acids, electrolytes, thiamine, vitamin B_{12}, and calcium also frequently occur.

Alcohol is fundamentally interrelated to nutritional status, because it displaces other forms of food with nutritional value. In addition, alcohol affects organ systems involved in the digestion and absorption of nutrients and produces deficiencies of folic acid, pyridoxine, thiamine, iron, zinc, and vitamins A, D, and K. In the past, little was known about the effects of a zinc-deficient diet in combination with alcohol intake during pregnancy. It is becoming clear, however, that pregnant women who are low in dietary zinc and who drink alcohol have substantially impaired ability to metabolize alcohol. Therefore, for these women the risks of fetal alcohol syndrome or fetal alcohol effects may be increased.[8]

Tremors resulting from alcohol withdrawal occur about 4 to 6 hours after the last drink ingested and may be accompanied by irritability, retching, nausea, vomiting, diaphoresis, and increased body temperature, heart rate, respirations, and blood pressure. The peak effects of minor withdrawal occur within 12 to 24 hours of the last drink. Alcoholic hallucinosis involving a confusional state in which the person misinterprets existing stimuli can occur in up to 25% of persons withdrawing from alcohol. Visual or tactile misinterpretation and disorientation give rise to restlessness and sometimes fearfulness with feelings of paranoia.

Some patients may experience hallucinations with alcohol withdrawal. Auditory hallucinations usually involve voices familiar to the patient and may often be threatening and guilt producing. The patient believes they are real and often acts on the hallucination, which can lead to self-injury or harm to others. Although they occur with alcohol withdrawal, auditory hallucinations are more commonly associated with cocaine and benzodiazepine withdrawal. Alcoholics are more prone to visual and tactile hallucinations during withdrawal. Seizures can also accompany alcohol withdrawal and usually occur within 48 hours of the last drink. Delirium tremens is the most serious form of alcohol withdrawal. *Delirium* refers to heightened autonomic nervous system activity, which produces tremors, agitation, and rapid pulse and fever and which may occur as early as 1 or 2 days or as late as 14 days after the last drink.

Smoking cigarettes decreases maternal calcium, zinc, and B vitamins and is associated with decreased infant birthweight. Smoking also doubles the effects of alcohol on infant birthweight so that the patient who drinks 10 alcoholic beverages per week and does not smoke can be compared with the patient who smokes cigarettes and drinks 5 drinks per week.

Current knowledge regarding illicit drug use in pregnancy indicates that substantial toxicity and long-term damage may occur. Marijuana is lipophilic, readily crosses the placenta, and can be detected for up to 30 days in maternal urine toxicologies. Marijuana increases maternal heart rate and blood pressure, impairs lung function, and may potentially cause fetal hypoxia.[9] Marijuana smoke contains more tar than high-tar tobacco cigarettes. Acute effects of the principal psychoactive ingredient in marijuana, tetrahydrocannabinol, include impairment of specific intellectual and psychomotor tasks and interference with transfer of data to long-term memory storage, which impedes acquisition of knowledge. Driving ability impairment occurs as well as loss of perspective, anxiety, and paranoia. Local irritation of the bronchial mucous membranes occurs, which leads to increased secretions and chronic bronchitis and lung inflammation and possible degeneration. In addition, shortening of the luteal phase of the menstrual cycle occurs, leading to potential infertility. Mild abstinence symptoms may be observed on discontinuance; these include anorexia, tremors, perspiration, irritability, cramps, diarrhea, nausea, and sleep disturbances.[10]

Cocaine, a powerful stimulant, frequently is classified as the most addicting substance known to man. It stimulates rapid release of norepinephrine, dopamine, and epinephrine in the brain, causing a "rush." Tolerance and craving occur quickly after initial use, and dependence can occur within a few weeks. Cocaine's anesthetic effect causes vasoconstriction and activates the sympathetic nervous system, which controls numerous functions of the brain and other organs, including blood pressure, heart rate, heart muscle contractility, blood glucose level, mood, and appetite. With use, blood pressure increases, as does temperature, physical activity, and mental alertness. Tachycardia and ventricular fibrillation may occur. Rapidly increasing blood pressure may lead to aneurysms with resulting hemorrhage—often fatal. Cocaine use also precipitates grand mal seizures at relatively low doses, and long-term use can sensitize the individual to seizures at lower doses (known as "kindling") occasionally resulting in status epilepticus. Cocaine decreases lung functioning and the ability to transport oxygen into the blood because of its powerful vasoconstrictive effects. Studies show free-basing cocaine leads to serious lung dysfunction after as little as 3 months exposure.[11] Cocaine also suppresses appetite and may cause weight loss and vitamin deficiency, particularly water soluble B and C vitamins, leading to malnutrition, anemia, and metabolic abnormalities. Other problems related to cocaine use are skin infections, edema, and redness related to vaginally administered cocaine, hepatitis, infection from human immunodeficiency virus, endocarditis, and burns caused by free-basing. An overdose is evidenced by irregular heart rate, ventricular tachycardia or fibrillation, cerebral hemorrhage, seizures, heat stroke, and respiratory failure. Symptoms of chronic use include nasal problems such as congestion and cold symptoms, frequent nosebleeds, ulcerations of the nose, and perforated nasal septum.

Opiates (narcotics), such as morphine, heroin, codeine, hydromorphone (Dilaudid), oxycodone (Percodan), meperidine (Demerol), methadone (Dolophine), and propoxyphene (Darvon), produce analgesia, drowsiness, euphoria, and respiratory depression. Occasionally dysphoria may result with morphine use, consisting of mild anxiety, fear, nausea, vomiting, inability to concentrate, apathy, decreased physical activity, and diminished visual acuity.

Chronic effects of narcotic dependence include decreased socialization and increased isolation, diminished libido, menstrual irregularities, and constipation. Because of ingredients frequently used to dilute narcotics for intravenous nonmedical administration, foreign substances may enter the lungs and cause acute embolic phenomenon or chronic granuloma formation. In addition, injection by unsterile methods may lead to infectious complications such as abscesses and cellulitis at the injection site, septic thrombophlebitis, serum hepatitis, septic arthritis, and, less commonly, tetanus, bacterial endocarditis, meningitis, and brain or spinal epidural abscesses. Acute intoxication includes varying degrees of unresponsiveness, shallow and slow respirations, miosis, bradycardia, and hypothermia. Unless treated, pupils dilate from severe cerebral hypoxia, skin becomes cyanotic, and circulation falls. Death may occur from respiratory depression and apnea.

Withdrawal syndrome is characterized by increased respiratory rate, diaphoresis, lacrimation, yawning, rhinorrhea, piloerection, tremors, anorexia, irritability, anxiety, and dilated pupils. These symptoms occur approximately 8 to 12 hours after the last dose is taken. Later signs occurring 24 to 48 hours after the last dose include insomnia, nausea, vomiting, diarrhea, weakness, abdominal cramps, tachycardia, hypertension, involuntary muscle spasms, and chills alternating with sweating and flushing. Symptoms gradually subside over 7 to 10 days, however, methadone withdrawal symptoms may last as long as 3 weeks.

Minor tranquilizers (anxiolytic or "antianxiety" agents) are more similar in action to sedative hypnotics than to major tranquilizers or neuroleptics. They suppress anxiety and easily produce dependence. There are two major classes of minor tranquilizers: propranedial and benzodiazepines. Meprobamate (Equanil), a propranedial, is a central nervous system depressant that sedates and tranquilizes. Effects include drowsiness, ataxia, slurred speech, weakness, fatigue, visual disturbances, syncope, and euphoria. Long-term effects include hematologic disorders, rapid eye movement suppression, and cardiac abnormalities. Acute intoxication or overdose produces stupor, coma, convulsions, and circulatory and respiratory collapse. Withdrawal can produce delirium, convulsions, tremors, ataxia, headache, and insomnia. Because of these complications, withdrawal should be medically supervised.

Diazepam (Valium) and alprazolam (Xanax) are two of the most widely prescribed and misused benzodiazepines. They are prescribed for insomnia, acute reactive anxiety, chronic anxiety, seizures, neuromuscular disorders, as a preanesthetic, and for alcohol withdrawal syndrome. All benzodiazepines increase the seizure threshold and are used as anticonvulsants. Side effects include drowsiness, ataxia, fatigue, slurred speech, and other indicators of central nervous system depression. Depending on the specific benzodiazepines misused, withdrawal symptoms begin to appear from 12 to 24 hours after cessation and peak within 5 to 8 days. If the patient is psychologically addicted, withdrawal must be initiated cautiously and under medical supervision, as respiratory arrest can occur. Overdose causes suppressed respirations and stupor.

Inhalants such as paint thinners (Toluene) and aerosols cause neurotoxicity and brain damage after chronic, long-term use.[12] Patients will often appear mentally slow or with depressed reaction time. Inhalants are most often used in conjunction with other illicit drugs.

Substance use increases maternal morbidity and mortality. The major contributing factor to death is drug overdose with cardiac or respiratory arrest. Status epilepticus may also lead to respiratory arrest and fatal cardiac arrhythmias. In susceptible patients, acute hypertension can lead to cerebral infarction and hemorrhage. Because alcohol and drugs impair fine motor coordination as well as judgment, the incidence of trauma increases substantially. It is estimated that approximately one half of all traffic accident fatalities in 1987 and between 20% to 40% of all trauma treated in hospital emergency rooms were alcohol related.[13–15] This includes falls, motor vehicle accidents, gunshot wounds, blunt trauma, and a spectrum of other violent occurrences.

Exposure to human immunodeficiency virus is greater among substance-dependent patients, especially those who use drugs intravenously and share needles or among women who prostitute to buy drugs. The pregnant patient may not engage in these behaviors but may be involved or living with a partner who uses drugs and who, therefore, substantially increases her risk for exposure. Hepatitis B or serum hepatitis is transmitted via blood or blood products, instruments (needles), or tattooing devices. Recovery is protracted and mortality is still appreciable, ranging from 0.1% to 5%, depending on the infective dose and the age and condition of the patient.[16] Vertical transmission of hepatitis B virus from mother to fetus at the time of delivery has serious health implications for the newborn. Mothers who are carriers of the hepatitis B surface antigen have as high as 90% probability of transmitting the hepatitis virus to their newborn. Therefore, routine blood testing must be conducted.[17]

Frequently, low socioeconomic status plays an important role in contributing to poor pregnancy outcomes in women who use drugs or alcohol. These women often lack social support, may live in a high-stress environment such as project housing where drug use and accessibility are more prevalent, have limited incomes, are single parents, and are unemployed. Depression is often a factor in women who are stressed and overwhelmed and, although the use of alcohol and drugs may momentarily alleviate these feelings, with continuing use of mood-altering addictive substances, depression most always occurs.

The developing fetus is not protected from the effects of maternal substance use. Most drugs used are lipophilic and of low molecular weight, allowing transfer across the placenta. Exposure to illicit drugs may potentially interfere with fetal development and can cause fetal demise. Delayed fetal metabolism and excretion of drugs occur because of immature hepatic and renal function. Drugs such as cocaine, marijuana, and cigarettes cause decreased uteroplacental blood flow and in turn may lead to intrauterine growth retardation and decreased birthweight. Intrauterine growth retardation is also the most frequent consequence of fetal exposure to alcohol.[18] Fetal dependence on drugs such as opiates can develop, and fetal withdrawal may subsequently occur if the mother experiences withdrawal.

The fetus of a woman using alcohol and other drugs is also at higher risk for congenital anomalies. Fetal alcohol syndrome affects 50,000 neonates each year, and 10% suffer irreversible birth defects. This preventable disorder is associated with maternal consumption of more than four drinks per day although the Seventh Special Report to the United States by the Congress on Alcohol and Health stated that no safe threshold has been identified.[19] Criteria for the diagnosis of fetal alcohol syndrome include demonstration of abnormalities in growth, central nervous system dysfunction, craniofacial abnormalities, and major organ system malformation. When only some of these criteria are met, a diagnosis of fetal alcohol effects can be made.

Researchers hypothesize that the vasoconstrictive action of cocaine may cause defects in the genitourinary system, gastrointestinal tract, and neural tube defects as well as cause limb reduction.[3] The following malformations are most commonly seen:

Prune belly syndrome	Anal atresia
First degree hypospadias	Missing digit three on left hand
Second degree hypospadias	Missing digit four on left hand
Hydronephrosis	Neural tube defects
Ileal atresia	

During the first trimester, maternal cocaine use is associated with an increased incidence of spontaneous abortion as a result of vasoconstriction of placental vessels. Abruptio placentae is also associated with cocaine use, presumably because of acute hypertension. Studies revealed that the rate of abruptio placentae did not decrease even when the patient abstained from cocaine use after the first trimester; this strongly suggests that permanent damage to placental and uterine vessels occurs with cocaine use.[20] Cocaine also induces uterine contractions, and preterm labor and precipitous delivery are associated with recent cocaine use.[21]

The potential fetal and neonatal risks encountered with polydrug abuse include stillbirths, sudden infant death syndrome, and cerebral infarctions. Maternal opiate and cocaine dependence increase the risk of sudden infant death syndrome by 5% to 10% over the general population.[21] Neonates passively exposed to opiates during pregnancy will generally experience withdrawal 24 to 72 hours after delivery. Neonatal abstinence syndrome, or neonatal withdrawal, consists of many symptoms, most commonly high-pitched crying, sweating, coarse flapping tremors, restlessness, and gastrointestinal upset. In addition, excoriation of knees, elbows, toes, and nose are frequently observed because of hyperactivity and excessive movement. Acute neonatal opiate withdrawal peaks at 3 or 4 days of age, frequently after hospital discharge. These symptoms can occur up to 3 weeks after delivery and last until 4 to 6 months after birth. The most severe neonatal reactions appear to be related to opiate and cocaine use. Neonates exposed to cocaine during pregnancy exhibit symptoms similar to classic withdrawal: irritability, fine tremors, poor feeding patterns, high respiratory and heart rates, poor sleep patterns, inconsolability, and poor state control. Maternal cocaine use during the first trimester of pregnancy as well as through the entire pregnancy places the neonate at risk for neurobehavioral abnormalities due to the effects of cocaine on the central nervous system. Maternal cocaine use is also associated with impaired neonatal motor development. During the initial Brazelton exam, the neonate may display hypertonicity, especially when placed in a supine position. At 4 months of age, the infant continues to display fine tremors of the upper extremities and increased extensor motor tone in the lower extremities.[22] Cocaine-exposed infants are at 40 times greater risk for motor development dysfunction than those babies not exposed to cocaine.[22]

Etiology

Existing theories of the etiology of substance misuse and dependence proliferate. As early as 1942, Jellinek suggested hereditary as well as environmental causes of alcoholism.[23] He observed that alcoholics with a family history of alcoholism had a poorer prognosis than alcoholics with no family history of alcoholism. The National Council on Alcoholism and the American Medical Society on Addiction Medicine in 1990 stated, "Alcoholism is a primary, chronic disease with genetic, psychosocial and environmental factors influencing its development and manifestations."[24] In the 1970s and 1980s, hormonal neurotransmitters were first implicated in the etiology of alcoholism and other data suggested a deficiency of naturally produced enkephalins in the brain of alcoholics.[25,26]

Since ancient writings, personality factors have been implicated in the development of alcoholism; however, treatment research has not substantiated these theories. Nevertheless, there is evidence to indicate that personality does play an important role in chemical dependence. Three central behaviors identified among the chemically dependent population were impulsivity, failing to inhibit behavior that previously led to negative consequences, and placing more value on immediate drug effects (*e.g.,* intoxication) than on long-term consequences (*e.g.,* liver damage).[27] In addition, genetic factors have been implicated in certain personality traits preceding the onset of alcohol and drug problems. Many alcohol and drug treatment researchers, however, believe the behaviors are most often identifiable after the onset of dependence.[28]

The evolvement of chemical dependence in a given individual is probably a combination of biologic and psychologic factors, as well as environmental and social factors that serve either to increase or decrease the likelihood for alcohol and other drug dependency. Biologic influences include individual responses to drugs (*i.e.,* sensitivity and qualitative effects). Some individuals may have inherently higher tolerance, thus placing the person at greater risk for dependence. Some of the environmental and social factors include drug availability, family and peer influences, culture, and initial experimentation or exposure.

Framework for Accepted Theory

Pregnant women who use alcohol and other drugs are at high risk because of the many potential complications of alcohol and drug use. Although the use of addictive substances is frequently the cause of the initial problem, it is too often identified only as an afterthought, sometimes too late to provide positive outcomes for mother and infant. Drugs misused include some over-the-counter medications, prescription medications, alcohol, tobacco, illicit drugs, hallucinogens, inhalants, and solvents. All of these substances produce mood-altering effects that impede the ability to make sound decisions and use good judgment.

Traditionally, substance misuse or abuse is defined as the use of alcohol and other drugs in a way that differs from approved medical or social practices.[29] Addiction or dependence infers a physiologic *or* psychologic need for the drugs, but not necessarily both. There is also an inability to stop using drugs without help. A diagnosis of chemical dependence can be made even in the absence of physiologic withdrawal symptoms.

Use of the term "abuse" in reference to the pregnant women implies control or an ability for the chemically dependent pregnant woman to decide behavior. This may further subject these women to mistreatment by health care professionals as well as law enforcement and judicial systems.

The use of alcohol and other drugs interferes with the ability of the chemically dependent pregnant woman to understand the impact of substance use on herself and her unborn fetus. It also interferes with the developmental tasks of pregnancy, disallowing the chemically dependent pregnant women the ability to progress through these stages, which can be described as follows:

1. Acceptance of the pregnancy.
2. Differentiation of herself from her fetus.
3. Adjustment to changes in her self-image.

4. Reflection and evaluation of her relationship with her own mother and working through these feelings.
5. Coming to terms with her dependency on others and the loss of certain freedoms.

Use of the term "chemically dependent" allows the health care professional to reframe thinking and past attitudes, and support this woman who is very needy and severely compromised. Taking this into account as well as the informal definition of chemical dependence: "Despite the negative consequences it creates, one continues to use alcohol and other drugs," it is not difficult to understand the rationale for approaching this patient population from a different frame of reference and treat accordingly.

Important to remember is that some women discontinue alcohol and drug use during pregnancy. This does not imply they are not dependent. Binge alcohol and drug use may be observed in all populations and still qualify the diagnosis of "dependence." Motherhood does not cure dependence, although in some cases it does delay progression of the disease.

With psychologic dependence, the drug is needed to feel "normal" and to cope with daily life events. Physical dependence includes tolerance and withdrawal. "Tolerance is the body's need for higher and higher doses to achieve the same effects. Withdrawal is the appearance of physiological symptoms when the drug is stopped too quickly."[29] In the late stages of dependence, the individual may exhibit decreased tolerance or the need for lower dosages of alcohol and other drugs because of the liver's inability to clear toxins as readily. Thus, the patient has already passed the point of tolerance (*i.e.,* needing higher and higher doses to achieve the same effects, see Figure 8-1). Characteristics of chemical dependence are directly proportional to the severity of the disease and include denial, minimizing, rationalizing, and blaming. The dependent person typically feels guilt and shame and may try to hide drug use, which leads to difficulty in obtaining an accurate history.

Physical symptoms of the disease include blackouts (*i.e.,* a period when the individual cannot remember what happened while using drugs or alcohol), tremors, hallucinations, seizures, weight loss, poor concentration, and sometimes physical illness directly related to use (*i.e.,* malnutrition and hepatitis B). Behavioral symptoms include preoccupation with use, attempts to cut down use, and feelings of guilt about use. The user frequently becomes annoyed when others mention that dependence may be a problem, often uses drugs or alcohol when awakening just to feel normal, and has irresponsible behaviors and difficulties with authority figures (*e.g.,* police, courts, and financial institutions). Problems with school, job, family members, relationships with significant others, and decreased spirituality usually occur.

Numerous myths have flourished surrounding dependence to alcohol and other drugs, which must be dispelled if the disease is to be clearly understood. Initially, these patients do not have to want help to receive help and they do not

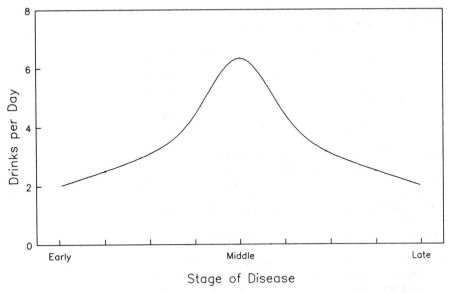

Figure 8-1. Tolerance occurs with alcohol and other drugs. It is the body's need for higher and higher doses to achieve the same effects.

have to hit bottom before beginning recovery. A common misconception is that people dependent on alcohol and other drugs lack will power; however, an effect of dependence is the loss of ability to abstain. Therefore, intervening for the patient is as appropriate as any other medical decision the health care team makes.

There are varied approaches for substance dependence treatment during pregnancy. Comprehensive chemical dependency programs may be designed for inpatient or outpatient treatment, and admission is always based on individual needs. Treatment ranges from 5 days of nonmedical detoxification in a free-standing facility to 28 to 30 days of hospital-based inpatient treatment, to a comprehensive outpatient chemical dependency program, depending on the patient's needs. Inpatient treatment is usually the treatment of choice for women with no support systems, or a home environment not conducive to recovery or medical requirements that necessitate hospitalization. After treatment, referral is sometimes made to a halfway house to continue treatment in a less-structured environment but with provisions for continuing support during recovery.

A multidisciplinary team of nurses, social workers, physicians, dieticians, spiritual counselors, and chemical dependence therapists should be available in the treatment setting. The goal of the model is to meet the physiologic, psychosocial, and chemical dependence treatment needs of the pregnant patient. Referral sites are located in major medical centers, social service agencies, and university hospital settings.

TABLE 8-1
The Twelve Steps of Alcoholics Anonymous

1. We admitted we were powerless over alcohol—that our lives had become un-manageable.
2. Came to believe that a Power greater than ourselves could restore us to sanity.
3. Made a decision to turn our will and our lives over to the care of God as we understood Him.
4. Made a searching and fearless moral inventory of ourselves.
5. Admitted to God, ourselves, and to another human being the exact nature of our wrongs.
6. Were entirely ready to have God remove all these defects of character.
7. Humbly asked Him to remove our shortcomings.
8. Made a list of all persons we had harmed, and became willing to make amends to them all.
9. Made direct amends to such people whenever possible, except when to do so would injure them or others.
10. Continued to take personal inventory and when we were wrong, promptly admit-ted it.
11. Sought through prayer and meditation to improve our conscious contact with God as we understood Him, praying only for knowledge of His will for us and the power to carry that out.
12. Having had a spiritual awakening as the result of these steps, we tried to carry this message to alcoholics, and to practice these principles in all our affairs.

Source: Alcoholics Anonymous: *The Story of How Many Thousands of Men and Women Have Recovered from Alcoholism* ("The Big Book") (3rd ed.). New York, Alcoholics Anonymous World Services, Inc., 1939.

Most widely recognized are treatment programs based on the 12-step philosophy of Alcoholics Anonymous (see Table 8-1). The 12-step philosophy is based on the 12 traditions (see Table 8-2). The overall goal is to provide an intensive setting that encourages abstinence in pregnancy and supports the patient's long-term recovery. Treatment assists the patient in understanding the disease of addiction, the impact of alcohol and other drugs on pregnancy, and explores the developmental tasks of pregnancy.

Treatment for pregnant women will explore the above tasks and assist the patient in understanding which tasks she has accomplished and how chemical dependence has interfered in this process. Once the patient is detoxified, the treatment process consists of group education concerning the disease, including films, lectures, readings, and audiotapes. At some point in the recovery process patients must realize the critical nature of their disease and become committed to recovery and "working the program." Those who are unable to do so are usually asked to leave. Once an educational basis for participation is established and motivation is observed, patients participate in individual and group therapy. Individual therapy provides a nurturing nonjudgmental relationship in which the patient can focus on drug use, recovery, and underlying psychopathology. Group psychotherapy provides peer support and an opportunity to work on interpersonal relationships and decreases the patient's isolation and sense of uniqueness. Feedback is given in an atmosphere of caring and concern and is

TABLE 8-2
The Twelve Traditions

One—Our common unity should come first; personal recovery depends upon AA unity.

Two—For our group purpose there is but one ultimate authority—a loving God as He may express Himself in our group conscience. Our leaders are trusted servants; they do not govern.

Three—The only requirement for AA membership is a desire to stop drinking.

Four—Each group should be autonomous except in matters affecting other groups of AA as a whole.

Five—Each group has but one primary purpose—to carry its message to the alcoholic who still suffers.

Six—An AA group ought never endorse, finance or lend the AA name to any related facility or outside enterprise, lest problems of money, power and prestige divert us from our primary purpose.

Seven—Every AA group ought to be fully self-supporting, declining outside contributions.

Eight—Alcoholics Anonymous should remain forever nonprofessional, but our service centers may employ special workers.

Nine—Alcoholics Anonymous, as such, ought never be organized; but we may create service boards or committees directly responsible to those they serve.

Ten—Alcoholics Anonymous has no opinion on outside issues; hence the AA name ought never be drawn into public controversy.

Eleven—Our public relations policy is based on attraction rather than promotion; we need always maintain personal anonymity at the level of press, radio and films.

Twelve—Anonymity is the spiritual foundation of all our Traditions, ever reminding us to place principles before personalities.

Source: Alcoholics Anonymous: *The Story of How Many Thousands of Men and Women Have Recovered from Alcoholism* ("The Big Book") (3rd ed.). New York, Alcoholics Anonymous World Services, Inc., 1939.

facilitated by a professional counselor. It is hoped that behavioral changes evolve as a result. Mandatory attendance at Alcoholics Anonymous, Narcotics Anonymous, or other 12-step meetings are required.

Additional group education classes provide a structured environment for understanding the impact of drug use on pregnancy, the fetus, and the newborn and acquiring parenting skills. An integral part of recovery are classes that focus on assertiveness, coping skills, problem solving, and conflict management.

Family therapy is also a crucial component of chemical dependence services. The family can potentially support the patient's recovery or they can interfere with her efforts to maintain sobriety. Addiction affects each family member, and therapy can help individuals to understand their roles and recognize unhealthy patterns of communication. A spiritual focus emphasizes balanced lifestyle and integration of concepts such as wholeness into daily life.

The comprehensive outpatient model provides a full range of medical and psychosocial support, the benefits of which are numerous. The model provides an integration of the patient's needs, decreases fragmentation of care, increases communication between service providers, and increases patient compliance because all services are centrally located.

Continuing chemical dependence services, also known as aftercare services, are critical because mothers dependent on alcohol and other drugs are at high risk for relapse after delivery. The return to drug use can be precipitated by the delivery, postpartum depression, adjustment to motherhood, and poor maternal–infant interactions.

Assessment

It is difficult to obtain accurate histories from patients using alcohol and other drugs because of the sensitive social nature of chemical dependence, even when examiner comfort exists. If patients suspect reprisal from answering questions honestly, they will be less likely to respond accurately. Patients with defensive postures brought on by accusatory perinatal staff may be anxious and attempt to mask substance use. It is difficult to elicit correct information when patients are anxious, defensive, or in crisis. Respondents vary their report of daily alcohol intake between 1 and 8 oz depending on how questions regarding use are worded.[31] Also, recall may be inaccurate due to denial, minimizing, level of alertness, or decreased memory retention related to a drug-induced state. Only through an understanding of this disease and how it affects the patient's ability to be honest, plus an acceptance that the patient is not being devious, will nurses be able to establish the trust required for an accurate assessment of alcohol and drug use.

Some states now have reactive laws pertaining to reports of maternal drug use and the rights of unborn children that impede obtainment of accurate histories. Women may fear reprisal and conceal drug use even when they are aware their urine is being tested for the presence of mood-altering substances. Assessing the patient's compliance with other recommendations made by the health care team in the past may be helpful for assessing present compliance or inability to comply. If obtaining information from the patient is difficult, other resources can be utilized, such as family members who accompany the patient and phone calls to previously used health care agencies (*i.e.,* with the permission of the patient).

Sources of Information for the History
Patient
Family members
Physical exam and laboratory results
Past medical history
Previously utilized health care agencies

Assessment of the patient begins with a medical and obstetric history. Here certain factors associated with drug and alcohol use may be identified and may alert the nurse to obtain comprehensive screening. Historical and psychosocial characteristics associated with chemical dependence follow.

Major depressive episodes
History of marked emotional deprivation
Poor relationships with family members
Family history of alcohol or drug use
Self-induced social isolation
Reference to drug-using partner
Minimal coping and communication skills
Secrecy or vagueness
Low self-esteem
Self-destructive behavior
Mistrust of authority figures or other professionals

Factors that may be revealed in the medical history that are associated with chemical dependence are as follows:

Cellulitis	Cirrhosis
Hepatitis	Depression
Bacterial endocarditis	Suicide attempt
Pancreatitis	Acute hypertension
Pneumonia	Acquired immunodeficiency syndrome
Multiple drug allergies	Sexually transmitted disease

The following factors may be exposed when taking the obstetric history and can signal chemical dependence:

Abruptio placentae	Amnionitis
Fetal death	Preeclampsia, eclampsia
Low birthweight infant	Gestational diabetes
Meconium staining	Placental insufficiency
Premature labor	Septic thrombophlebitis
Premature rupture of membranes	Sexually transmitted disease
Spontaneous abortion	Sudden infant death syndrome

Physical assessment is integral with the history and should begin with an assessment of the following aspects of the patient's physical appearance which may be associated with chemical dependence:

Patient looks physically exhausted
Pupils are extremely dilated or constricted
Appearance of pregnancy fails to coincide with stated gestational age
Track marks, abscesses, or edema are visible in upper or lower extremities
Nasal mucosae are inflamed or indurated
Patient is not well oriented

The skin is examined for integrity, bruises, cellulitis, open sores, and lesions. Physical findings consistent with substance use may lead the practitioner to consider further screening for those patients who deny use. For example, the pregnant patient with middle-to-late-stage alcoholism may have facial angiomata and other skin lesions, increased blood pressure, and an enlarged liver. Past or present drug users may have thrombophlebitis or sclerosed veins on hands, arms, legs, ankles, or feet. Changes in pupillary size may be noted, or complaints of sleep difficulty, early morning awakenings, and associated feelings of anxiety and depression may be present. Lethargy, fatigue, weight loss, perforated nasal septum (as a result of insufflated cocaine), rhinitis, congested lungs, or decreased breath sounds may be noted. In addition, cardiac arrhythmias, tender abdomen or abnormal liver size, and vaginal redness or edema (related to vaginally administered cocaine) may be observed. The following are obstetric factors related to substance use:

> Early contractions
> Spotting or vaginal bleeding
> Inactive or hyperactive fetus
> Poor weight gain
> Sexually transmitted disease
> No prenatal care

Routine laboratory tests such as those that follow should be considered in addition to the urine toxicology.

Blood type and screen	Tuberculin skin test
Complete blood count	Human immunodeficiency virus antibody screen
Platelet count	
SMA-6	Pap smear
Rubella titer	Cervical culture for *Neisseria gonorrhoeae*
Serologic tests	
Hepatitis B surface antigen	Chest x-ray with shielded abdomen
Blood alcohol level	Urine culture and sensitivities
Liver function tests	Urine toxicology

Elevations in liver function studies (*e.g.,* GGTP, SGOT, SGPT, LDH, MCV, and triglycerides) and decreased levels of white and red blood cell counts and platelet count may be indicative of chronic alcohol or drug use.[32]

To encourage patient compliance, it is helpful to explain that an accurate intake history of alcohol and other drug use is necessary for a clear picture of all factors affecting the pregnancy. Teaching the patient first about the damaging effects of alcohol and other drugs on the unborn child only increases the patient's sense of guilt and shame, and she may be less likely to answer honestly. Feelings of low self-esteem, guilt, and, most especially, shame occur with chemical dependence. Therefore, education about drug effects on the fetus is helpful only after rapport has been established and the patient has been open about her drug use.

The educational focus should be placed on the maternal effects of drug and alcohol use. This accomplishes several goals: It encourages the patient to take care of herself, it establishes the nurse's primary interest in the patient, and it acknowledges her as an individual separate from her unborn child. This is important as acceptance of the unborn fetus may or may not have been consciously established.

It is important to maintain a caring, sincere, and nonjudgmental attitude in questioning patients about substance use to facilitate rapport and increase the patient's responsiveness and honesty. Symptoms of the disease are denial, minimizing, rationalizing, and blaming; thus, open, honest answers cannot be expected immediately. Often, information must be pieced together to give a clearer picture of chemical dependence.

All potential substances of misuse during the assessment must be discussed (see Table 8-3). The same question format is repeated for each chemical, and it is important to be as accurate as possible regarding amount, method, and frequency of drug use. Substance misuse varies individually from experimental use to use a few times a week or month, weekend use only, daily use, or binge use.

TABLE 8-3
Potential Substances of Abuse

Psychoactive Substances with *Known-Dependence Liability*

Central Nervous System Depressants

Alcohol

Minor tranquilizers

Atarax	Serax
Ativan	Softran
Donnatol	Valium
Equanil (meprobamate, Miltown, Milpath)	Vistaril
Librax	Xanax
Librium	

Hypnotic sedatives and barbiturates

Ambar	Nytol
Amytal	Paraldehyde
Chloral hydrate	Pentothal
Compoz	Phenobarbital
Dalmane	Placidyl
Doriden	Quaalude (Sopor)
Luminal	Seconal
Mebaral	Sleep-Ez
Nembutal	Sominex
Noludar	Tuinal

Cough medicine and other alcohol-based medication

Antihistamines—cold medications

(continued)

TABLE 8-3 (*Continued*)

Psychoactive Substances with *Known-Dependence Liability*

Central Nervous System Stimulants

Benzedrine (Bennies)	Dexamyl	Nicotine
Caffeine	Dexaspan	Preludin
Cocaine (crack, snow, blow, free-base)	Dexedrine	Ritalin
Desbutal	Methamphetamine (crystal meth, ice, crank)	Tenuate
Desoxyn	Methedrine	

Analgesics

Narcotic		*Nonnarcotic*	
Codeine	Nisentil	Aspirin	Mydol
Demerol	Pantopon	Cope	Phenaphen
Dilaudid	Paregoric	Darvon	Ponstel
Heroin	Prinadol	Emperin compound	Soma
Levo-Dromoran	Talwin	Equagesic	Vanquish
Lomotil		Excedrin	
Methadone		Florinal	
Morphine			

Hallucinogens
DMT—Dimethyltryptamine
Ecstacy
LSD—Lysergic acid diethylamide
MDA—Methylenedioxyamphetamine
Mescaline
Morning glory seeds
Peyote
Psilocin
Psilocybin
STP (DOM)—2,5-Dimethoxy-4-methylamphetamine

THC—Tetrahydrocannabinol
Marijuana
Hashish

Muscle Relaxants

Psychoactive Substances without *Known-Dependence Liability*

Major Tranquilizers

Compazine	Stelazine
Haldol	Taractan
Mellaril	Thorazine
Pacatal	Trilafon
Sparine	Vesprin

Antidepressants

Aventyl	Parnate
Elavil	Sinequan
Lithium	Tofranil
Morpramin	Triavil
Nardil	Vivactil

It is important to ask the least invasive questions first to lower the patient's defenses and increase her comfort. It is also helpful to word questions in such a way as to imply drug use is expected, for example: "When was the last time you used a narcotic?" For many patients this would be the last time they had surgery or severe pain and used a prescription medication according to the physician's instructions. With this type of questioning, no judgments about substance use are made. Since cigarettes, over-the-counter drugs, prescription medications, and alcohol use are legal and socially acceptable, it is helpful to begin questioning about these substances and then proceed to illicit drugs.

Obtaining information about past use first and then present use is best. This can be accomplished by inquiring about each month of gestation beginning with the month before the last menstrual period.

1. When did you first start smoking?
2. How many cigarettes a day did you smoke at that time?
3. When did you notice an increase in your smoking?
4. At present, how many cigarettes a day do you smoke? Has this changed throughout your pregnancy?
5. Are there times when you smoke more?

Next, proceed to questions concerning over-the-counter medications. "Doctor shopping" occurs when the patient consults more than one physician for the same complaint without the knowledge of the physicians involved in an effort to obtain medications. The following questions assist in identifying the practice of doctor shopping, as well as in assessing patient compliance to prescribed health practices. The same questions may be used for prescription medicines.

1. When as the last time you used an over-the-counter medication in this pregnancy?
2. What did you use the medication for?
3. Did you take it as directed or did you find taking an extra dose helped?
4. How many tablets (doses) did you take daily, weekly, and monthly?
5. What over-the-counter medications are you now taking?
6. How many different physicians are prescribing these medications for you?
7. Were these medications prescribed for you specifically?

In obtaining a history about alcohol use, the nurse must be very specific and definitive about what constitutes alcohol (*e.g.,* beer, light beer, malt, wine, champagne, coolers, Champale, liqueurs such as Kahlua or schnapps, spirits, or mixed drinks containing hard alcohol).

1. How many drinks does it take to make you high?
2. When did you first start drinking alcohol?
3. How much did you drink at that time?

4. What alcoholic beverages did you drink then?
5. How often did you drink at that time: weekly, daily, and monthly?
6. Were there times when you drank more?
7. How much are you now drinking?
8. Is this more or less than you used to drink?
9. Has anyone in your family ever had a problem with alcohol or drugs? If so, who?

Questions 1 and 8 may help determine tolerance. Most women will reply with two or less drinks. If they respond with more than two drinks, a higher tolerance to alcohol is indicated. If alcohol use increases over time, there is tolerance (*i.e.,* more and more of the same is required to achieve the same effects). Patients who once were able to drink a certain amount of alcohol but find they now tolerate less may not be exhibiting an ability to decrease intake; instead they may be experiencing progression of the disease to late-stage alcoholism.

Once alcohol use is discussed, illicit drug use should be the next topic (see Table 8-3). If the patient denies use of one drug, questioning should proceed to the next drug. Examiners must remember to be nonjudgmental and matter of fact. Because drugs of misuse vary in different areas of the country, it is helpful to be familiar with the drugs particular to that community. Questioning can proceed as follows:

1. When was the first time you used cocaine?
2. Did you snort it, free-base, or use it intravenously—"shoot it"?
3. How much did you use in one day?
4. How many days of the week did you use it?
5. In this pregnancy, has your use remained the same as we have talked about?
6. If it is different, what amount are you now taking? How often? What route?

With cocaine you may have to interpret the amount used based on cost, as some women cannot tell you the amount or sometimes even the cost.

After all drugs are discussed, it is a good idea to ask, "Have you used any other drug we have not talked about?" The following four questions are helpful in determining a problem with substance use. Called the CAGE, it consists of the following:

1. **C** Have you ever tried to **c**ut down on your use?
2. **A** Have you ever been **a**nnoyed when someone mentioned that your alcohol or drug use was a problem?
3. **G** Do you ever feel **g**uilty about your use?
4. **E** Do you ever use an **e**ye opener in the morning to feel better after using the night before?

One of four positive answers indicates there might be a problem, two of four positive is indicative of chemical dependence. The test has been found to be up to 62% reliable with all populations and, although first used to determine alcohol misuse and dependence, is also applicable to other drug use.[33]

A similar but longer instrument, the Michigan Alcoholism Screening Test, has been studied and applied extensively. It is a 24-item questionnaire requiring yes–no responses correctly identifying 87% to 95% of the population (see Table 8-4).[33]

TABLE 8-4
Michigan Alcoholism Screening Test

Carefully read each statement and decide whether your answer is yes or no. Please give the best answer or the answer that is right most of the time. Circle the appropriate response.

Circle Yes or No

1.	Do you feel you are a normal drinker? (By normal we mean you drink less than or as much as most other people.)	Yes No
2.	Have you ever awakened the morning after some drinking the night before and found that you could not remember a part of the evening?	Yes No
3.	Does your wife, husband, a parent, or other relative ever worry or complain about your drinking?	Yes No
4.	Can you stop drinking without a struggle after one or two drinks?	Yes No
5.	Do you ever feel guilty about your drinking?	Yes No
6.	Do friends or relatives think you are a normal drinker?	Yes No
7.	Are you able to stop drinking when you want to?	Yes No
8.	Have you ever attended a meeting of Alcoholics Anonymous?	Yes No
9.	Have you ever gotten into physical fights when drinking?	Yes No
10.	Has drinking ever created problems between you and your wife, husband, a parent, or other near relative?	Yes No
11.	Has your wife, husband, a parent, or other near relative ever gone to anyone for help about your drinking?	Yes No
12.	Have you ever lost friends because of your drinking?	Yes No
13.	Have you ever been in trouble at work because of your drinking?	Yes No
14.	Have you ever lost a job because of drinking?	Yes No
15.	Have you ever neglected your obligations, your family or work for two or more days in a row because you were drinking?	Yes No
16.	Do you drink before noon fairly often?	Yes No
17.	Have you ever been told you have liver trouble? (Cirrhosis?)	Yes No
18.	After heavy drinking have you ever had delirium tremens (DTs) or severe shaking or heard or seen things that weren't really there?	Yes No
19.	Have you ever gone to anyone for help about your drinking?	Yes No
20.	Have you ever been in a hospital because of drinking?	Yes No
21.	Have you ever been a patient in a psychiatric hospital or on a psychiatric ward of a general hospital where drinking was part of the problem that resulted in hospitalization?	Yes No
22.	Have you ever been seen at a psychiatric or mental health clinic or gone to any doctor, social worker, or clergyman for help with any emotional problem, where drinking was part of the problem?	Yes No
23.	Have you ever been arrested for drunken driving under the influence of alcoholic beverages?	Yes No
24.	Have you ever been arrested, even for a few hours, because of other drunken behaviors?	Yes No

(continued)

TABLE 8-4 (*Continued*)

MAST Scoring Key

Item					
1.	Yes—0	No—2	13.	Yes—2	No—0
2.	Yes—2	No—0	14.	Yes—2	No—0
3.	Yes—1	No—0	15.	Yes—2	No—0
4.	Yes—0	No—2	16.	Yes—1	No—0
5.	Yes—1	No—0	17.	Yes—2	No—0
6.	Yes—0	No—2	18.	Yes—2	No—0
7.	Yes—0	No—2	19.	Yes—5	No—0
8.	Yes—5	No—0	20.	Yes—5	No—0
9.	Yes—1	No—0	21.	Yes—2	No—0
10.	Yes—2	No—0	22.	Yes—2	No—0
11.	Yes—2	No—0	23.	Yes—2	No—0
12.	Yes—2	No—0	24.	Yes—2	No—0

Total possible: 53 points
Score: 0–4 nonalcoholic; 5–6 suggestive of alcoholism; 7 or more definite alcoholism.
Positive response to 8, 19, or 20 considered diagnostic.

Nursing Diagnoses

- Potential for sensory–perceptual alterations related to intoxication or withdrawal manifested by maternal drug dependence (*e.g.,* alcohol, cocaine, opiates, and sedative-hypnotics)
- Anxiety related to indefinite outcome of newborn
- Potential for impaired skin and tissue integrity related to maternal intravenous drug dependence as manifested by evidence of cellulitis and thrombosis of veins
- Potential for altered health maintenance related to maternal drug dependence as manifested by spontaneous abortion, abruptio placentae, precipitous delivery, and fetal distress.
- Potential for infections related to maternal intravenous drug use and multiple sexual contacts as manifested by sexually transmitted diseases, human immunodeficiency virus infection, and premature rupture of membranes
- Pain related to maternal tolerance to narcotics secondary to chemical dependence
- Potential for ineffective coping related to guilt regarding maternal drug use as manifested by increased anxiety and defensive behaviors
- Knowledge deficit regarding impact of drug use during pregnancy related to lack of knowledge regarding drug use in pregnancy

Theoretical Basis for the Plan of Nursing Care and Intervention

The patient who is both pregnant and chemically dependent often experiences a heightened sense of anxiety as labor begins and often fears that analgesia or anesthesia will be withheld. This fear of potential pain and increased anxiety may lead to self-medication with alcohol or drugs at the time of labor. The use of illicit drugs at the onset of labor may prolong the latent phase until the drugs are cleared, and progression into active labor may then occur. Pain medications should never be withheld because a pregnant patient is chemically dependent; instead regional anesthetics (epidural or pudendal block) are generally recommended. It is important to obtain blood alcohol and urine toxicology on all patients suspected of chemical use to assess level of intoxication and rule out the presence of other drugs.

The intoxicated intrapartum patient with a history of heavy alcohol use will be likely to have established tolerance and should be closely monitored for withdrawal symptoms. Vital signs are monitored regularly. Injury during intoxication (*e.g.,* falls, burns, and other accidents) is possible, thus patient safety is an important nursing activity. Symptoms of alcohol intoxication include slurred speech, increased blood pressure, rapid pulse, increased respirations, constricted pupils, and lethargy or hyperactivity.

Alcohol overdose is characterized by various levels of anesthesia and decreased central nervous system, cardiac, and respiratory functioning. Pupils may be slowly reactive and at midpoint with depressed tendon and pain reflexes. Cardiac arrhythmias may be present, and lungs may be congested. Nursing management includes establishing an airway, checking frequently for vital signs, evaluating cardiovascular status, controlling shock, establishing a means of measuring urinary output, frequently making neurologic assessments, and maintaining adequate intravenous intake. If the patient is alert, oriented, and can take oral fluids, electrolyte solutions such as Gatorade should be encouraged, unless the patient is on a sodium-restricted diet. In addition, vitamin and thiamine supplements are usually administered to patients with chronic alcoholism.

The patient experiencing alcohol withdrawal may have any of the following symptoms: anxiety; increased blood pressure, pulse, respirations, temperature; tremors; nausea; vomiting; diarrhea; decreased appetite; sleep disturbance; poor proprioception; auditory, visual, or tactile hallucinations; and a decreased ability to distinguish reality from fantasy. The patient in withdrawal should be monitored at least hourly until vital signs are stable and symptoms have subsided (see Table 8–5). The usual drug of choice for alcohol withdrawal is diazepam. Maternal vital signs and fetal heart rate are taken each hour prior to administration of additional doses of diazepam. If the patient is stuporous or if the fetal heart rate is nonreassuring, diazepam is withheld. Diazepam loading is effective because of its long half-life (*i.e.,* 20 to 50 hours), which provides tapering of blood levels and ensures smooth withdrawal, increased patient comfort, and decreased anxiety. Patients should be restrained only if absolutely necessary.

TABLE 8-5
Clinical Institute Withdrawal Scale for Alcohol

Temperature (per axilla)
1. 98.7–99.5
2. 99.5–100.4
3. Greater than 100.4

Pulse (beats per minute)
1. 90–95
2. 95–100
3. 100–105
4. 105–110
5. 110–120
6. Greater than 120

Respiration Rate (inspirations per minute)
1. 20–24
2. Greater than 24

Blood Pressure (diastolic)
1. 95–100 mmHg
2. 100–103 mmHg
3. 103–106 mmHg
4. 106–109 mmHg
5. 109–112 mmHg
6. Greater than 112 mmHg

Nausea and Vomiting: Ask "Do you feel sick to your stomach? Have you vomited?" (Observation)
0. No nausea and no vomiting
2. Mild nausea with no vomiting
4. Intermittent nausea with dry heaves
6. Constant nausea, dry heaves and vomiting

Tremor: Arms extended and fingers spread apart. (Observation)
0. No tremor
2. Not visible, but can be felt finger tip to finger tip
4. Moderate with patient's arms extended
6. Severe, even with arms not extended

Paroxysmal Sweats (Observation)
0. No sweat visible
2. Barely perceptible sweating, palms moist
4. Beads of sweat obvious on forehead
6. Drenching sweats

Tactile Disturbances: Ask "Have you any itching, pins and needles sensations, any burning, any numbness, or do you feel bugs crawling on or under your skin?" (Observation)
0. None
2. Mild itching, pins and needles, burning, or numbness
4. Intermittent tactile hallucinations (*i.e.,* bugs crawling)
6. Continuous tactile hallucinations

Auditory Disturbances: Ask "Are you more aware of sounds around you? Are they harsh? Do they frighten you? Are you hearing anything that is disturbing to you? Are you hearing things you know are not there?" (Observation)
0. Not present
2. Mild harshness or ability to frighten (increased sensitivity)
4. Intermittent auditory hallucinations (appears to hear things you cannot)
6. Continues auditory hallucinations (shouting, talking to unseen persons)

Visual Disturbance: Ask "Does the light appear to be too bright? Is its color different? Does it hurt your eyes? Are you seeing anything that is disturbing to you? Are you seeing things you know are not there?" (Observation)
0. Not present
2. Mild sensitivity (bothered by lights)
4. Intermittent visual hallucinations (occasionally sees things you cannot)
6. Continuous visual hallucinations (seeing things constantly)

Hallucinations: Ask "Are you hallucinating?" (Observation)
0. None
1. Auditory, tactile or visual only
2. Non-fused auditory and visual
3. Fused auditory and visual

Clouding of Sensorium: Ask "What day is this?" "Where are you?" "Who am I?"
0. Oriented
2. Disoriented for date by no more than 2 calendar days
3. Disoriented for date by more than 2 calendar days
4. Disoriented for place and/or person. Reorient to time, place, and person, if necessary

Quality of Contact (Observation)
0. In contact with examiner
2. Seems in contact, but is unaware or oblivious to environment
4. Periodically appears to become detached
6. Makes no contact with examiner

Anxiety: Ask "Do you feel nervous?" (Observation)
0. No anxiety. At ease
2. Appears anxious
4. Moderately anxious, or guarded
6. Overt anxiety (equal to panic)

TABLE 8-5 (*Continued*)

Agitation (Observation)
0. Normal activity
2. Somewhat more than normal activity
4. Moderately fidgety and restless
6. Paces back and forth during most of the interview, or constantly thrashes about

Thought Disturbances (Flight of Ideas) (Observation)
0. No disturbance
2. Does not have much control over nature of thoughts
4. Plagued by unpleasant thoughts continuously
6. Thoughts come quickly and in disconnected fashion

Convulsion (Observation) In progress notes, note duration, extent, and type.
0. No   6. Yes

Headache, Fullness in Head: Ask "Does your head feel different?" "Does it feel like there is a band around your head?" Do not rate for dizziness or light-headedness. Otherwise, rate severity.
0. Not present
2. Mild
4. Moderately severe
6. Severe

Flushing of Face (Observation)
0. None
1. Mild to moderate
2. Severe

Total CIWA Score   _____

Rater   _____

Clinical Observations Related to Detox (*i.e.,* evaluate mental status including mood, thought processes, perceptions, cognitive functions.)

Treatment Protocol
  Assessments will be done on admission and every 4 hours (while awake) by the nurse for the first 48 hours. If the CIWA score at any time is greater than 10, the assessment will be done every two hours and if greater than 15, assessments will be done every hour. Treatment will be instituted if the CIWA score is greater than 15 on two consecutive occasions or above 20 once. The treatment will be diazepam 20 mg p.o. × 1, then 10 mg every hour until the score falls to 10 or less on two occasions. (The physician may instead elect to administer hourly doses of 20 mg until the CIWA score falls to 10 or less if clinically indicated.)

Source: Sellers, E. The Addiction Research Foundation, Toronto, Canada.

  The patient experiencing cocaine intoxication may have increased blood pressure, rapid pulse, increased respirations, dilated pupils, elevated temperature, hyperactivity, and tremors. Cocaine acts as a central nervous stimulant and causes stimulation of the pregnant uterus and vasoconstriction of placental and uterine vessels. The complications seen in the intrapartum period are abruptio placentae, precipitous delivery, preterm labor, and premature rupture of membranes. There may be fetal hyperactivity, bradycardia, meconium-stained amniotic fluid, and late or variable decelerations. Medications are not usually given to assist in detoxification of cocaine.

  The patient experiencing opiate intoxication may have constricted pupils and lethargy. Withdrawal symptoms include dilated pupils, rhinorrhea, lacrimation, piloerection, nausea and vomiting, diarrhea, yawning, abdominal cramps, and restlessness. Sclerotic veins may necessitate insertion of a central intravenous line for vascular access. The patient may also have hepatitis or cellulitis, and extreme caution should be taken in handling blood and body fluids because of the increased risk of human immunodeficiency virus and hepatitis B in these patients.

  The patient experiencing opiate withdrawal may require methadone, especially if greater than 20 weeks pregnant. If the patient is already receiving methadone maintenance, the last administered dose must be confirmed. If the mother experiences withdrawal, the fetus may become hyperactive and also experience withdrawal. A urine toxicology will confirm opiate use as well as the presence of polydrug use. With opiate-dependent patients, it is important to avoid administration of butorphanol (Stadol), pentazocine (Talwin), and other narcotic antagonists for pain management as these drugs will precipitate withdrawal and increase risk of harm to mother and fetus.

Use of benzodiazepines such as diazepam, alprazolam (Xanax), and oxazepam (Serax) and barbiturates such as thiopental (Pentothal), pentobarbital (Nembutal), along with other barbiturate-like drugs such as methaqualone (Quaalude), ethchlorvynol (Placidyl), and chloral hydrate (Noctec), cause central nervous system depressive symptoms in the intoxicated patient. These drugs are frequently used in combination with other substances. The patient may have slurred speech, drowsiness, ataxia, weakness, fatigue, visual disturbances, syncope, and euphoria. Occasionally in withdrawal, hallucinations may be present.

Many women also use hypnotics or antianxiety drugs, and complications include accidental or deliberate overdose.[34] The toxic reaction develops over a period of several hours, and the patient may or may not have evidence of recent drug ingestion. This usually occurs when the patient mixes depressants together (such as alcohol and hypnotics). A confused organic state may occur, and more of the same drugs may be inadvertently taken. Heart rates of the mother and fetus should be monitored closely. The patient should also be closely observed to prevent injury or accidents and should be restrained only if necessary. Evidence of withdrawal includes hyperactivity, anxiety, seizure activity, confusion, disorientation, and hallucinations. If the patient exhibits any seizure activity, behavior that would require restraint, or becomes disoriented, phenobarbital is generally administered (see Table 8-6). This drug is highly effective in the management of withdrawal from barbiturates and other hyposedatives and is practical and safe.[35] Loading involves hourly administration of 120 mg of phenobarbital to accomplish several goals, including patient comfort and sedation, prevention of seizures or respiratory arrest, and patient's orientation to time, place, and person. It is similar to the diazepam load described earlier for alcohol withdrawal and is equally efficient as it produces smooth withdrawal because of a long drug half-life. Often chemically dependent patients require high doses of drugs for detoxification as a result of tolerance and a phenomenon known as "cross-tolerance." Cross-tolerance is exhibited when the pregnant patient who is dependent on one substance can ingest other drugs in unusually high doses without appearing to be overdosed.

Toxic overdose, withdrawal, and temporary psychosis are the most common acute problems seen in patients who use central nervous system depressants. Naloxone (Narcan), a narcotic antagonist, is *not* effective for treatment of central nervous system depressant overdose. Symptoms of overdose include abnormal vital signs, confusion, impaired memory, disorientation, and, potentially, coma. The patient should be closely observed, and drug administration should be avoided.

TABLE 8-6
Phenobarbital Loading Guidelines

Use for hypnosedatives, short-acting benzodiazpines (Halcion, Xanax) or barbiturate withdrawal. Individualize for each patient. Draw blood levels and urine drug screen on admission to establish baseline.

Withdrawal Symptoms (subjective):
- (1) anxiety, apprehension
- (2) insomnia
- (3) visual hallucinations (severe)
- (4) tactile hallucinations (severe)
     (sense of insects on skin)

Withdrawal Symptoms (objective):
- (1) course tremor (mainly hands and fingers)
- (2) anorexia, nausea and vomiting
- (3) tachycardia
- (4) increased B.P. and orthostasis on standing
- (5) disphoresis
- (6) increased temperature
- (7) hyperreflexia
- (8) fasiculations (muscle twitching)

Patients in suspected withdrawal should be assessed and vital signs obtained hourly for the above symptoms.

At the first sign of **two or more signs or symptoms** (one must be objective) house officer should be notified and phenobarbital load should be instituted:

120–240 mg p.o. first dose (1.8–2.4 mg/kg) **then** 120 mg p.o. q 1 hr is given until patient is intoxicated and displays at least **two** of the following symptoms:
- (1) patient is asleep and arousable
- (2) ataxic
- (3) dysarthric
- (4) nystagmus and constricted pupils
- (5) labile mood

Patient should continue to be observed and vital signs recorded hourly during phenobarbital load. Hold for pulse <60, systolic blood pressure <90, or diastolic blood pressure <60, respirations <12. Phenobarbital blood level should be measured at exactly eight hours after the load has been stopped.

Acute physical symptoms may obscure immediate identification of the patient who is either in withdrawal or overdosed from drugs and alcohol. The following are some acute emergencies where substance use may be suspected.

Common Emergencies Related to Substance Use
Acute bacterial endocarditis
Aneurysm
Bleeding
Cardiac arrythmias
Cerebral infarct
Coma
Diabetic ketoacidosis
Eclampsia
Paralysis
Paresthesia
Psychiatric emergencies (*e.g.,* psychosis and attempted suicide)
Pulmonary embolus
Recurrent acute pancreatitis
Respiratory distress
Sepsis
Seizures
Abruptio placentae
Severe malnutrition
Trauma

When a patient has an acute emergency, a urine drug screen and blood alcohol level should be ordered immediately. If the patient is alert and oriented, an attempt to obtain an alcohol and drug history should be made. The potential for acute life-threatening illness mandates that care be managed on a unit that provides intensive perinatal nursing. For all emergency admissions where overdose or severe withdrawal is present, an intravenous line should be established and the patient placed on cardiac and fetal monitoring.

All efforts should be made to address alcohol and drug use while the patient is still in the hospital. Consultation with an alcohol and drug treatment professional is warranted, and hospitals with an inpatient alcohol and drug treatment facility can usually provide in-house consultations. If there is no hospital-based treatment program for chemical dependency, consultation may be sought from a local treatment facility while the patient is still hospitalized. The patient should be assessed by a chemical dependency counselor who will conduct a thorough history and recommend referral resources or treatment depending on the patient's medical and psychosocial situation.

If admission on the inpatient antepartum unit is planned, education of the patient regarding effects of substance use on her health and that of the fetus should be implemented. Once delivered, treatment options become limited because of child care issues and many patients will be less compliant with treatment suggestions. If inpatient or outpatient treatment is recommended but the patient declines, other resources for assessment, referral, and home health care should be planned.

A proactive approach to the chemically dependent woman using alcohol and other drugs is more effective than a reactive approach and will facilitate better communication and an understanding by the patient that the health care team is most concerned about her welfare.

Expected Outcomes

MATERNAL STABILITY

The patient will do the following:

1. Demonstrate decreased signs of intoxication from polydrug use as evidenced by stable vital signs and mental status
2. Avoid opiate withdrawal after methadone administration as evidenced by absence of signs and symptoms of withdrawal
3. Identify anxiety and verbalize concerns for well-being of the newborn
4. Identify causes of obstetric complications and the need for drug abstinence
5. Demonstrate knowledge of risk factors associated with potential for infection (*e.g.,* human immunodeficiency virus, sexually transmitted diseases, and hepatitis)
6. Verbalize that others validate existence of pain and will relate a decrease in pain after relief measures have been initiated
7. Verbalize guilt feelings regarding alcohol or drug use and demonstrate a decrease in anxiety and defensive behaviors
8. Verbalize a need for abstinence and chemical dependence treatment

FETAL WELL-BEING

The fetus will do the following:

- Remain stable as evidenced by heart rate within normal limits (*i.e.,* 110 to 160 beats per minute) and normal fetal activity

References

1. Quellette EM: A report on fetal alcohol syndrome. Testimony before the House Select Committee on Children, Youth and Families. Waltham, MA, June 30, 1983.
2. Clayton RR: Cocaine use in the U.S.: In a blizzard or just being snowed. *NIDA Res Monograph* 65:8, 1986.
3. Van Bremen, J: A first national hospital incidence study. *Perinat Addict Res Ed Update.* June 1991.
4. Rosner M, Keith L, Chasnoff I: The Northwestern University drug dependence program: The impact of intensive prenatal care on labor and delivery outcomes. *Am J Obstet Gynecol* 144:23, 1982.

5. Schenker S, Speeg KV: The risk of alcohol intake in men and women: All may not be equal. *N Engl J Med* 322(2):127, 1990.

6. Tuyns AJ: Cancer of the esophagus: Further evidence of the relation to drinking habits in France. *Intern J Cancer* 5:151, 1970.

7. Williams RR, Horn JW: Association of cancer sites with tobacco and alcohol consumption and socioeconomic status of patients: Interview study from the Third National Cancer Society. *J Nat Cancer Inst* 58:547, 1977.

8. Cefalo RC, Moos MK: *Preconceptional Health Promotion.* Rockville, MD, Aspen, 1988.

9. Zuckerman B, Frank DA, Hingson R, et al: Effects of maternal marijuana and cocaine use on fetal growth. *N Engl J Med* 320:762, 1989.

10. Denber HC: *Clinical Psychopharmacology.* New York, Stratton Intercontinental Medical Book Corp., 1979.

11. Weiss RD, Mirin SM: *Cocaine.* Washington, DC, Psychiatric Press, 1987.

12. Filey CM, Heaton RK, Rosenberg NL: White matter dementia in chronic toluene abuse. *Neurology* 40:532, 1990.

13. Burke TR: The economic impact of alcohol abuse and alcoholism. *Pub Health Rep* 103:564, 1988.

14. National Highway Traffic Safety Administration, National Center for Statistics and Analysis: *Drunk Driving Facts.* Washington, DC, NHTSA, 1988.

15. Roizen J: Alcohol and trauma, in Giesbrecht N, Gonzales R, Grant M, et al. (eds): *Drinking and Casualties: Accidents, Poisonings and Violence in an International Perspective.* London, Routledge, 1988.

16. Petersdorf RG, Adams RD, Braunwald A, et al: *Harrison's Principles of Internal Medicine* (10th ed.). New York, McGraw-Hill, 1983.

17. Butterfield CR, Shockley M, San Miguel G, Rosa C: Routine screening for hepatitis B in an obstetric population. *Obstet Gynecol* 76:25, 1990.

18. Chasnoff IJ: Drugs and women: Establishing a standard of care. *Ann NY Acad Sci* 562:203, 1989.

19. Seventh Special Report to the U.S. Congress on Alcohol and Health, Rockville, MD, U.S. Department of Health and Human Services, January 1990.

20. Chasnoff IJ, Griffith DR, MacGregor S, et al: Temporal patterns of cocaine use in pregnancy. *J Am Med Assoc* 261(12):1741, 1989.

21. Chasnoff IJ, Burns KA, Burns WJ: Cocaine use in pregnancy: Perinatal morbidity and mortality. *Neurotoxicol Teratol* 9:291, 1987.

22. Schneider JW, Griffith D, Chasnoff I: Infants exposed to cocaine in utero: Implications for developmental assessment and intervention. *Inf Young Children* 2(11):25, 1989.

23. Jellinek EM: Alcohol addiction and chronic alcoholism. Research Council on Problems of Alcohol, Scientific Committee. New Haven, Yale University Press, 1942.

24. National Council on Alcoholism and the American Medical Society on Addiction Medicine: Editorial: The disease of alcoholism. Part VIII: Is alcoholism really a disease? *Med/Scientif Advis* 5(4):7, 1990.

25. Blum K, Frachtenberg M: New insight into the causes of alcoholism. *Profess Couns* Mar./Apr.:433, 1987.

26. Cohen S: *The Chemical Brain: The Neurochemistry of Addictive Disorders.* Minnesota, CompCare Publishers, 1988.

27. Khantzian EJ, Treece C: DSM III psychiatric diagnosis of narcotic addicts: Recent findings. *Arch Gen Psych* 42:1067, 1985.

28. Flores PJ: *Group Psychotherapy with Addicted Populations.* New York, Haworth Press, 1988.

29. Schuckit MA: *Drug and Alcohol Abuse: A Clinical Guide to Diagnosis and Treatment.* New York, Plenum Press, 1985.

30. Alcoholics Anonymous: *The Story of How Many Thousands of Men and Women Have Recovered from Alcoholism ("The Big Book")* (3rd ed.). New York, Alcoholics Anonymous World Services, Inc., 1939.

31. Knuppel RA: "Alcohol and Pregnancy." Paper presented at National Association for Perinatal Addiction Research and Education National Conference. Miami, Sept. 16, 1989.

32. Mendelsohn JHH, Mello NK: *The Diagnosis and Treatment of Alcoholism* (2nd ed.). New York, McGraw-Hill, 1985.

33. Hays, JT, Spickard WA: Alcoholism: Early diagnosis and intervention. *J Gen Intern Med* 2:424, 1987.

34. Cohen S: Valium: Its use and abuse. Drug Abuse and Alcoholism Newsletter, vol. 5. San Diego, Vista Hill Foundation, 1976.

35. Martin PR, Bhushaw KM, Whiteside EA, Sellers, EM: Intravenous phenobarbital therapy in barbiturate and other hypnosedative reactions: A kinetic approach. *Clin Pharmacol Therapeut* 26:256, 1979.

36. Finnegan LP (ed.): *Drug Dependence in Pregnancy: Clinical Management of Mother and Child.* National Institute of Drug Abuse, Service Research Monograph Series. Rockville, MD: U.S. Government Printing Office, 1978.

9.
◆ ◆ ◆

Hypertensive Disorders in Pregnancy

Carol J. Harvey
Mary Ellen Burke

Supportive Data

Incidence

It is estimated that hypertension complicates approximately 7% of all pregnancies, although the incidence varies by region, country, and patient population.[1] *Hypertensive disorders* refers to a variety of conditions in which blood pressure is elevated and maternal or fetal condition may be compromised. The following shows a clinical classification of hypertensive disorders in pregnancy.[1–3]

Pregnancy-induced hypertension (PIH)
    Hypertension
    Preeclampsia
        Mild
        Severe
    Eclampsia
Chronic hypertension
Chronic hypertension with superimposed PIH
    Superimposed preeclampsia
    Superimposed eclampsia

Pregnancy-induced hypertension may be subdivided into three categories: hypertension alone, preeclampsia, and eclampsia. *Hypertension* is defined as a systolic pressure ≥140 mmHg or a diastolic pressure ≥90 mmHg; or a 30 mmHg or greater rise in systolic pressure or 15 mmHg or greater rise in diastolic pressure above baseline values measured on at least two occasions 6 hours or more apart. *Preeclampsia* is a term describing hypertension with proteinuria, generalized edema, or both. Symptoms most often appear after the twentieth week of gestation. The following are criteria for severe preeclampsia:

- Blood pressure ≥160 mmHg systolic, or ≥110 mmHg diastolic, on at least two occasions 6 hours apart with the patient at bed rest
- Proteinuria ≥5 g in 24 hours or 3+ to 4+ on qualitative assessment
- Oliguria (≤400 ml in 24 hours)
- Cerebral or visual disturbances
- Epigastric pain
- Pulmonary edema or cyanosis
- Impaired liver function of unclear etiology
- Thrombocytopenia

Eclampsia refers to the development of seizures or coma without an underlying neurologic or febrile origin in a patient with preeclampsia.

The specific incidence of PIH is unknown. Many variables, such as underlying medical disorders, limited prenatal care, and confusing clinical presentation, may make identification difficult. However, it is generally acknowledged that the incidence is higher in nulliparous women and women under 20 or over 35 years of age.[4] Occasionally, it may be seen in the multipara with multiple gestation, renal or vascular disease, or fetal hydrops. Both its incidence and severity have been shown to increase in women with multiple gestation or hydatidiform molar pregnancies.[2] The reported incidence of eclampsia has ranged from 1 in 147 to 1 in 1228 pregnancies with an incidence of 1.5% in twin gestation.[1] It is primarily a disease of the young primigravida but is also increased in women over 35 years of age.

Chronic hypertension is defined as a blood pressure of 140/90 mmHg or greater prior to pregnancy, before the twentieth week of gestation in the absence of a hydatidiform mole, or that persists for more than 42 days postpartum. Many causes of chronic hypertension in pregnancy have been documented:[1]

Primary essential hypertension
Secondary hypertension
   Renal
      Acute glomerulonephritis
      Chronic nephritis
      Lupus nephritis
      Diabetic nephropathy
   Endocrine
      Cushing syndrome
      Primary aldosteronism
      Pheochromocytoma
      Thyrotoxicosis
   Neurologic disorders
      Quadriplegia

The incidence is unknown as diagnosis is often difficult, especially when prenatal care is initiated after 20 weeks gestation.

Chronic hypertension with superimposed preeclampsia is characterized by the following specific diagnostic criteria:[2,5]

- Documentation of chronic hypertension
- Evidence of a superimposed, acute process characterized by an increase in systolic blood pressure of at least 30 mmHg or diastolic blood pressure of at least 15 mmHg above baseline on two occasions at least 2 hours apart
- Development of proteinuria, gross edema, or both

The HELLP syndrome refers to a subset of patients with a severe form of PIH who develop multiple organ damage. *HELLP* stands for *h*emolysis, *e*levated *l*iver enzymes, and *l*ow *p*latelet count. The reported incidence ranges from 2% to 12%, but the true incidence remains unknown because of differences in diagnostic criteria.[6–9]

Significance

Hypertensive disorders are relatively common during pregnancy and remain a significant cause of maternal morbidity and mortality. Associated complications are dependent on the specific disorder, maternal organ system affected, and severity of the disease process.

In women with preeclampsia, the renal, hematologic, and hepatic systems are most likely to be involved. A study of 303 patients with severe PIH showed that 17% had thrombocytopenia, 8.5% had HELLP syndrome, 7.3% developed disseminated intravascular coagulation, and 5% manifested pulmonary edema.[10] The incidence of placental abruption is increased significantly in women with hypertensive disorders during pregnancy. Abdella and co-workers reported an incidence of placental abruption of 4% in patients with chronic hypertension, 10.2% in patients with severe preeclampsia, and 15.1% for those with chronic hypertension and superimposed preeclampsia or eclampsia.[11] Cerebral causes of maternal death in women with PIH include cerebral edema, focal anemia, thrombosis, and vascular accidents ranging from petechiae to frank bleeding.[12] Maternal complications associated with HELLP syndrome include acute renal failure, hepatic rupture, adult respiratory distress syndrome, and disseminated intravascular coagulation. Mortality ranges from 2% to 24% of women with the syndrome.[6–8] Maternal complications associated with eclampsia include pulmonary edema, intracranial hemorrhage, renal failure, disseminated intravascular coagulation, postpartum hemorrhage, HELLP syndrome, placental abruption, and death.

Perinatal morbidity and mortality are also increased in pregnancies complicated by hypertensive disorders and are primarily dependent on gestational age at onset and severity of the disease. Much of the mortality is a consequence of prematurity related to early spontaneous labor or therapeutic interruption necessitated by worsening maternal disease. Hypertensive disorders of pregnancy place the fetus at increased risk for intrauterine growth retardation, hypoxia, and intrauterine demise. The presence of HELLP syndrome is associated with perinatal mortality between 7.7% and 60%.[6–8,13]

Etiology

Pregnancy-induced hypertension has been called the "disease of theories," for over the past 200 years numerous potential causes have been proposed but none have been well established. Theories have included maternal dietary considerations, genetic factors, and even the presence of a worm (*Hydatoxi lualba*) in maternal serum. Each theory has been contested, and even the worm proved to be lint artifact on the specimen slide. Pregnancy-induced hypertension affects multiple organ systems and is manifested in a variety of clinical presentations affecting a large cross-section of women and its etiology may be multifactorial.

A large data base accumulated over 200 years from observing women with this disorder supports the following:[14–15]

1. Chorionic villi must be present in the uterus for a diagnosis of PIH to be made.
2. Women exposed for the first time to chorionic villi are at increased risk for developing PIH.
3. Women exposed to an increased amount of chorionic villi (*e.g.,* multiple gestation or hydatidiform mole) are at greater risk for developing PIH.
4. Women with a history of PIH in a previous pregnancy are at increased risk for developing PIH.
5. Women who change partners are more likely to develop PIH in a subsequent pregnancy.
6. There is a genetic predisposition for the development of PIH which may be single gene or multifactorial.
7. Vascular disease places the patient at greater risk for developing superimposed PIH.

These established observations have provided a base for the development of theories and research questions about the etiology of PIH.

Although PIH is probably of multifactorial origin, many theories are under investigation. A genetic theory is supported by sociological data as well as by research in the field of genetics.[15,16] A single gene responsible for the development of PIH may be existent, although multifactorial inheritance remains possible, and the relationship between chronic hypertension, superimposed PIH, and genetics is still under investigation. Dietary factors in the development of preeclampsia have been considered for at least 100 years.[17] Calcium deficiency was first associated with the development of PIH in an epidemiological study.[18] Since then two other studies support the role of calcium deficiency as a potential cause, however, large randomized studies are needed to further clarify the relationship.[19,20]

Framework for Accepted Therapy

In addition to an ill-defined cause of PIH, the pathophysiology of this disorder is not fully understood. The intrapartum nurse must understand the various processes involved in the disorder to provide supportive and coordinated care. Currently two models have been proposed: One is based on early hemodynamic alterations, and the other on a vasospastic process. Proposed first, the vasospasm model has been the traditionally accepted process associated with PIH. The hemodynamic hypothesis was postulated following institution of research concerning obstetric hemodynamic status.

Both models incorporate data obtained from research based on the response pattern of patients to infusion of pressor agents. In normal pregnancy, the patient becomes refractory to the pressor effects of angiotensin II, which leads to a decrease in blood pressure beginning in the late first trimester. Women who subsequently develop PIH demonstrate an opposite response and are more susceptible to the effects of infused pressor agents such as angiotensin II or norepinephrine. The response to infusion of pressor agents is linked with the production of prostaglandins and the ratio between vasodilative and vasoconstrictive types of prostaglandins.

Plasma blood volume, renal perfusion, and cardiac output are all increased in normal pregnancy. The hemodynamic model suggests that an early high cardiac output state, above that which is associated with normal pregnancy, is the cause of long-term end-organ damage observed in patients with preeclampsia or eclampsia. This high cardiac output state occurs early in the pregnancy of women who later have preeclampsia prior to the development of clinical symptoms of the disease. Early in pregnancy hormonally mediated vasodilation acts as a compensatory mechanism so that the patient maintains a normal blood pressure. As the disease process progresses, the increase in cardiac output leads to an increase in blood pressure. In some patients, the systemic vascular resistance may increase to protect the end organs and subsequently reduce cardiac output, leading to a low-output–high-resistance state.

The early high cardiac output state is hypothesized to cause damage to the endothelium over time via exposure to increased pressures and flow rates. Damage to the endothelium is followed by platelet adherence to the damaged area, which leads to platelet aggregation and a decrease in the serum platelet count. It is hypothesized that platelet aggregation may in turn have an effect on the ratio of prostacyclin to thromboxane, vasoactive prostaglandins that play an important role in the disease process.[21] Prostacyclin is a vasodilator prostaglandin, while thromboxane is a vasoconstrictive prostaglandin. The interplay between these agents is hypothesized to have a cause and effect on the course of the disease.[21,22]

It was in 1918 that PIH was first characterized by vasospasm.[12] The currently suggested mechanisms for this process include an increased responsiveness of vascular smooth muscle to pressor substances and an imbalance of vasoactive prostaglandins.[14,21] Vasospasm occurs when arterial and venous circulation is disrupted by segmental cyclic vasoconstriction. This dynamic process is unpredictable and may affect any or all organ systems. Patients with PIH may have vasospasm so severe that it can be observed in the patient's nail beds.

The vasospasm model suggests that blood flow is impeded through arteries, leading to arterial hypertension. Vasospasm may affect every artery and organ system in the body, including the uterus and placenta, with vascular endothelium damaged by the vasospasm. Disruption of the endothelium leads to an early step in the coagulation process, which is platelet adherence and aggregation at the site of vessel damage. The cyclic vasospasm process may affect various sites leading to increased endothelial damage, use of large numbers of platelets, and decreased circulating platelets. Severely damaged endothelium may allow for the escape of platelets, fibrinogen, and other blood components to the interendothelium and interstitial spaces.[9,23] Serum fibrinogen levels may be decreased. Microangiopathic hemolytic anemia may result from fibrin deposited at the damaged sites. The red blood cells are then destroyed as they move through the narrowed vessels.

Vasospasm may lead to increased complications among patients with chronic hypertension and superimposed PIH. Chronic hypertension is associated with constriction of blood vessels throughout the entire body. As these narrowed blood vessels are subjected to the vasospasm associated with PIH, the result may be a dangerously constricted blood vessel, decreased flow, injury to the endothelium, and destruction of blood components. Vascular constriction associated with vasospasm may in turn further increase the blood pressure and may contribute greatly to severe end-organ damage. Patients with chronic hypertension and superimposed PIH are at greater risk for intrauterine growth retardation, intrauterine fetal demise, and worsening of renal, vascular, and cardiac diseases than those with either disorder alone.

Normal pregnancy results in a 40% to 50% increase in circulating plasma fluid volume; however, patients who develop PIH have a decrease in circulating volume. This decreased plasma volume may be dramatic, especially in those patients with chronic hypertension who develop superimposed preeclampsia. Patients with chronic hypertension are at increased risk for having a circulating volume less than that of a normal pregnancy. This is associated with an increased risk of perinatal morbidity and mortality in the absence of superimposed PIH.[24] Chronic hypertension with superimposed PIH may result in an even more dramatic decrease in circulating volume.

Hemoconcentration is another common occurrence. Normally, the pregnant patient experiences a decrease in hemoglobin and hematocrit levels as the plasma fluid volume increases with gestation. Normal hemoglobin for pregnancy is 10 to 12 mg/dl, due to dilution of red blood cell mass with the increase in plasma blood volume.[12,25] The hematocrit level is also normally decreased from prepregnant levels. Patients with PIH experience an increase in hemoglobin and hematocrit levels above normal prepregnant values, and plasma volume levels decrease, with fluid shifted to the extravascular space.

Patients with PIH may, paradoxically, have anemia, which results from destruction of red blood cells as they pass through spasmed sections within blood vessels. A peripheral blood smear may provide documentation of such changes in the form of Burr cells or schistocytes. Some patients may initially have elevated hemoglobin and hematocrit counts, which decrease dramatically with the infusion of crystalloid solutions or with mobilization of excess extravascular fluid, such as occurs with lateral positioning and bed rest. A drop in hematocrit with no evidence of bleeding internally or externally usually signifies worsening of the disease process.[23,25]

Thrombocytopenia is another common occurrence in patients with PIH and may develop secondary to damage to the intravascular integument. The segmental vasospasm, high cardiac output state, and possibly increased thromboxane activity associated with PIH cause damage to the internal wall of the blood vessel, resulting in a platelet response to the injury.[26] Platelets are then mobilized to the damaged areas, with the resultant decrease in platelet number and impaired response to the overwhelming damage throughout the maternal vasculature.

Thrombocytopenia places the patient at risk for developing an inability to clot effectively, especially at delivery. These patients are at increased risk for developing disseminated intravascular coagulation and hemorrhagic shock. Thrombocytopenia associated with PIH has not been shown to have an effect on the fetal platelet count[26] and does not require percutaneous umbilical blood sampling prior to delivery.

Renal blood flow increases by 40% to 50% in normal pregnancy by the third trimester with a resultant increase in the glomerular filtration rate and renal plasma flow in evidence by the end of the first trimester.[28,29] Serum blood urea nitrogen, creatinine, and uric acid levels are decreased secondary to the increased glomerular filtration rate. Concomitantly, creatinine and uric acid excretion is elevated. The development of a glomerular lesion—capillary endotheliosis—has been associated historically with the development of proteinuria in the patient with preeclampsia. It has been hypothesized that vasospasm and the increased hypercoagulability of pregnancy result in a partial obstruction and ischemia of the lumen by the formation of fibrin–fibrinogen immunoglobulins.[30] More recent research suggests that the damage and proteinuria associated with preeclampsia may be the result of a high cardiac output state which damages capillary endothelium and end-organ systems, notably in the kidneys.[31]

Patients with PIH, especially those with preeclampsia and/or eclampsia, demonstrate a decrease in plasma blood volume, glomerular filtration rate, and renal plasma flow. This decrease may be more evident in the patient with chronic hypertension complicated by superimposed PIH, especially if the underlying reason for the chronic hypertension is renal disease. Laboratory analysis reveals a rise in serum blood urea nitrogen, creatinine, and uric acid levels. Urine creatinine clearance may decrease, and oliguria may develop as the disease process worsens.[32,33]

Oliguria is not a common occurrence in preeclampsia, even though each patient should be assessed for this complication, but it is considered a severe manifestation of the disease. Oliguria may result from three underlying mechanisms.[34] The first subset includes patients whose oliguria is secondary to a relative intravascular fluid volume depletion. Hemodynamic monitoring in this subset characteristically demonstrates a low wedge pressure, moderately increased systemic vascular resistance, low-to-normal cardiac output, and hyperdynamic left ventricular function. Volume infusion raises the wedge pressure and cardiac output, decreases systemic vascular resistance, and may increase urine output. Approximately 56% of patients in one study on oliguria were included in this group.[34] The second subset includes patients with isolated renal arterial spasm. These patients demonstrate a persistent oliguria when the measured intravascular volume would normally be sufficient to perfuse the kidneys. The systemic vascular resistance measurements remain in the normal range. The third subset includes patients with the least common complication of preeclampsia. These patients demonstrate a dramatically increased systemic vascular resistance, elevated wedge pressure, and a low cardiac output. Oliguria in this case is hypothesized to develop from the vasospasm associated with preeclampsia, in addition to a low cardiac output. This low cardiac output is the result of depressed left ventricular function secondary to the severe vasospasm that increases the systemic vascular resistance. These patients are fluid restricted, with the goal of therapy to reduce the systemic vascular resistance and thus reduce left afterload. Unless severe renal cortical damage occurs, or the pregnancy complicates underlying renal disease, renal function usually returns to normal by the end of the postpartum period.[33] Hematuria may be noted, especially in a patient with disseminated intravascular coagulation. Hematuria results from red blood cell destruction, giving the urine a characteristic cranberry juice appearance. The presence of hematuria warrants further evaluation.

Hepatic complications occur in response to a high cardiac output state, endothelial damage, and/or vasospasm, which result in ischemia and, possibly, necrosis. Hepatic damage is one of the myriad complications that may occur in preeclampsia or eclampsia, even in those patients who do not have the classic triad of symptoms. It may also occur in patients experiencing chronic hypertension with superimposed PIH.

The earliest sign of hepatic damage may be an increase in liver function tests, especially the SGOT. Therefore, serial studies are indicated to monitor the patient for increased liver impairment. Symptoms of hepatic damage include substernal right upper quadrant or epigastric pain and tenderness of the liver on palpation. Hemorrhagic necrosis may occur along the edge of the liver. Since the liver is encapsulated, a subcapsular hematoma may result which may be noted on ultrasound examination. Rupture of the liver, a rare but often fatal complication, may occur if bleeding is extensive. Immediate surgery is necessary in this critical condition.

Pulmonary complications associated with PIH include dramatic alterations in colloid osmotic pressure, as shown in the following list:

Nonobstetric   25.4 ± 2.3 mmHg
Obstetric
   Antepartum   22.4 ± 0.54 mmHg
   Postpartum   15.4 ± 2.1 mmHg
Pregnancy-induced hypertension
   Antepartum   17.9 ± 0.68 mmHg
   Postpartum   13.7 ± 0.46 mmHg

Colloid osmotic pressure is the pressure gradient that controls fluid movement between the capillary space and the interstitial space. It is normally decreased in pregnancy due to hormonally mediated changes and may be further decreased by the infusion of crystalloids, hemorrhage, and a supine position in labor.[35,36]

Colloids are a group of plasma protein molecules that include albumin, globulin, and fibrinogen. Albumin accounts for 75% of the colloid particles, globulin accounts for most of the remaining particles, and fibrinogen accounts for the least amount. The actual number of these molecules in the plasma is responsible for the osmotic pressure. Colloids are large molecules that do not cross uninjured capillary membranes. If there is damage to the capillary wall and colloid particles escape to the interstitial space, plasma fluid will follow. Conversely, if colloids such as albumin or fresh frozen plasma containing colloid particles are administered intravenously to the patient, fluid will move from the interstitial space to the capillaries, increasing the plasma fluid volume.[37] This is known as Starling's law of the capillary: Fluid will move in or out of a capillary when an imbalance of colloid to fluid occurs.[38] Every capillary has these permeability characteristics.

Patients with PIH are at increased risk for developing pulmonary edema because of damage of the pulmonary capillaries from high cardiac output, endothelial damage, and decreased colloid osmotic pressure. This risk is increased with the infusion of large amounts of crystalloid solution. One liter of normal saline solution causes a 12% decrease in colloid osmotic pressure, a change that may be measured for 3 to 5 days after delivery.[36] During the intrapartum period, patients may receive a considerable volume of intravenous fluid, especially if epidural anesthesia is employed. Patients with PIH may also receive fluid boluses to temporarily increase circulating volume. The infusion of colloids, such as a solution of albumin, in patients with severe PIH is generally not recommended as damaged capillaries may allow for passage of the infused colloids into the interstitial space, carrying even more intravascular volume into the interstitial space, which compounds the problem.

Cerebral vascular resistance is increased in PIH secondary to vasospasm, though cerebral blood flow remains normal.[39] The pathophysiology of cerebral edema is unclear, though it has been hypothesized that it may develop during hypertensive crisis when the ability of the brain to autoregulate cerebral blood flow is diminished or may result from cerebral anoxia during eclamptic seizures.[39] Use of large amounts of crystalloid solutions may also contribute to the development of cerebral edema.[36,39]

Visual disturbances, associated with severe preeclampsia, range from patients seeing "spots" or "spiderwebs" in front of their eyes to blindness. Patients often report blurred vision. Physical assessment may reveal atrioventricular nicking, retinal edema, or a detached retina. Prognosis for full recovery is excellent if delivery is immediate, though symptoms may persist for several days postpartum.

Cerebral changes may also include headache, hyperreflexia, clonus, and altered level of consciousness. The headache associated with severe PIH is not relieved by acetaminophen or comfort measures. The presence of altered consciousness, especially in conjunction with any other cerebral change, is considered ominous and may be associated with eclampsia.[23] Patients with eclamptic seizures may have evidence of hypodense areas on computed tomography scans, reflecting hemorrhage or infarction. These lesions have been noted in approximately 50% of patients with eclamptic seizures and may be better detected with advanced equipment and assessment skills.

Hemodynamic values in patients with PIH have been studied, with varied results reported.[40–49] (A complete discussion of invasive hemodynamic assessment is presented in Chapter 11, page 197–201.) Cardiac function of the normal heart is such that information obtained from the right side of the heart may not correlate with information regarding the function of the left side of the heart. In patients with severe PIH, the two sides often have widely divergent conditions and values. There may be a variety of reasons why such differences exist, including the degree of severity of the disease process, the presence of underlying chronic vascular disease affecting the system, or treatment with volume or antihypertensive agents affecting one system more than another.

Studies have been inconsistent with respect to specific conclusions. They report a range of hemodynamic findings that support the theory of an initial hyperdynamic model with high cardiac output and a late or end stage model of low cardiac output and high systemic vascular resistance. There is also a demonstrated lack of correlation between the central venous pressure and the pulmonary capillary wedge pressure.

Uteroplacental perfusion is also decreased in women with PIH. Oligohydramnios, intrauterine growth retardation, fetal stress, and intrauterine fetal demise are all associated with PIH. The spiral artery, which communicates between the maternal circulation and the placental intervillous space, is subject to vasospasm and high cardiac output.[50] A lesion may develop in the spiral artery further impeding blood flow, the mechanism for which is not clearly understood at this time. Treatment of PIH may also affect placental blood flow. For example, bed rest in the lateral position increases blood flow, while antihypertensive medications may decrease blood flow. Hydralazine has been demonstrated to decrease placental perfusion, even with intermittent administration.[51] A decrease in the diastolic pressure to less than 90 mmHg in the patient with severe hypertension will decrease placental flow, often with a concomitant decrease in the fetal heart rate. This is associated with vasodilation in the face of insufficient intravascular volume. Vasodilative antihypertensives, regional anesthesia, and supine hypotensive syndrome of pregnancy may all contribute to decreased flow in these instances.

The historic basis for therapy relies on the clinical observation that bed rest in the lateral position promotes blood pressure reduction and increased renal and placental flow and may also prolong gestation. Bed rest, therefore, remains an important part of therapy. In addition, a variety of pharmacologic agents have been used for control of hypertension and prevention of seizures. New modalities that address prevention of PIH are currently under investigation.

Treatment of hypertension in pregnancy is directed toward reduction of blood pressure by decreasing the systemic vascular resistance or cardiac output, increased blood volume and flow, and prevention of hypertensive crisis. Hypertensive crisis places the patient at risk for cerebral vascular accidents, myocardial ischemia and infarction, renal damage, liver hematoma and rupture, placental infarction, abruptio placentae, and intrauterine fetal demise.

Antihypertensive treatments include pharmacologic agents and bed rest. Lateral positioning results in increased blood flow to the kidneys and uterus, movement of interstitial fluid back into the intravascular space, and reduction in blood pressure and endogenous catecholamine production.[52] The goal of antihypertensive treatment in patients with mild-to-moderate PIH is to reduce the blood pressure to baseline. In the ambulatory setting, patients with chronic hypertension are treated to maintain a diastolic pressure of less than 90 mmHg. Patients with severe PIH or PIH superimposed on chronic hypertension, however, are treated to maintain a diastolic pressure between 90 and 100 mmHg. Patients with severe PIH, especially those in hypertensive crisis, may not tolerate a decrease in diastolic pressure to less than 90 mmHg. Such patients may require intravascular volume expansion before drug administration to prevent maternal hypotension. A variety of agents are available. The most commonly used antihypertensive agents in pregnancy are vasodilating agents, centrally acting adrenergic blockers, and calcium channel blockers.

Hydralazine hydrochloride is the first-line antihypertensive agent of choice for treating pregnant women in the United States.[27,51,52] Hydralazine acts by relaxing arteriolar smooth muscle, which results in vasodilation. Vascular resistance decreases throughout the body with the greatest benefit experienced by cerebral, coronary, renal, and splanchnic circulations. Patients may experience increased heart rate, cardiac output, and oxygen consumption; therefore, patients with myocardial ischemia may not be candidates for hydralazine therapy. No long-term fetal effects have been demonstrated, though fetal bradycardia and decelerations have been reported when the diastolic pressure decreases below 90 mmHg.[52]

Labetalol hydrochloride is a beta-blocking agent. It acts by both alpha and beta blockade, causing vasodilation without significant change in cardiac output or heart rate. It has not been associated with adverse effects on the fetus as have other beta blockers such as propranolol. The onset of action is rapid, though the duration of action is variable. It is another first-line agent for the treatment of severe hypertension or may be used as a second agent for hypertension refractory to hydralazine.[53]

Sodium nitroprusside is the first-line drug of choice for severe hypertension or hypertensive crisis in nonpregnant patients. It is a rapid-acting agent, with an extremely short half-life. It is suggested for use in patients whose pressure remains refractory to other hypertensive agents, including hydralazine, labetalol, and diazoxide, and who may have left ventricular failure or pulmonary edema. Use of sodium nitroprusside in pregnancy is controversial. The agent breaks down into a variety of metabolites, including cyanide. Animal data have suggested that fetal cyanide toxicity may occur without the mother experiencing any symptoms of toxicity.[54] Therefore, sodium nitroprusside is limited to postpartum use and in the antepartum patient in whom delivery is imminent.

Diazoxide, another first-line agent used in the nonpregnant population, has also been studied in pregnancy. It is a potent vasodilator that decreases blood pressure by decreasing the systemic vascular resistance and increases cardiac output and heart rate. The vasodilatory effect is almost immediate and results in a rapid drop in blood pressure, often to diastolic pressures of 60 to 70 mmHg. This may be accompanied by shocklike symptoms in the mother and by fetal bradycardia. Therefore, intravascular volume expansion is often indicated prior to drug administration. Diazoxide causes maternal and fetal hyperglycemia, as well as inhibits uterine contractions. Its use in pregnancy remains under investigation.[55]

Nitroglycerin, a potent agent, causes venous vasodilation by acting on smooth muscle. It decreases blood pressure by decreasing cardiac output. Its effect on blood pressure is associated with the patient's fluid volume status.[56] Fetal stress may be noted with a mean arterial pressure of less than 106 mmHg, and fetal heart rate variability may be diminished as cerebral autoregulation is decreased and cerebral volume increased.[56]

Anticonvulsant agents are administered for the prevention or control of eclamptic seizures. They are administered when a patient has increased central nervous system responses. Agents include magnesium sulfate ($MgSO_4$) and phenytoin. Magnesium sulfate is a first-line agent for the prevention or treatment of eclamptic seizures. Though not an antihypertensive agent, it does relax smooth muscle and, therefore, may be associated with a transient decrease in maternal blood pressure. Magnesium sulfate reduces the amount of acetylcholine at the synaptic junction, causing a decrease in the number of impulses carried through the neuromuscular junction. Magnesium sulfate has not been shown to affect fetal heart rate variability significantly.[57–59]

Phenytoin has been used as an anticonvulsant agent for a number of years in patients with neurologic seizures. It acts by blocking the spread of electrical activity at the neuronal membrane and preventing posttetanic potentiation, thereby preventing the seizure focus from traveling through the central nervous system.[60] It is currently under investigation for use in preeclampsia and eclampsia. Studies have indicated that the dosage is dependent on patient weight and that larger doses may be needed during pregnancy because of the increased intravascular volume.[60–62] Such dependency on intravascular volume for dosage might be misleading for the preeclamptic patient with a decreased intravascular volume and renal clearance.

Low-dose aspirin therapy has been used prophylactically to prevent proteinuric hypertension in patients at risk for preeclampsia.[63,64] Low-dose aspirin decreases the amount of thromboxane, a potent vasoconstrictor produced by platelets which leads to platelet aggregation. Prostacyclin, a potent vasodilator produced by the endothelium, inhibits platelet aggregation. The ratio of thromboxane to prostacyclin is affected by low-dose aspirin. Questions remain whether low-dose aspirin administered on a daily basis is associated with an increase in maternal or perinatal bleeding problems.

Assessment

Initial clinical assessment of the intrapartum patient with hypertension begins with a thorough history. The patient's chief complaint should be determined and documented. History of her present hypertensive disorder should be elicited, and the patient should be questioned regarding presence of symptoms such as headache, vision changes, shortness of breath, chest pain, or epigastric tenderness. Past medical history should also be reviewed including presence of associated collagen vascular disorders, previous hospitalizations, and treatment modalities. Family history should be evaluated including presence of disorders related to the cardiovascular system.

General physical assessment involves use of inspection, palpation, percussion, and auscultation to determine the presence or absence of signs and symptoms associated with hypertension during pregnancy. (See "Protocol for the Nursing Management of the Patient with Pregnancy-Induced Hypertension," page 289.) Other noninvasive assessment parameters include level of consciousness, blood pressure, hemoglobin oxygen saturation, electrocardiographic findings, and urine output. Invasive hemodynamic monitoring may be indicated for selected patients with severe PIH such as those with refractory hypertension, oliguria unresponsive to intravenous fluid challenge, or pulmonary edema. Nurses caring for such patients are responsible for gathering and preparing equipment, assisting the physician during insertion, and patient support. It is also necessary for nurses to thoroughly understand the principles of hemodynamic monitoring in order to interpret patient data and plan care and initiate appropriate interventions. (See Chapter 11, pages 197–201, for a discussion of invasive hemodynamic monitoring.)

Following initial history and physical assessment, laboratory tests may include hemoglobin, hematocrit, blood urea nitrogen, serum creatinine, and uric acid levels; peripheral smear; and liver function tests.

Hypertension during pregnancy is considered a high-risk condition and, therefore, encompasses all of the special psychosocial problems discussed previously (see Chapter 4). In addition, fear, anxiety, and pain associated with labor and delivery may further compromise maternal status. Psychosocial assessment should include evaluation of maternal anxiety level and availability of support resources.

Nursing Diagnoses

Nursing diagnoses specific to patients with hypertension are generally physiologic problems, complications of hypertension, and knowledge deficits. Selected diagnoses include the following:

- Alteration in multisystem tissue perfusion, decreased, related to:
    Altered arterial pressure
    Cyclic vasospasm
    Cerebral edema and/or hemorrhage
- Potential for pulmonary edema related to:
    Increased afterload
    Pulmonary vascular endothelial damage
    Decreased colloid osmotic pressure
- Potential for impaired gas exchange related to:
    Decreased central nervous system function
    Ventilation/perfusion imbalance
    Pulmonary edema
- Potential for alteration in cardiac output, decreased, related to:
    Increased afterload
    Excessive antihypertensive therapy
    Ventricular dysfunction
- Potential for infection related to:
    Hospital environment
    Invasive hemodynamic monitoring
- Potential for placental abruption related to:
    Vasospasm
    Decreased uteroplacental perfusion
- Altered comfort level and anxiety
- Potential for fetal hypoxia

Theoretical Basis for the Plan of Nursing Care and Intervention

Thorough nursing assessment of the intrapartum patient with hypertension is particularly important as the patient and her fetus are at risk for significant multisystem compromise. Initial assessment includes evaluation of the patient's general appearance and vital signs. The presence or absence of symptoms of PIH should be determined and documented, followed by system-specific assessment.

Neurologic assessment should include evidence of alterations in central nervous system function. Postictal patients or those with cerebral edema may have alterations in level of consciousness. Should seizures occur, documentation should include time of onset, associated symptoms, and duration. Magnesium sulfate is administered to prevent or control eclamptic seizures. During $MgSO_4$

infusion, the patient should be carefully monitored for signs of toxicity such as decreased respiratory rate, absence of deep tendon reflexes, and decreased muscle strength. Toxicity is treated with intravenous administration of calcium gluconate.

Pulmonary assessment should include frequent auscultation of breath sounds and evaluation for evidence of pulmonary edema. Signs and symptoms include presence of a cough, distended jugular veins, tachypnea, tachycardia, orthopnea, decreased arterial hemoglobin oxygen saturation, and anxiety. Invasive hemodynamic monitoring is utilized in the patient with respiratory distress, and evaluation of systemic vascular resistance, pulmonary capillary wedge pressure, and cardiac output determine immediate interventions.

Assessment of the adequacy of cardiac output to meet the demands of pregnancy, labor, and delivery is especially important. In addition to noninvasive evaluation, invasive hemodynamic monitoring via pulmonary artery catheterization may be indicated. Electrocardiographic monitoring may also be utilized, especially if other evidence of cardiovascular compromise is present.

Renal function may be assessed via evaluation of hourly intake and urinary output. Those patients receiving $MgSO_4$ should have an indwelling urinary catheter inserted to facilitate more accurate assessment. All intravenous fluid should be regulated by an infusion pump. Urinary output that is less than 30 cc/hour should be reported to the patient's physician. Renal damage may be manifested by the inability to concentrate urine. Qualitative urine assessment should include assessment for proteinuria or hematuria.

Expected Outcomes

During the intrapartum period, the patient with a hypertensive disorder will do the following:

1. Maintain adequate cardiac output
2. Maintain optimal hemodynamic parameters
3. Maintain adequate gas exchange and tissue perfusion
4. Exhibit no signs or symptoms of infection
5. Maintain reassuring fetal heart rate responses

References

1. Anderson GD, Sibai BM: in Gabbe SG, Niebyl JR, Simpson JL (eds.): *Obstetrics: Normal and Problem Pregnancies*. New York, Churchill Livingstone, 1986, pp. 819–863.
2. Gant NF, Pritchard JA: in Eden RD, Boehm FH (eds.): *Assessment and Care of the Fetus*. Norwalk, CT, Appleton & Lange, 1990, pp. 711–723.
3. American College of Obstetricians and Gynecologists: Management of preeclampsia. *ACOG Tech Bull* Feb. 91:1–5, 1986.

4. Chesley LC: Diagnosis of preeclampsia. *Obstet Gynecol* 65:423, 1985.

5. Chesley LC: *Hypertensive Disorders in Pregnancy.* New York, Appleton-Century-Crofts, 1978.

6. Weinstein L: The HELLP syndrome: A severe consequence of hypertension in pregnancy. J Perinatol 6:316, 1982.

7. VanDam P, Reener M, Baekelandt M: Disseminated intravascular coagulation and the syndrome of hemolysis, elevated liver enzymes and low platelets in severe preeclampsia. *Obstet Gynecol* 73:97, 1989.

8. Moodley J, Pillay M: The HELLP syndrome in severe hypertensive crisis of pregnancy: Does it exist? *S Afr Med J* 67:246, 1985.

9. Thiagarajah S, Bourgeosis FJ, Harbert GM: Thrombocytopenia in preeclampsia: Associated abnormalities and management principles. *Am J Obstet Gynecol* 150:1, 1984.

10. Sibai BM, Spinnato JA, Watson DL, et al: Pregnancy outcome in 303 cases with severe preeclampsia. *Obstet Gynecol* 64:319, 1984.

11. Abdella TN, Sibai BM, Hays JM, et al: Relationship of hypertensive disease to abruptio placentae. *Obstet Gynecol* 63:365, 1984.

12. Cunningham F, MacDonald P, Gant N: *Williams' Obstetrics.* Norwalk, CT, Appleton & Lange, 1989.

13. Sibai B, Taslimi M, El-Naser A: Maternal-perinatal outcome associated with the syndrome of hemolysis, elevated liver enzymes, and low platelets in severe preeclampsia–eclampsia. *Am J Obstet Gynecol* 155:501, 1986.

14. Chesley L (ed.): *Hypertensive Disorders in pregnancy.* New York, Appleton-Century-Crofts, 1978.

15. Chesley L, Cooper D: Genetics of hypertension in pregnancy: Possible single gene control of preeclampsia and eclampsia in the descendants of eclamptic women. *Br J Obstet Gynaecol* 155:501, 1986.

16. Kilpatrick D, Gibson F, Liston W, et al: Association between susceptibility to pre-eclampsia within families and HLA DRA. *Lancet* 11:1063, 1989.

17. Williams J: *Obstetrics.* New York: D. Appleton & Company, 1908.

18. Belizan J, Villar J: The relationship between calcium intake and edema-proteinuria and hypertension-gestosis. *Am J Clin Nutr* 33:2202, 1980.

19. Belizan J, Villar J, Repik J: The relationship between calcium intake and pregnancy-induced hypertension: Up-to-date evidence. *Am J Obstet Gynecol* 158:898, 1988.

20. Lopez-Jaramillo P, Navarez M, Weiger R, et al: Calcium supplementation reduces the risk of pregnancy-induced hypertension in an Andes population. *Br J Obstet Gynaecol* 96:96, 1989.

21. Walsh S: Preeclampsia: An imbalance in placental prostacyclin and thromboxane production. *Am J Ostet Gynecol* 152:335, 1985.

22. Gant N, Daley G, Chand S, et al: A study of angiotensin II pressor response throughout primigravid pregnancy. *J Clin Invest* 52:2682, 1973.

23. Pritchard J: in Hypertensive disorders of pregnancy, 17th ed. Pritchard J, MacDonald P, Gant N (eds.): *Williams' Obstetrics.* Norwalk, CT, Appleton-Century-Crofts, 1985, pp. 525–560.

24. Zuspan F: Chronic hypertension in pregnancy. *Clin Obstet Gynecol* 27:854–873, 1984.

25. Coustan D, Plotz R: The laboratory in diseases associated with pregnancy. *Laboratory Medicine in Clinical Practice,* H. Mandell (ed.). Philadelphia, John Unger Publishing, Inc. 1983.

26. Burrows R, Hunter D, Andrew M, et al: A prospective study investigating the mechanism of thrombocytopenia in preeclampsia. *Obstet Gynecol* 70:334–338, 1987.

27. Pritchard J, MacDonald P, Gant N: Medical and surgical illnesses during pregnancy and the puerperium in Pritchard J, MacDonald P, Gant N (eds.): *Williams' Obstetrics.* Norwalk, CT, Appleton-Century-Crofts, 1985, pp. 561–640.

28. McCarthy E, Pollak V: Maternal renal disease. *Clin Perinatol* 8:307–319, 1981.

29. Gabert H, Miller J: Renal disease in pregnancy. *Obstet Gynecol Surv* 40:449–460, 1985.

30. Arias F, Maricella-Jiminez R: Hepatic fibrinogen deposits in preeclampsia: Immunofluorescent evidence. *N Eng J Med* 295:578–582, 1976.

31. Easterling T, Benedetti T: Preeclampsia: A hyperdynamic disease model. *Am J Obstet Gynecol* 160:1447, 1989.

32. Lee W, Gonik B, Cotton D: Urinary diagnostic indices in preeclampsia-associated oliguria: Correlation with invasive hemodynamic monitoring. *Am J Obstet Gynecol* 156:100–103, 1987.)

33. Sibai B, Villar M, Mabie B: Acute renal failure in hypertensive disorders of pregnancy. *Am J Obstet Gynecol* 162:777–783, 1990.

34. Clark S, Greenspoon J, Aldahl D: Severe preeclampsia with persistant oliguria: Management of hemodynamic subsets. *Am J Obstet Gynecol* 154:490–494, 1986.

35. Moise K, Cotton D: The use of colloid osmotic pressure in pregnancy. *Clin Perinatol* 13:827–842, 1986.

36. Benedetti T, Carlson R: Studies of colloid osmotic pressure in pregnancy-induced hypertension. *Am J Obstet Gynecol* 135:308, 1978.

37. Gonik B, Cotton D, Spellman T, et al: Peripartum colloid osmotic pressure changes: Effects of controlled fluid management. *Am J Obstet Gynecol* 151:812–815, 1985.

38. Starling EH: On the absorption of fluids from the connective tissue spaces. *J Physiol* 19:312, 1896.

39. Benedetti T, Quilligan E: Cerebral edema in severe pregnancy induced hypertension. *Am J Obstet Gynecol* 137:860, 1980.

40. Benedetti T, Cotton D, Read J, et al: Hemodynamic observations in severe preeclampsia with a flow directed pulmonary artery catheter. *Am J Obstet Gynecol* 136:465, 1980.

41. Rafferty T, Berkowitz R: Hemodynamics in patients with severe toxemia during labor and delivery. *Am J Obstet Gynecol* 138:263, 1980.

42. Phelan J, Yurth D: Severe preeclampsia. I: Peripartum hemodynamic observations. *Am J Obstet Gynecol* 144:17, 1982.

43. Hankins G, Wendel G, Cunningham G, et al: Longitudinal evaluation of hemodynamic changes in eclampsia. *Am J Obstet Gynecol* 150:506, 1984.

44. Benedetti T, Kates K, Williams V: Hemodynamic observations in severe preeclampsia complicated by pulmonary edema. *Am J Obstet Gynecol* 152:330, 1985.

45. Wasserstrum N, Cotton D: Hemodynamic monitoring in severe pregnancy-induced hypertension. *Clin Perinatol* 13:781, 1986.

46. Henderson D, Vilos G, Milne K, et al: The role of Swan–Ganz catheterization in severe pregnancy-induced hypertension. *Am J Obstet Gynecol* 148:570, 1984.

47. Clark S, Cotton D: Usual indications for pulmonary artery catheterization in the patient with severe preeclampsia. *Am J Obstet Gynecol* 158:453, 1988.

48. Cotton D, Gonik B, Dorman K, et al: Cardiovascular alterations in severe pregnancy induced hypertension: Relationship of central venous pressure to pulmonary capillary wedge pressure. *Am J Obstet Gynecol* 151:762, 1985.

49. Cotton D, Lee W, Huhta J, et al: Hemodynamic profile of severe pregnancy-induced hypertension. *Am J Obstet Gynecol* 158:523, 1988.

50. Brosens I, Roberts MW, Dixon H: The role of spiral arteries in the pathogenesis of preeclampsia. *Obstet Gynecol* 1:177, 1972.

51. Cotton D, Gonik B, Dorman K: Cardiovascular alterations in severe pregnancy-induced hypertension seen with an intravenously given hydralazine bolus. *Surg Gynecol Obstet* 161:240, 1985.

52. Doany W, Brinkman C: Antihypertensive drugs in pregnancy. *Clin Perinatol* 14:783, 1987.

53. Mabie W, Gonzalez A, Sibai B, et al: A comparative trial of labetolol and hydralazine in the acute management of severe hypertension complicating pregnancy. *Obstet Gynecol* 70:328, 1987.

54. Berkowitz D, Coustan D, Moyoshiko T (eds.): *Handbook of Drugs in Pregnancy.* Toronto, Churchill Livingstone, 1986.

55. Neuman T, Weiss B, Rabello Y, et al: Diazoxide for the acute control of severe hypertension complicating pregnancy: A pilot study. *Obstet Gynecol* 53:50S, 1979.

56. Cotton D, Longmire S, Jones M, et al: Cardiovascular alterations in severe pregnancy induced hypertension: Effects of intravenous nitroglycerin coupled with blood volume expansion. *Am J Obstet Gynecol* 154:1053, 1986.

57. Flowers C: Magnesium sulfate in obstetrics. *Am J Obstet Gynecol* 91:763, 1965.

58. Stone S, Pritchard J: Effect of maternally administered magnesium sulfate on the neonate. *Obstet Gynecol* 137:574, 1970.

59. Stallworth J, Yeh S, Petrie R: The effect of magnesium sulfate on fetal heart rate variability and uterine activity. *Am J Obstet Gynecol* 140:702, 1981.

60. Ryan G, Lange I, Navgler M: Clinical experience with phenytoin prophylaxis in severe preeclampsia. *Am J Obstet Gynecol* 161:1297, 1989.

61. Appleton M, Kuehl T, Raebel M, et al: Magnesium sulfate vs. phenytoin in pregnancy induced hypertension—preliminary report. *Am J Obstet Gynecol* (Supplement) 164:273, 1991.
62. Freidman S, Lim K, Baker B, et al: A comparison of phenytoin infusion vs. magnesium sulfate infusion in preeclampsia. Society of Perinatal Obstetricians' Annual Meeting. Houston, TX, 1990.
63. Sibai B, Mirro R, Chesney C: Low-dose aspirin in pregnancy. *Obstet Gynecol* 74:551, 1989.
64. Wallenburg H, Dekker G, Makovitz J, et al: Effect of low-dose aspirin on vascular refractoriness in angiotensin-sensitive primigravid women. *Am J Obstet Gynecol* 164:1169, 1991.

10

Diabetes Mellitus in Pregnancy

Lisa K. Mandeville

Supportive Data

Incidence

In 1989 the Centers for Disease Control estimated there were approximately 6 million persons in the United States with diabetes mellitus and 500,000 new cases are diagnosed each year.[1] In 1987 the national health cost for care of patients with diabetes was $20.4 billion.[1] Type I (insulin-dependent) and type II (non-insulin dependent) diabetes were estimated to affect 0.3% of all pregnant women in 1986.[2] Each year 15,000 infants are born to women with diabetes mellitus.[1]

Type I accounts for 5% to 10% of all persons with diabetes but has a prevalence peak of diagnosis at 11 to 15 years.[3] The larger group with type II diabetes has a peak of diagnosis at 51 to 55 years of age. Thus, even though there are more people with type II diabetes than there are with type I, pregnant women are more likely to have type I diabetes.

Type I diabetes is characterized by a lack of adequate insulin production with loss of pancreatic beta cells. The type I patient requires diet therapy and exogenous insulin to control blood glucose. Those with type II diabetes generally have normal numbers of insulin-producing beta cells but exhibit a failure of appropriate release (often delayed) and abnormal response at the tissue level to insulin. Thus, insulin release may or may not be normal but appropriate reactions in peripheral tissues do not occur. The person with type II diabetes generally responds well to diet therapy and may even improve blood glucose control with exercise and weight reduction if obese.

Gestational diabetes is defined as abnormal carbohydrate metabolism first diagnosed during pregnancy. Women with gestational diabetes usually require

TABLE 10-1
Diabetes in Pregnancy Classification

Class	Age at Onset	Duration	Vasculopathy
A*(Gestational)	During Pregnancy	Variable	None
B**	>20 Years old	<10 Years	None
C**	<20 Years old	10–19 Years	None
D**	<10 Years old	>20 Years	None
F**	Any	Variable	Diabetic nephropathy
H**	Any	Variable	Cardiomyopathy
R**	Any	Variable	Proliferative retinopathy

*May or may not require insulin.
**Insulin dependent.

treatment with diet therapy alone but occasionally may need insulin administration to control hyperglycemia. Although rare, the patient may have had preexisting but undiagnosed diabetes (either type I or II) prior to conception. Gestational diabetes occurs 10 times more frequently than overt type I or type II diabetes and affects 2% to 3% of all pregnancies.[2]

In 1949 Priscilla White developed a classification scheme for diabetes in pregnancy for the purpose of identifying risk categories.[4] The system was revised in 1978 and is still used today for descriptive as well as prescriptive purposes (see Table 10-1).[5]

Significance

Both mother and baby are at increased risk of morbidity when diabetes is present. Maternal morbidity is increased among women with types I and II but probably not for those with gestational diabetes when compared with the diabetes-free population. Treatment goals during pregnancy include achievement and maintenance of euglycemia, which places the patient with diabetes at risk for hypoglycemia. Insulin reactions or hypoglycemia occur variably from one individual to the next but are estimated to occur once each week for those receiving conventional insulin management; it is estimated as twice each week among patients receiving intensified insulin therapy such as with those during pregnancy.[6] Insulin reactions account for 4% of deaths among people having type I diabetes.[6] Further morbidity may be encountered as diabetic ketoacidosis (DKA) is increased among pregnant women with diabetes because of increased ketone body formation from fat breakdown. Even those with gestational diabetes may be at risk for DKA during beta agonist therapy for preterm labor as a result of the hyperglycemic effects of this drug. Its overall incidence during pregnancy is 9.3%.[4] Infectious processes such as urinary tract and upper respiratory infections predispose the pregnant woman to DKA. There is a significant risk for perinatal mortality during an acute episode of DKA, thereby making prevention an important management goal.

The progression of diabetic-related vasculopathies during pregnancy has been well established. Once thought to affect only severe proliferative retinopathy, pregnancy is now known to potentially advance even milder forms of background retinopathy, although the reasons for this increase are not known.[7,8] Although pregnancy-induced hypertension traditionally has been said to be increased among all people with diabetes, it is not more likely to occur among those with gestational, class B, or class C diabetes. The incidence does seem to be increased, however, in classes D, F, and R.[9] There is evidence to suggest that hypertension may be worsening of preexisting nephrotic syndrome, the symptoms of which are similar to pregnancy-induced hypertension.[10] If diabetic nephropathy is accompanied by hypertension or renal insufficiency, early delivery may be indicated as with pregnancy-induced hypertension; this results in a preterm birth which leads to further perinatal morbidity.

Maternal mortality among pregnant women with types I and II diabetes is increased tenfold over the general population, although this estimate may not be representative of an increase over the rate expected of a nonpregnant population with diabetes of the same age group. Maternal mortality for pregnant women with diabetes is estimated as 0.115% or 115 per 100,000 women.[11]

Fetal and neonatal morbidity and mortality are increased among infants of diabetic mothers (IDM) when compared with the general population. Historic trends reveal a decrease in overall perinatal mortality from 20% as recently as 1969 to a current estimate of 5%.[12] This decrease can be attributed to improvements in antepartum care, including better methods of maintaining euglycemia and enhanced fetal surveillance, and advances in neonatal health care. Intra-uterine fetal demise continues to occur more frequently among women with diabetes, although the cause is usually unknown. Congenital anomalies are increased among IDM and occur in 6% to 8% of all pregnant women with diabetes. These anomalies have been attributed to a hyperglycemic state at the time of fetal organogenesis. It is widely purported that achievement and maintenance of euglycemia among people having types I and II diabetes prior to conception and during the first 6 weeks of gestation can reduce the incidence of congenital anomalies among IDM to rates approaching the 2% to 3% incidence observed among the general population and those with gestational diabetes.[13–17]

Fetal macrosomia is a common complication of types I and II diabetes, as well as gestational diabetes, and may lead to shoulder dystocia and potential injury at birth. Thus, cesarean delivery may be indicated when estimated fetal size is excessive. Controversy exists as to any absolute maximum weight necessitating operative delivery, but it is generally considered when estimates are over 4000 g. Of course, reliability of ultrasound measurements and maternal clinical status will play a role in this decision.

Despite attempts to normalize blood glucose in the antepartum and even intrapartum periods, neonatal hypoglycemia still occurs in 15% of IDM.[18] Past theories, which suggest that fetal hyperglycemia during the third trimester and the intrapartum period leads to fetal hyperinsulinemia and subsequent hypoglycemia at birth when maternal glucose supplies are withdrawn, may not totally explain this phenomenon. The fetal pancreas is responsive to glucose prior to 20 weeks gestation and may establish insulin production at that time.[19] Later attempts to correct maternal hyperglycemia might then fail to eliminate neonatal hyperinsulinemia and subsequent hypoglycemia at birth. Other metabolic derangements are more frequently seen among IDM, such as polycythemia presumably due to diminished intravascular volume secondary to fetal hyperglycemia. Hyperbilirubinemia may also occur more often as the excess red blood cells are broken down. Less common but also recognized is an increased incidence of hypocalcemia due to fetal hyperglycemia.

The phenomenon of delayed fetal lung maturation is clearly recognized among IDM although its cause is unknown. Although not at increased risk of spontaneous preterm labor by virtue of their diabetes, these patients are at greater risk for an indicated early delivery if antepartum testing results indicate fetal compromise. Both respiratory distress syndrome and hyaline membrane disease occur more frequently at later gestational ages than are observed among infants of nondiabetic mothers.

Etiology

The cause of type I diabetes, characterized by loss of pancreatic beta cells, remains unknown. Etiologic speculation has included inheritance, autoimmune response, and viral causes and may, in fact, be multifactorial. A study of twins revealed that only 50% of monozygotic twins are concordant for type I diabetes, suggesting that there is a familial tendency.[20] Interestingly, the same study revealed 90% of twins with type II diabetes were concordant for the disease, supporting the commonly held theory that type II diabetes has a stronger familial etiologic pattern than does type I. Viral infections such as Coxsackie virus, mumps, and congenital rubella have been associated with the development of type I diabetes but probably occur in genetically susceptible individuals only.[21] The bulk of evidence suggests that type I diabetes is associated with certain human leukocyte system A antigens that are found on the short arm of chromosome 6. Depending on which antigen is present, the risk for type I diabetes can be increased from two- to fortyfold.[22]

The etiology of type II diabetes also remains elusive, although it has been suggested that inheritance occurs as a dominant trait.[23] Obesity also plays some causative or possibly additive role occurring in 80% of type II patients.[24]

Insulin antagonism caused by the placental hormones, human placental lactogen, progesterone, cortisol, and prolactin, leads to gestational diabetes. As greater amounts of lactogen, in particular, are produced with advancing gestation, the "diabetogenic" effect of pregnancy becomes more pronounced, reaching significant levels around 26 weeks.[25] Yet all pregnant women do not experience this disorder. Some women with gestational diabetes may have human leukocyte system A antigens similar to those with type I diabetes.[26] Additionally, women with gestational diabetes are at risk for later development of type I and, even more commonly, type II diabetes. Thus, gestational diabetes may be the expression of pregnancy-induced stresses on carbohydrate metabolism in the immunogenetically predisposed patient. Risk factors for gestational diabetes include maternal age greater than 30 years and obesity, both factors associated with type II diabetes.

Framework for Accepted Therapy

Provision of acute or intrapartum nursing care for the patient with diabetes requires a working knowledge of the disease process and management methods. Labor and delivery do not occur as isolated events but are part of a natural progression, and continued care of diabetes must occur. The nurse integrates intrapartum care within the larger framework of care of the patient with diabetes. Similarly, other indications for admission to labor and delivery such as diabetic ketoacidosis should be regarded as an interim within the patient's total care. Physiology of diabetes and pregnancy is discussed as are general management principles appropriate for long-term self-care, intrapartum management, or acute care for other problems.

In individuals who do not have diabetes, blood glucose levels are normally maintained between 60 and 110 mg/dl of blood through the actions of glucagon and insulin. Both hormones are secreted by pancreatic islet cells: A cells secrete glucagon and B cells secrete insulin. The catabolic (energy-releasing) hormone glucagon functions to free glucose, while insulin, an anabolic (energy-requiring) hormone, actively transports glucose across cell membranes for use as an essential fuel source. Insulin also acts to cause storage of glucose and protein and to increase fat formation.

Insulin is synthesized in the endoplasmic reticulum and stored in granules in the B cells. On stimulation, the granules move to the cell membrane and are released by exocytosis. Those with type I diabetes exhibit decreased insulin release, and most have a complete absence of B cells. Type II diabetes has traditionally been attributed to insulin resistance, thus, although normal or even elevated insulin levels are present, hyperglycemia still occurs.

Normal individuals exhibit a state of hyperinsulinemia in very early pregnancy. Progesterone and estrogen work in concert to stimulate B cells and increase insulin production, thus decreased circulating glucose levels and increased fat deposition occur. As pregnancy progresses, the placental hormones (*i.e.,* human placental lactogen, progesterone, cortisol, and prolactin) act to antagonize insulin. The net result is enhanced storage during the fed state and enhanced metabolism during the fasting state.

In early pregnancy, women with type I diabetes usually require no increase and sometimes a decrease in their insulin dose. Women with type II diabetes may often continue with diet therapy alone. There is a small subgroup of patients treated with oral antihyperglycemics prior to pregnancy. Once pregnancy is diagnosed, the medication is discontinued and insulin therapy started. Gestational diabetes is rarely manifest in early pregnancy, but if occurring, preexisting type I or type II diabetes is suspected.

As pregnancy continues and placental mass increases, a corresponding increase in placental hormone production is seen, which results in elevated blood glucose levels. Increased insulin dosages are required to achieve euglycemia in women with type I diabetes, and insulin therapy may be required for women with type II or gestational diabetes despite careful attention to diet. The goals for patient management include screening for gestational diabetes among the general population; achievement and maintenance of euglycemia for all those with type I, type II, and gestational diabetes; and screening for maternal and neonatal complications.

Since 1980 the International Workshop-Conference on Gestational Diabetes has recommended universal screening for gestational diabetes.[27] This conference was sponsored jointly by the American Diabetes Association, the American College of Obstetricians and Gynecologists, the National Institutes of Health, and the Centers for Disease Control. Screening consists of a blood glucose level obtained 1 hour after ingestion of a 50-g oral glucose load. The screen can be done without regard to time of day or last oral intake.[28] Different centers may use varying maximal cutoffs for determining a positive screen. The 1986 ACOG Technical Bulletin recommended a plasma threshold of 140 mg/dl, although 135 mg/dl may also be used.[29,30] If the screen is positive, a 3-hour oral glucose tolerance test is ordered. Patients should be placed on a 3-day carbohydrate loading diet prior to the test. A fasting blood glucose level is drawn and then a 100-g oral glucose solution ingested. Blood glucose determinations are then drawn at 1, 2, and 3 hours. To constitute a positive test, two or more values must meet or exceed the maximal values established by the National Diabetes Data Group (see Table 10-2).[31]

Derangements of carbohydrate metabolism are the probable cause of the maternal and fetal complications seen with diabetes mellitus. Hyperglycemia during the critical period of early organ formation has been linked to the development of congenital anomalies among IDM.[13–17] Thus, high blood glucose levels in the first 7 weeks of pregnancy should be avoided. Many women with diabetes do not plan their pregnancies and, therefore, progress through the early weeks unaware of pregnancy, sometimes after a malformation has already occurred. Control of blood glucose level should still be attempted to avoid other fetal/neonatal complications such as macrosomia, intrauterine fetal demise, and neonatal metabolic abnormalities. In addition, careful attention to blood glucose normalization may assist in the prevention of maternal complications such as symptomatic hypoglycemia, which may lead to accidents and trauma. Diabetic ketoacidosis is an essentially preventable complication of pregnancy and it occurs most often when the patient has an upper respiratory or urinary tract infection. It can be life-threatening to mother and fetus and thus rigorous treatment of all infections and careful urine screening for ketones are advocated. The

TABLE 10-2
Criteria for Gestational Diabetes

	Venous Plasma	Whole Blood
Fasting	105	90
1 Hour	190	170
2 Hours	165	145
3 Hours	145	125

patient with euglycemia because of a stable blood glucose level may be better able to forestall DKA as blood glucose will be easier to control during times of infection than will the patient whose baseline glucose is erratic or high. Certainly, patients frequently monitoring their own blood glucose levels and checking for ketonuria will detect rising blood glucose and ketones earlier and may be able to seek treatment to prevent DKA.

Screening for fetal/neonatal complications includes routine maternal serum alpha fetoprotein levels to assess risk for neural tube defects and ultrasound to rule out fetal structural anomalies. Ultrasound may also identify the macrosomic infant and can detect the presence of hydramnios, which is associated with maternal diabetes mellitus. It is important to note that macrosomia and hydramnios often may occur when only gestational diabetes is present. Hydramnios is thought to be a result of excessive fetal urination because of fetal hyperglycemia. Genetic studies are usually not offered as IDMs are not at risk for chromosomal abnormalities by virtue of diabetes. Only when other indications are present (*e.g.,* maternal age ≥35 years) are genetic counseling and discussion of genetic testing indicated.

Because of the risk of unexplained intrauterine fetal demise, antepartum testing is recommended during the third trimester. The nonstress test is recommended for this purpose and should be given at 30 weeks gestation.[29] There is no consensus regarding the ideal form of antepartum testing, thus the nonstress test, contraction stress test, and biophysical profile are all used. It is, however, important to remember that although once- or twice-weekly testing may be adequate for the stable patient, the unstable patient may require more intensive monitoring (*i.e.,* daily or more frequent intervals).

The increased incidence of immature fetal lungs at greater gestational ages may predispose IDMs to hyaline membrane disease and respiratory distress syndrome even when delivered near term. Thus, lung maturity studies are frequently performed prior to delivery. Amniocentesis is performed, and the fluid is tested for lecithin-to-sphingomyelin ratios and presence or absence of phosphatidylglycerol.

Screening for maternal complications includes careful attention to blood glucose levels as well as to the presence or progression of diabetic vasculopathies. Blood glucose target values should be established for each patient. Recommended goals as promulgated by the American College of Obstetricians and Gynecologists are listed in Table 10-3.[29] For some patients these goals may be unrealistic. As many as 22% of those with diabetes may have hypoglycemia unawareness, a condition that involves the loss of normal hypoglycemic warning signs (*i.e.,* shaking, sweating, and dizziness).[6] For these patients severe hypoglycemia develops before the individual recognizes the problem, and they are therefore unable to treat it. Thus, target blood glucose levels may need to be raised with these patients to prevent frequent hypoglycemic episodes. Screening for hypoglycemia is therefore accomplished by careful review of the patient's blood glucose levels and discussion of low values. Questions regarding the presence of hypoglycemic symptoms, the dietary pattern (*i.e.,* timing and con-

TABLE 10-3
Goals for Glycemic Control for Pregnant Women with Diabetes[29]

	Fasting	*Before Other Meals*	*Postmeal*	*2–6* AM
Type I and Type II	60–90 mg/dl	60–105 mg/dl	120 mg/dl	60–90 mg/dl
Gestational diabetes	105 mg/dl			120 mg/dl

tent), and treatment of hypoglycemia should be asked, and all episodes of hypoglycemia explained.

Diabetic ketoacidosis is generally avoided with careful control of blood glucose levels and aggressive treatment of all infections, but screening for it involves urine testing for ketones. All patients should check each morning's first voided specimen for ketones and should upgrade testing when infected. Sometimes testing three or four times a day will be advised, especially when blood glucose values are elevated.

Pregnant women with diabetes are screened for vasculopathies including retinopathy and nephropathy. Retinopathy is a complication of diabetes whereby the eye develops lesions as a result of abnormal blood vessels. The cause is unknown, but this disorder accounts for the increased risk of blindness in those with diabetes. Retinopathy is divided into two categories: background nonproliferative retinopathy and the more severe proliferative diabetic retinopathy. Fundus photos should be taken by an ophthalmic photographer and read by a qualified ophthalmologist or retinologist during pregnancy. When diagnosed during pregnancy, proliferative retinopathy is treated with laser panretinal photocoagulation. Control of maternal hypertension is generally advised to prevent further damage to blood vessels in the eye.

Women with diabetic nephropathy are at risk for progression of renal decompensation as well as perinatal risks such as intrauterine fetal demise, neonatal death, and intrauterine growth retardation. The acceleration of nephropathy to nephrotic syndrome seen in the late trimester may have traditionally been diagnosed as pregnancy-induced hypertension, as symptoms and laboratory values are similar. Patients who have had diabetes for 10 years or longer or who have proteinuria are at risk for nephropathy and are screened during pregnancy. Proteinuria and hypertension generally increase during gestation. The reasons for increased proteinuria are not known, but reversion to prepregnancy levels are seen after delivery.[32] Screening is accomplished in the first trimester via creatinine clearance and 24-hour total urine protein level. Creatinine clearance is designated as normal (≥90 ml/minute), moderately reduced (60 to 89 ml/minute), and severely reduced (<60 ml/minute).[33] The presence of 300 to 500 mg of protein in a 24-hour urine sample is diagnostic of diabetic nephropathy during pregnancy.[34] Once detected, the patient is observed for worsening nephrotic syndrome or superimposed pregnancy-induced hypertension (*i.e.*, elevated uric acid). Bed rest is advised for the nephrotic patient beginning in the second trimester to increase renal as well as uterine blood flow. Ultrasound and early antepartum testing are indicated to screen for intrauterine growth retardation and uteroplacental insufficiency. Early delivery may become necessary if renal function deteriorates, thus patients with nephropathy are counseled about preterm delivery.

Methods for achievement and maintenance of euglycemia for pregnant women with diabetes involve self-care practices. Patients must monitor blood glucose levels, administer insulin, and maintain an appropriate diet. For some patients regular, planned exercise may also be helpful.

The Consensus Development Conference on Self-Monitoring of Blood Glucose recommended that pregnant women with diabetes monitor their own blood glucose levels.[35] Modern management of pregnancy complicated by type I diabetes mandates this practice. Patients generally check blood glucose levels prior to meals and at bedtime every day. The use of a device designed to read oxidase reagent strips is most helpful. Patients should maintain careful and accurate records of blood glucose values and should especially document periods of hypoglycemia, noting time, symptoms, blood glucose level, and type and amount of treatment.

Once the pattern of blood glucose values is noted, insulin dose, dietary intake, and exercise periods are manipulated to obtain euglycemia without periods of hypoglycemia. Insulin is most often given as a mixture of NPH or lente and regular insulin in split-dose form (*i.e.,* morning and evening), but it may also be given as longer acting ultralente insulin (*i.e.,* either one or two injections each day) with regular at breakfast, lunch, and dinner. Insulins may be mixed in the same syringe but should be given within 5 minutes of mixing. Random rotation is no longer recommended as absorption rates differ within each area of the body. The following areas are in order of *decreasing* absorption: abdomen, arms, thighs, and buttocks.[36] Thus, patients are advised to restrict rotation to one area at a time (see Figure 10-1). Insulin should be administered 30 minutes before each meal.[36]

Pregnant women with diabetes should be regularly seen by a registered dietitian for prescription and dietary teaching. It is virtually impossible to expect patients to carefully and meticulously follow a diet plan without seeing a registered dietitian for assistance with problems, ongoing teaching, and motivation. The diet plan will also require changes as pregnancy progresses. Most patients find it difficult to eat large meals in late gestation and will require multiple small feedings to ensure adequate caloric intake. A diet planned for those with diabetes contains 50% carbohydrates, 30% fats, and 20% proteins. The meal plan should include three meals and a bedtime snack. Additional morning and evening snacks may be required. The pregnant woman requires about 300 calories per day more than she does when she is not pregnant to meet increased metabolic demands.[37] The normal adult with diabetes requires approximately 16.4 cal/lb/day. For the pregnant adolescent, the overweight adult, and the underweight adult, these requirements should be adjusted (see Table 10-4).

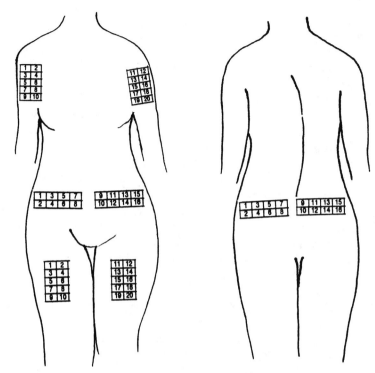

Figure 10-1. Method of restricted rotation for insulin self-administration. All insulin injection sites within one region (arms, abdomen, hips, and thighs) should be used before proceeding to the next region.

The role of exercise for pregnant women with diabetes remains unknown and controversial. Some regard diabetes as a relative contraindication to exercise.[38] Those with type I diabetes who are in poor control may exhibit a *rise* in blood glucose levels following exercise.[39] In well-controlled diabetes, symptomatic hypoglycemia may be a problem; therefore 15 g of glucose should be

TABLE 10-4
Recommended Caloric Intake for Pregnancy
Complicated by Diabetes

	Cal/lb/day	Total Weight Gain Goal
Adult (normal)	16.4	
Adolescent	20.5	30 lb
Underweight	22.7	30 lb
Obese	13.6	20 lb

taken before or 15 to 30 g after moderate exercise.[40] It has been suggested that exercise may be of the most benefit to those with well-controlled type I diabetes and to those with type II and gestational diabetes, although these women may be at slightly increased risk for preterm labor.[41] Women with diabetes who have hypoglycemia unawareness, diabetic vasculopathies, hypertension, or multiple gestation or who have not engaged in some form of physical exercise should not exercise during pregnancy.

Whether women with diabetes have spontaneous labor or have labor induced, the goals for care include maintenance of euglycemia and screening for complications. Often induction of labor is attempted as soon as mature lung indices are obtained to prevent the occurrence of unexplained intrauterine fetal demise. The nursing implications of induction of labor are then added (see Chapter 7).

A common plan of management includes withholding insulin and diet on the morning of induction. An intravenous line is started in the early morning and 5% dextrose solution administered at 125 cc/hour. Intravenous insulin is administered to maintain blood glucose levels at 60 to 110 mg/dl. Intravenous insulin is used because of its rapid half-life (3 minutes), making timely normalization and careful titration of blood glucose possible. Often, the well-controlled diabetic does not require insulin during labor. Thus, careful attention to blood glucose monitoring is important to determine the need for insulin and appropriate dosages. When cesarean section is planned, the morning insulin is withheld and intravenous insulin administered if necessary to maintain blood glucose levels at 60 to 110 mg/dl.

Assessment

The physical assessment specific to pregnant women with diabetes should include height, weight, and vital signs. Thyroid palpation is important as thyroid disorders are commonly associated with diabetes. Cardiac examination is also performed, with careful attention to the evaluation of pulses. Lower extremity pulses extending down to the ankle should be evaluated and documented. The feet must be carefully examined for lesions, ulcers, or ingrown toenails, which could lead to infection.

Patients are screened for diabetic neuropathy. Beginning symptoms include either a pattern of decreased foot sensation of pain or temperature or a pattern of foot pain and parasthesias. Once diabetic neuropathy is present, patients are at great risk for foot injury. They should be taught to check their shoes carefully for objects that they may not feel once their shoes are on, and they should examine their feet daily for lesions or injuries they cannot feel.

The skin is carefully examined especially over insulin injection sites. Bruising or hypertrophic areas are documented. Those with diabetes are at risk for delayed healing, and areas of lesions and injuries should be examined periodically.

The blood glucose levels is checked on admission. The most convenient method is by bedside blood glucose monitoring.[42] The usual patterns of glycemic control should be ascertained; this is most easily accomplished by a review of self-monitored blood glucose values. Patients may have a daily log of values they document or they may be documented in the prenatal record. These values should be reviewed, and the pattern established. Patients may exhibit normal values (see Table 10-3), or they may have frequent episodes of hypoglycemia. A pattern of erratic blood glucose values may be displayed, with wide swings between high and low numbers. Some patients remain very stable, but their overall pattern is high. This is fairly typical of those with uncontrolled type II or gestational diabetes. Even if no low numbers appear, the patient is questioned as to the occurrence of hypoglycemia. Some episodes may occur between testing times and may not be recorded. Other patients may have symptoms of hypoglycemia at "normal" blood glucose levels. The rate of fall of blood glucose can produce insulin reactions even when the absolute blood glucose value is normal. These episodes should be treated seriously and as though the patient had a low blood glucose value, as loss of consciousness and subsequent injury can occur.

Glycosylated hemoglobin, or HbA_{1c}, is a laboratory test that is loosely related to the glycemic control over the 4 to 8 weeks before determination. Glycosylation results from enzymatic bonding of glucose to hemoglobin A amino acids. The test is not reliable for screening for gestational diabetes or fine tune control, but is useful as an indicator of overall blood glucose control. When performed serially (*i.e.,* generally every 6 to 8 weeks), the trend of glycemic control may be determined.

The American Diabetes Association recommends the following laboratory tests be performed at initial evaluation for all those with diabetes.[43]

- Fasting blood glucose level
- HbA_{1c}
- Lipid profile (high-density lipoprotein cholesterol, low-density lipoprotein cholesterol, and triglycerides)
- Serum creatinine
- Urinalysis
- Urine culture
- Thyroid function tests (T_4 or thyroid-stimulating hormone)
- Electrocardiogram

These tests are generally included at the first prenatal visit along with routine prenatal laboratory evaluation, but may be ordered on admission to labor and delivery if they have not been previously obtained. Within the early prenatal period 24-hour urine collection is accomplished to assess for protein and creatinine and for comparison if renal decompensation occurs. During the antepartum period, serial screening for urinary tract infections is done even when patients are symptom free. Bacteria greater than 100,000 colony count are treated. Urine culture and sensitivity are obtained if patients complain of symptoms or if infection is suspected.

Assessment of pregnant women with diabetes includes a review of diabetes self-care knowledge. If patients are acutely ill or in labor, this assessment may be postponed. Evaluation includes knowledge of self-administered blood glucose monitoring, insulin administration, diet, prevention and treatment of hypoglycemia, and prevention of DKA. Method of monitoring, either visually read reagent strips or blood glucose meter, is documented. It is preferable that those with type I diabetes perform glucose level monitoring with a blood glucose meter to improve accuracy. The meter should be in good working order and should be calibrated in accordance with the manufacturer's recommendations. It is helpful to observe patients during performance of self-monitoring to assess technique and correct problems.

Insulin self-administration should be observed and documented in the medical record. Occasionally even persons with long-standing diabetes will exhibit deterioration of careful technique. A review of storage, mixing, injection, and site selection and rotation is appropriate. Timing of injection prior to meals and daily time variations should be discussed.

Knowledge of diet is briefly assessed, and daily caloric intake and meal timing should be reviewed. The number of snacks prescribed and how regularly they are eaten are discussed. Often patients may skip snacks if they do not feel hungry. Nurses should explore how comfortable patients feel with their intake. They should feel ready to eat at mealtime but without symptoms of hypoglycemia. Similarly, when too many calories are prescribed, patients frequently omit snacks or even meals. Consistency with meal planning and timing are stressed. A dietary consultation is indicated for all pregnant women with diabetes at each admission. Registered dietitians can assist with diet manipulation and ongoing teaching.

Nurses determine patients' overall blood glucose control by a review of the blood glucose daily log; however, they should always question patients about hypoglycemia. Patients may have different symptoms of hypoglycemia, and specific symptoms each patient experiences should be assessed and documented. When patients cannot identify symptoms or have frequent severe reactions with no warning signs, hypoglycemia unawareness should be suspected. If present, increased self-monitoring for blood glucose levels is indicated to prevent hypoglycemia. Patients should be able to describe methods of treatment for hypoglycemia. Frequently, overtreatment with subsequent hyperglycemia is observed. Adequate treatment can usually be achieved with 20 g of carbohydrate (*e.g.,* 13.3 fl oz cola, 14.5 fl oz whole milk, or 12 fl oz orange or apple juice), but symptoms do not generally decrease until 20 minutes following treatment.[44] Thus, patients often continue eating until their symptoms disappear and should be encouraged to have 20 g of carbohydrate, wait 20 minutes, and then retest the blood glucose level. If hypoglycemia continues, an additional 20 g of carbohydrate can be taken.

Knowledge of urine testing for ketones is assessed. Patients should demonstrate adequate technique and knowledge of normal and abnormal results. Testing is generally performed daily on the first voided specimen and, if negative, no further testing may be indicated. Indications for upgrading testing (*e.g.,* upper respiratory, urinary tract, or other infection) and when to call health care providers must be taught.

Diabetes-complicating pregnancy is classified as high risk and thus includes all the special psychosocial problems seen with these groups of patients (see Chapter 4). In turn, psychological stress associated with childbearing has been found to adversely affect blood glucose control.[45] Diabetes is a unique disease in that care is largely performed at home by the patient. Knowledgeable patients with diabetes can be quite adept with their self-care and may often be reluctant to "give up" control of their diabetes to any health care provider. For these patients who may be used to manipulating their own insulin dosages, pregnancy may represent a significant loss of control of self and body. Encouraging discussion between patients, physicians, and nurses is important. Although it is reasonable to assume the diagnosis of diabetes made during pregnancy might cause acute stress, one study found that most patients experienced no adverse emotional status.[46] Another study found that women with gestational diabetes responded more stressfully than did those with preexisting diabetes to procedures and prescribed treatments associated with high-risk pregnancy.[47]

Newly diagnosed patients with diabetes or patients with long-standing disease and knowledge deficits are often very distressed and may operate under myths of diabetes and childbirth. Education often allays many misconceptions and fears. The increased risk of congenital anomalies among IDM predisposes pregnant women with diabetes to stressful pregnancies as the outcome of their pregnancies and health of their newborns remain uncertain. Prenatal diagnosis and antepartum testing techniques should be carefully explained, and the abilities and limitations of the tests discussed.

Of course, patients with diabetes and their families suffer from added fears of maternal morbidity and often worry about maternal death. Given the increased risks of pregnancy to women with diabetes, these fears are quite appropriate.

It seems pregnant women with diabetes may be at increased risk for anxiety and depression.[48] It has been suggested that due to the antepartum goals associated with "control," patients with diabetes may have increased fears of loss of control during labor.[49] Anxiety and fears of congenital anomalies, problems at birth such as lung disease or hypoglycemia, and intrauterine fetal demise suggest heightened sources of stress during the intrapartum period.

Women with diabetes are at increased risk for intrauterine fetal demise and congenital anomalies and, when either is diagnosed during the antepartum period, anticipatory grieving can be expected. Grief related to an anomalous infant may be related to the "loss" of a normal child. If the anomaly is lethal or severely threatens quality of life, the grieving period may be prolonged and difficult.

Psychosocial assessment includes evaluating maternal stress level and availability of support resources. Maternal stress level can be evaluated by discussing patients' identified sources of stress. Areas for exploration include family and home life, outside employment, medical problems associated with diabetes, other medical problems, financial concerns, past obstetric history, and legal problems. Support resources may be easily identified and available to patients, or avenues for support may need to be developed. The psychosocial assessment, devised jointly with the patient, should include a list of all areas of stress and lack of support sources. A plan designed to address needs is then developed. For example, a source of stress may be identified as a partner who is overly concerned about the patient's weight gain during pregnancy, claiming that she'll be "fat" by term. The patient can identify no sources of support. The plan to address the need identified might include diabetes and pregnancy teaching about normal weight gain during pregnancy and counseling with the couple.

Nursing Diagnoses

The nursing diagnoses specific to patients with diabetes mellitus are generally physiologic problems, complications of diabetes and pregnancy, or knowledge deficits. A list of potential diagnoses follows:

NUTRITION
- Altered nutrition: More than body requirements*
- Altered nutrition: Less than body requirements*
- Altered nutrition: Potential for more than body requirements*
- Knowledge deficit: Diabetic diet*

SELF-MONITORING FOR BLOOD GLUCOSE LEVELS
- Skill deficit: Self-monitoring for blood glucose levels
- Knowledge deficit: Self-monitoring for blood glucose levels*

INSULIN ADMINISTRATION
- Skill deficit: Insulin administration
- Knowledge deficit: Insulin administration*

HYPOGLYCEMIA
- Potential for trauma secondary to hypoglycemia*
- Knowledge deficit: Prevention, recognition, and treatment of hypoglycemia*

DIABETIC KETOACIDOSIS
- Hyperglycemia
- Ketonuria
- Potential for altered tissue perfusion (maternal and fetal)
- Potential for hypoglycemia due to inadequate glucose replacement

- Potential for shock or pulmonary edema due to inappropriate fluid replacement
- Potential for infection*
- Potential for cardiac or respiratory arrest due to hypo- or hyperkalemia
- Knowledge deficit: Prevention and recognition of DKA

NEUROPATHY
- Potential for skin integrity impairment related to neuropathy leading to loss of limb sensation

IN LABOR
- Potential for altered tissue perfusion: Uteroplacental
- Altered tissue perfusion: Uteroplacental*
- Hypoglycemia
- Hyperglycemia
- Pain*
- Anxiety*
- Fear*
- Powerlessness*
- Potential for infection*

PSYCHOSOCIAL
- Self-concept disturbance
- Altered parenting*
- Potential altered parenting*
- Parental role conflict*
- Ineffective individual coping*
- Ineffective denial*
- Noncompliance*
- Body image disturbance*
- Personal identity disturbance*
- Anticipatory grieving*

Theoretical Basis for the Plan of Nursing Care and Intervention

Nursing care during labor includes careful monitoring of blood glucose at 1- to 2-hour intervals to detect hypoglycemia or hyperglycemia. Target ranges for blood glucose are 60 to 110 mg/dl to minimize the incidence of neonatal hyperglycemia. Glucose utilization during labor is 2.5 mg/kg/minute.[51] Intravenous fluids are given at 125 cc/hour, and 5% dextrose is generally ordered. Patients must have nothing orally, because of the increased risk of cesarean delivery indicated by uteroplacental insufficiency and fetal stress.

---

*Official diagnostic categories approved by North American Nursing Diagnosis Association.[50]

Intravenous insulin is initiated when blood glucose levels exceed 110 mg/dl. The dose can vary from 0.2 to 6.0 units of insulin per hour and is based on hourly blood glucose determinations; it is carefully titrated with glucose containing intravenous fluids to maintain target blood glucose values. An intravenous control device is always used with insulin solutions. Only regular insulin is administered intravenously because of its rapid half-life. The insulin should be discontinued immediately prior to delivery to prevent postpartum hypoglycemia.

The use of oxytocin for induction or augmentation should follow appropriate protocols (see "Protocol for the Nursing Management of the Patient Requiring Oxytocin for Induction and Augmentation of Labor," page 287). When used concomitantly with insulin, oxytocin should be mixed in a separate intravenous fluid bag from insulin. Two separate infusion control devices will be necessary: one for the insulin containing fluid and one for the oxytocin-containing fluid.

During labor careful attention to fetal heart rate monitoring must be accomplished because of the increased risk of uteroplacental insufficiency. The guidelines for high-risk patients should be followed for all those who are insulin dependent.

Diabetic ketoacidosis represents a state of acutely decompensated diabetes and is classified as mild, moderate, or severe (see Table 10-5). Immediate goals include replacement of insulin, fluids, and electrolytes. Preliminary assessment is made as quickly as possible with particular attention to maintaining an airway. The patient may have an altered level of consciousness and may be alert, obtunded, stuporous, or comatose. Labored breath sounds, called Kussmaul's respirations, are typical of the patient with DKA as is fruity-smelling breath. Initial blood glucose level is usually in excess of 300, and ketonuria is present. A clear airway is established. Oxygen is administered via tight face mask at 8 to 10 liters/minute; however, intubation may be necessary.

After the patient is rapidly assessed and blood glucose and urine ketones evaluated, large amounts of intravenous fluids *without glucose* are rapidly administered to reduce dehydration and replace electrolytes. Normal saline is the usual fluid of choice, and 1 to 2 liters are administered over 30 minutes. Intravenous fluids are then administered at 200 to 250 cc/hour while assessment continues for intravascular volume. Invasive hemodynamic monitoring is often required to monitor fluid replacement and to prevent shock from decreased intravascular volume or pulmonary edema from excessive replacement. Glucose-containing fluids (*e.g.,* 5% to 10% dextrose in water) are administered when blood glucose falls to 200 mg/dl to prevent hypoglycemia.

TABLE 10-5
Diabetic Ketoacidosis Classification

	Total CO_2		pH
Mild	21–28 mEq/liter	and/or	≥7.30
Moderate	11–20 mEq/liter	and/or	7.10–7.30
Severe	≤10 mEq/liter	and/or	<7.10

Intravenous insulin is administered concomitantly with a usual starting dose of 12 U/hour but must be titrated to blood glucose. Once blood glucose falls to 200 mg/dl, intravenous insulin is continued at a lower infusion rate.

Cardiac monitoring and fetal monitoring are necessary during treatment of DKA. Potassium replacement is almost always required and should be started if potassium levels are less than 3.0 mEq/L. Potassium replacement should be discontinued if urinary output is less than 40 cc/hour. Cardiac or respiratory arrest may occur due to either hyper- or hypokalemia. Bicarbonate replacement is often necessary and started if the *p*H is less than 7.10. When *p*H reaches 7.20, bicarbonate may be discontinued. Most common complications of DKA include hypoglycemia and cerebral edema from excessive insulin therapy or inadequate glucose administration once blood glucose levels fall to 200 mg/dl.

Most often DKA develops in the pregnant patient as a result of infection, thus rigorous evaluation should occur at admission. Urine for culture and sensitivity is obtained and other cultures may be indicated (*i.e.,* blood and sputum). Broad spectrum antibiotics are administered even when little or no evidence exists to support a diagnosis of infection.

When DKA occurs during treatment of preterm labor, beta agonists are discontinued. Other tocolytic agents may be used, which do not have hyperglycemic effects such as magnesium sulfate.

Expected Outcomes

The patient with complications of diabetes and pregnancy will do the following:

1. Be euglycemic
2. Demonstrate appropriate self-monitoring technique of blood glucose levels
3. Verbalize understanding of when to check blood glucose level
4. Verbalize understanding of her specific diabetic diet
5. Demonstrate appropriate insulin administration
6. Verbalize understanding of insulin dosages and injection timing
7. Verbalize understanding of prevention, recognition, and treatment of hypoglycemia
8. Verbalize understanding of prevention and recognition of DKA
9. Have appropriate weight gain
10. Be without symptomatic hypoglycemia
11. Be free of infection
12. Have negative antepartum testing results (if appropriate gestational age)
13. Have appropriate fetal growth

During the intrapartum period, the patient with diabetes will do the following:

1. Have blood glucose levels range from 60 to 100 mg/dl
2. Be without symptomatic hypoglycemia
3. Have normal fetal heart rate findings

The patient with DKA will do the following:

1. Be euglycemic
2. Have normal respiratory function
3. Establish normal fluid and electrolyte balance
4. Be without urinary ketones
5. Be alert and oriented
6. Have normal fetal heart rate findings

References

1. Centers for Disease Control: *Health Objectives Planning for the Year 2000.* Atlanta, CDC, 1989.
2. U.S. Department of Health and Human Services, Public Health Service, Centers for Disease Control, Center for Prevention Services, Division of Diabetes Control. *Public Health Guidelines for Enhancing Diabetes Control through Maternal and Child Health Programs.* Atlanta, CDC, 1986.
3. Gamble DR, Taylor KW: Seasonal incidence of diabetes mellitus. *Brit Med J* 3:631–633, 1969.
4. White P: Pregnancy complicating diabetes. *Am J Med* 7:609–616, 1949.
5. White P: Classification of diabetes. *Am J Obstet Gynecol* 2:228–230, 1978.
6. Cryer PE, Binder C, Geremia BB, et al: Hypoglycemia in IDDM. *Diabetes* 38:1193–1199, 1989.
7. Rodman HM, Singerman LJ, Aiello LM: Diabetic retinopathy: Effects of pregnancy and laser therapy (abstract). *Diabetes* 29:1A, 1980.
8. Klein BEK, Moss SE, Klein R: Effect of pregnancy on progression of diabetic retinopathy. *Diabetes Care* 13(1):34–40, 1990.
9. Cousins L: Pregnancy complications among diabetic women: Review 1965–1985. *Obstet Gynecol Surv* 42(3):140–149, 1987.
10. Kitzmiller J, Cloherty J, Younger M, et al: Diabetic pregnancy and perinatal morbidity. *Am J Obstet Gynecol* 131:560, 1978.
11. Buehler J, Kaunitz A, Hogue C, et al: Maternal mortality in women aged 35 years or older: United States. *JAMA* 255:53, 1986.
12. Coustan DR: Diabetes mellitus, in Eden RD, Boehm FH (eds.): *Assessment and Care of the Fetus: Physiological, Clinical and Medicolegal Principles.* Norwalk, CT, Appleton & Lange, 1990.
13. Mills JL, Baker L, Goldman AS: Malformations in infants of diabetic mothers occur before the seventh gestational week. *Diabetes* 28:292–293, 1979.
14. Miller EM, Hare JW, Cloherty JR, et al: Major congenital anomalies and elevated HgbA$_1$c in early weeks on diabetic pregnancy. *N Engl J Med* 22:1331–1334, 1981.
15. Steel JM, Johnston FD, Smith AF, Duncan LJP: Five years' experience of a prepregnancy clinic for insulin-dependent diabetics. *Brit Med J* 285:353–356, 1982.
16. Fuhrmann K, Reiher H, Semmler K, et al: Prevention of congenital malformations in infants of insulin-dependent diabetic mothers. *Diabetes Care* 3:219–223, 1983.
17. Goldman JA, Dicker D, Feldberg D, et al: Pregnancy outcome in patients with insulin-dependent diabetes mellitus with preconceptual diabetic control: A comparative study. *Am J Obstet Gynecol* 2:293–297, 1986.
18. Coustan DR: Hyperglycemia–hyperinsulinemia: Effect on the infant of the diabetic mother, in Jovanovic L, Peterson CM, Fuhrmann K (eds.): *Diabetes and Pregnancy: Teratology, Toxicity and Treatment.* New York, Praeger, 1986.
19. Otonkoski T, Andersson S, Knip M, Simell O: Maturation of insulin response to glucose during human fetal and neonatal development. *Diabetes* 37:286–291, 1988.
20. Barnett AM, Eff C, Leslie RD, et al: Diabetes in identical twins: A study of 200 pairs. *Diabetologia* 7:46–49, 1971.

21. Cahill GF, McDevitt HO: Insulin-dependent diabetes mellitus: The initial lesion. *N Engl J Med* 304:1454–1465, 1981.

22. Mann JI, Houston AC: Genetic factors in diabetes mellitus, in Davidson JK (ed.): *Clinical Diabetes Mellitus: A Problem Oriented Approach.* New York, Thieme, 1986.

23. Ginsberg-Fellner F: Epidemiology, genetics and immunology, in Reece EA, Coustan DR: *Diabetes Mellitus in Pregnancy: Principles and Practice.* New York, Churchill Livingstone, 1988.

24. Bortz WM: Metabolic consequences of obesity. *Ann Intern Med* 71:833, 1969.

25. Kyle GC: Diabetes and pregnancy. *Ann Intern Med* 5:1–82, 1963.

26. Rubinstein P, Walker M, Krassner J, et al: HLA antigens and islet cell antibodies in gestational diabetes. *Hum Immunol* 3:271, 1981.

27. American Diabetes Association Workshop-Conference on Gestational Diabetes. Summary and recommendations. *Diabetes Care* 3:499–501, 1980.

28. Coustan DR, Widness JA, Carpenter MW, et al: Should the fifty-gram one hour plasma glucose screening test for gestational diabetes be administered in the fasting or fed state? *Am J Obstet Gynecol* 5:1031–1035, 1986.

29. American College of Obstetricians and Gynecologists. Management of diabetes mellitus in pregnancy. *ACOG Tech Bull* 92, 1986.

30. Carpenter MW, Coustan DR: Criteria for screening tests for gestational diabetes. *Am J Obstet Gynecol* 7:768–773, 1982.

31. National Diabetes Data Group: Classification and diagnosis of diabetes mellitus and other categories of glucose intolerance. *Diabetes* 28:1039–1057, 1979.

32. Kitzmiller JL, Brown ER, Phillippe M, et al: Diabetic nephropathy and perinatal outcome. *Am J Obstet Gynecol* 141:741, 1981.

33. Kitzmiller JL: Diabetic nephropathy, in Reece EA, Coustan DR: *Diabetes Mellitus in Pregnancy: Principles and Practice.* New York, Churchill Livingstone, 1988.

34. Jovanovic R, Jovanovic L: Obstetric management when normoglycemia is maintained in diabetic pregnant women with vascular compromise. *Am J Obstet Gynecol* 149:617, 1984.

35. American Diabetes Association: Consensus statement: Self-monitoring of blood glucose. *Diabetes Care* 10:95–99, 1987.

36. American Diabetes Association: Position statement: Insulin administration. *Diabetes Care* (supplement) 13:28–31, 1990.

37. Committee on Dietary Allowances, Food and Nutrition Board, National Academy of Sciences: *Recommended Dietary Allowances* (9th ed.). Washington, DC, U.S. Government Printing Office, 1980.

38. American College of Obstetricians and Gynecologists: Women and exercise. *ACOG Tech Bull* 87, September 1985.

39. Berger M, Berchtold P, Cuppers HJ, et al: Metabolic and hormonal effects of muscular exercise in juvenile type diabetes. *Diabetologia* 13:355, 1977.

40. Schiffrin A, Parikh S: Accommodating planned exercise in Type I diabetic patients on intensive treatment. *Diabetes Care* 8:337, 1985.

41. Hollingsworth DR: Exercise in normal and diabetic pregnancies, in Reece EA, and Coustan DR (eds.): *Diabetes Mellitus in Pregnancy: Principles and Practice.* New York, Churchill Livingstone, 1988.

42. American Diabetes Association: Position statement: Bedside blood glucose monitoring in hospitals. *Diabetes Care* 9:89, 1986.

43. American Diabetes Association: Position statement: Standards of medical care for patients with diabetes mellitus. *Diabetes Care* 12:365–368, 1989.

44. Brodows RG, Williams C, Amatruda JM: Treatment of insulin reactions in diabetics. *JAMA* 252:3378–3381, 1984.

45. Barglow P, Hatcher R, Berndt D, Phelps R: Psychosocial childbearing stress and metabolic control in pregnant diabetics. *J Nerv Mental Dis* 173:615–620, 1985.

46. Spirito A, Williams C, Ruggiero L, et al: Psychosocial impact of the diagnosis of gestational diabetes. *Obstet Gynecol* 73:562–565, 1989.

47. Zigrossi ST, Riga-Ziegler M: The stress of medical management on pregnant diabetics. *MCN* 11:320–323, 1986.

48. Barglow P, Hatcher R, Wolston J, et al: Psychiatric risk factors in the pregnant diabetic patient. *Am J Obstet Gynecol* 140:46, 1981.
49. Furlong-Lind R, Beck-Black L: Psychosocial implications, family planning and emotional support, in Reece EA, Coustan DR: *Diabetes Mellitus in Pregnancy: Principles and Practice.* New York, Churchill Livingstone, 1988.
50. North American Nursing Diagnosis Association: *Taxonomy I: Revised 1989 with Official Diagnostic Categories.* St. Louis, NANDA, 1989.
51. Jovanovic L, Druzin M, Peterson CM: Effect of euglycemia on the outcome of pregnancy in insulin-dependent diabetic women as compared with normal control subjects. *Am J Med* 71:921–927, 1981.

11
◆ ◆ ◆

Cardiac Diseases in Pregnancy

Nan H. Troiano

Supportive Data

Incidence

Cardiac disease occurs in approximately 1% of all pregnancies and remains the most important nonobstetric cause of maternal death.[1,2] It is the most common indirect cause of maternal mortality and, following hypertension, hemorrhage, and infection, the fourth most common direct cause.[3] Specific cardiac diseases that complicate pregnancy may be subdivided into those that are congenital, acquired, or ischemic in nature.

Congenital cardiac disease is becoming the most common cardiac problem in pregnant women. Two factors have contributed to this increased incidence. First, tremendous improvements in diagnostic, medical, and surgical capabilities have allowed women who otherwise might have died because of their cardiac abnormality to reach childbearing age. Second, the decreased incidence in many societies of rheumatic fever and associated cardiac sequelae has made congenital cardiac disease in pregnancy relatively more common. Though the exact incidence of pregnant women with uncorrected heart lesions is unknown, it is estimated that 1% of all liveborn infants have congenital cardiac disease.[4,5] The ratio of rheumatic cardiac disease to congenital cardiac disease seen during pregnancy—approximately 20:1 in the early 1950s—decreased to 3:1 by the late 1970s and has now approached unity in certain populations.[6–8] The most common lesions reported in pregnancy are atrial septal defect, ventricular septal defect, patent ductus arteriosus, pulmonary stenosis, aortic stenosis, coarctation of the aorta, and tetralogy of Fallot.[9]

Acquired cardiac disease is most often rheumatic in origin, though infective endocarditis secondary to intravenous drug use may also be encountered. With the decrease in incidence of acute rheumatic fever, rheumatic cardiac disease in pregnancy has declined as well. However, both are sufficiently common and, coupled with reports of resurgence, constitute a serious medical complication of pregnancy.[10] Significant rheumatic cardiac lesions are predominantly valvular in nature with the mitral valve most commonly affected. Approximately 90% of patients with rheumatic cardiac disease have mitral stenosis, 6.6% have mitral regurgitation, 2.5% have aortic regurgitation, and 1% have aortic stenosis.[11] It is uncommon to see isolated right-sided valvular lesions of rheumatic origin, yet such lesions are seen with increasing frequency as a result of valvular endocarditis.

Coronary artery disease and myocardial infarction in pregnancy are rare. However, ischemic cardiac disease is the leading cause of death in the United States, and, with the trend toward childbearing later in life, it is reasonable to predict such complications may increase in incidence. It has been estimated that myocardial infarction occurs in 1 out of every 10,000 pregnancies.[12] In a review by Hankins and colleagues, 70 well-documented cases in the world literature were analyzed.[13] Of those patients, only 13% had known coronary artery disease antedating their pregnancy. Two thirds had an infarct in the third trimester with a mortality rate of 45%. When delivery occurred within 14 days of infarction, mortality was greatly increased. Thus, hemodynamic demands associated with pregnancy may serve as a stress to the coronary circulation, thereby producing ischemia in patients with previously asymptomatic disease.

Other cardiac diseases, complex in nature, have been documented during pregnancy. Included in this group are peripartum cardiomyopathy and inherited, developmental conditions. *Peripartum cardiomyopathy* is defined as cardiomyopathy that develops between the last month of pregnancy and five months postpartum—only after other causes of cardiac failure have been eliminated. It occurs in approximately 1 per 1300 to 1 per 4000 pregnancies.[14] The peak incidence in the United States is during the second month postpartum. It occurs with greater frequency in underdeveloped areas, such as certain tribal populations within Africa, where the incidence is as high as 10%.[15] However, such high frequency may be due to cultural customs associated with pregnancy involving unusually high sodium intake thereby precipitating fluid overload. Inherited developmental conditions involving cardiac abnormality include Marfan's syndrome and idiopathic hypertrophic subaortic stenosis. Marfan's syndrome, characterized by general weakness of connective tissues, occurs in approximately 1 out of 10,000 people.[16] The syndrome is inherited in 65% to 75% of patients as an autosomal dominant disorder with 60% of affected children manifesting cardiac involvement. Idiopathic hypertrophic subaortic stenosis, primarily an autosomal dominant inherited condition, involves hypertrophy of the left ventricular wall. It represents a form of hypertrophic cardiomyopathy, a primary myocardial disease, that is most often clinically apparent during the childbearing years. Though the exact incidence in pregnancy is not known, the prevalence is increasing.

TABLE 11-1
Mortality Risk Associated with Pregnancy

Group I: Mortality <1%
  Atrial septal defect
  Ventricular septal defect (uncomplicated)
  Patent ductus arteriosus
  Pulmonic and tricuspid disease
  Corrected tetralogy of Fallot
  Biosynthetic valve prosthesis (porcine and human allograft)
  Mitral stenosis, NYHA class I and II
Group II: Mortality 5%–15%
  Mitral stenosis with atrial fibrillation
  Mechanical valve prosthesis
  Mitral stenosis, NYHA class III or IV
  Aortic stenosis
  Coarctation of the aorta (uncomplicated)
  Uncorrected tetralogy of Fallot
  Previous myocardial infarction
  Marfan's syndrome with normal aorta
Group III: Mortality 25%–50%
  Pulmonary hypertension
  Coarctation of the aorta, complicated
  Marfan's syndrome with aortic involvement

Significance

Additional risk accompanies women with cardiac disease as they undergo the physiologic stress of pregnancy. Perinatal morbidity and mortality are dependent on the specific cardiac lesion and the functional derangement of the lesion, as well as development of pregnancy-related complications.[17] It is important that issues addressed in counseling women with cardiac disease include review of the specific type of disease, its significance, and potential maternal and fetal risks.

A classification system describing the risk of maternal mortality associated with specific cardiac lesions during pregnancy has been described by Clark and is presented in Table 11-1.[18] Included in group I are conditions posing a risk of mortality under 1% when properly managed. Risk of mortality increases to between 5% and 15% for lesions included in group II. Despite the worse prognosis, some women, following appropriate counseling, find such risk acceptable. Patients with lesions in group III have up to a 50% risk of mortality. In addition, some conditions within this group, such as those leading to hemodynamically significant pulmonary hypertension, have as high as a 70% risk of functional morbidity during pregnancy.[17] This risk is generally unacceptable to the patient with prevention or termination of pregnancy considered.

Functional derangement also influences pregnancy outcome. The New York Heart Association (NYHA) system of classifying cardiac disease according to patient functional ability is often utilized in discussions of the pregnant cardiac patient. Guidelines for each class follow:[19]

Class I
  No limitation of physical activity
  Asymptomatic
Class II
  Slight limitation of physical activity
  Asymptomatic at rest
  Symptomatic with heavy physical activity
Class III
  Considerable limitation of physical activity
  Asymptomatic at rest
  Symptomatic with minimal physical activity
Class IV
  Severe limitation of physical activity
  Symptomatic with any physical activity
  May be symptomatic at bed rest

Patients with NYHA class I or II disease prior to pregnancy generally do well during pregnancy. Those with class III or class IV disease have approximately a 30% to 50% risk of significant hemodynamic morbidity and a 25% to 50% risk of mortality.[20] Limitations of this classification system during pregnancy should be noted. For example, up to 40% of women who develop congestive heart failure and pulmonary edema late in pregnancy are labeled as "functional class I."[18] The system has been expanded to include anatomic, physiologic, and etiologic principles that may influence prognosis. However, the earlier system is still widely used.

Development of other specific pregnancy-related complications may produce additional cardiovascular stress thereby altering patients' functional classifications. Such conditions include pregnancy-induced hypertension, anemia, bleeding, and infection. Association of these complications with significant cardiac disease may worsen prognosis.

Significant fetal morbidity and mortality may also accompany pregnancy complicated by cardiac disease. Outcome tends to correlate with maternal functional capacity. As maternal Po_2 falls below 70, decreased fetal oxygen saturation ensues, increasing the risk of hypoxic insult.[21] In cases of cyanotic congenital cardiac disease, there is increased risk of spontaneous abortion, intrauterine growth retardation, prematurity, and stillbirth. The fetus is also at increased risk for congenital cardiac anomalies. Most congenital cardiac lesions are multifactorial in origin with a 2% to 5% risk of fetal cardiac malformations. However, a range of 1.1% to as high as 14% has been reported.[8,22] With rheumatic cardiac disease, fetal complications are related to the mother's prepregnant functional classification. In women with class I or II disease, there is no significant increase in fetal mortality. However, fetal mortality increases to approximately 12% with class III disease and 30% with class IV, the latter including therapeutic abortions.[23] There is no increase in incidence of congenital anomalies in patients with rheumatic heart disease.

In inherited, developmental cardiac conditions, fetal risk is variable. For example, fetal mortality exceeds 10% in cases of women with Marfan's syndrome and 50% of liveborn infants are affected with this disorder.[24] However, in cases of women with idiopathic hypertrophic subaortic stenosis, risk of fetal mortality does not increase, though the risk of inheritance may be as high as 50% in families with high gene penetrance and autosomal dominant inheritance patterns.[25]

In pregnant women with prosthetic cardiac valves, fetal risk is influenced by the specific type of prosthesis. Spontaneous abortion has been noted in up to 60% of pregnancies with a mechanical valve prosthesis.[24] This may be related to use of warfarin derivatives for anticoagulation. In addition, infants of women who have taken warfarin have up to a 25% risk of having congenital abnormalities, including nasal hypoplasia, optic atrophy, mental retardation, and dwarfism. As many as 20% of pregnancies end in spontaneous abortion with tissue prosthesis.

Congenital cardiac lesions are thought to be multifactorial in 90% of cases, whereby effects of a number of genes coupled with an environmental catalyst result in genetic predisposition.[26] Such lesions may also be associated with maternal disease, viral infection, and drug or alcohol ingestion. In addition, cardiac disease may represent a component of other genetic syndromes such as trisomy 21.

Etiology

Maternal diseases that increase the risk of fetal cardiac disorders include diabetes mellitus, lupus erythematosus, and phenylketonuria. For example, infants of insulin-dependent diabetic mothers have a 3% to 5% risk of congenital cardiac defects including ventricular septal defects, coarctation of the aorta, and transposition of the great vessels.[27] Maternal systemic lupus erythematosus is associated with fetal cardiac abnormalities, most commonly complete heart block. Infants of mothers with phenylketonuria are at a 25% to 50% risk of cardiac lesions including ventricular and atrial septal defects and tetralogy of Fallot.[27] Infants exposed to rubella *in utero* have approximately a 35% incidence of cardiac defects, including ventricular and atrial septal defects as well as patent ductus arteriosus.[26] It has also been reported that mothers who use alcohol during pregnancy have a 25% to 50% risk of fetal cardiac anomalies such as septal defects and patent ductus arteriosus.[27]

Acquired cardiac disease is most often rheumatic in origin but may also be related to bacterial endocarditis. Acute rheumatic fever is caused by the Lancefield group A streptococcus, *Streptococcus pyogenes*.[28] The most common sites of streptococcal infection are the oropharynx, nasopharynx, and the skin. Cutaneous streptococcal infection has never been shown to cause acute rheumatic fever. The mechanism by which group A streptococci spread beyond the pharynx to cause the disease is not understood. The leading theory is that acute rheumatic fever is an autoimmune disorder in which tissue damage is mediated by the host's own hyperimmune response to the antecedent streptococcal infection.[29]

The acute phase of this disorder is characterized by inflammatory reactions in connective tissue, especially the heart, joints, skin, and subcutaneous tissue. Initial myocardial abnormalities consist of edema of the ground substance, fragmentation of collagen fibers, cellular infiltration, and fibrinoid degeneration.[30] Following the initial 2- to 3-week phase, Aschoff nodules, the most characteristic lesion of acute rheumatic fever, develop. These persist for many years and are associated with progressive fibrosis and stenosis of the mitral valve. Interstitial myocarditis, diffuse cellular infiltrates in interstitial tissues adjacent to Aschoff bodies, plays an important role in the development of heart failure. Coronary arteritis is also a common finding in this disorder and may be important in producing permanent myocardial damage.

Infective endocarditis refers to microbial infection of the heart valves due to either bacteria or fungi. Until recently, infective endocarditis most often occurred in association with congenital or rheumatic cardiac defects. However, use of illicit drugs intravenously has become a significant new cause. Acute bacterial endocarditis, including infection from *Staphylococcus aureus, Streptococcus pyogenes, Streptococcus pneumoniae, Neisseria gonorrhoae,* and group B streptococcus, often involves normal heart valves. The associated clinical course is usually fulminant. In contrast, subacute bacterial endocarditis, a result of valvular vegetations induced by *Streptococcus viridans,* occurs in association with preexisting cardiac defects. The clinical course is typically indolent. Transient and asymptomatic bacteremia is the primary cause in the development of endocarditis. Blood-borne bacteria adhere to endothelium at sites of high blood flow, which become covered with platelets and fibrin, thus forming vegetations.

Ischemic cardiac disease is usually associated with atherosclerosis, the primary cause of progressive coronary artery disease and myocardial infarction in the general population. However, vascular occlusion is no longer thought to be solely responsible, especially in women of childbearing age. Other, less common causes of ischemic heart disease that may be seen in young women follow:[31,32]

> Coronary atherosclerosis
> Congenital lesions
> > Anomalous origins of coronary arteries
> > Aortic valvular stenosis
> Inflammatory disease of the coronary arteries
> > Kawasaki's disease
> > Connective tissue syndromes
> Hypertrophic cardiomyopathy
> Vasospastic phenomena
> > Primary idiopathic
> > Secondary to drugs or pregnancy-induced hypertension

Spontaneous coronary artery dissection
Metastatic carcinoma
Impaired hemoglobin oxygen diffusion
Polycythemia

Framework for Accepted Therapy

Provision of intrapartum nursing care for the pregnant woman with cardiac disease requires a working knowledge of normal cardiac function, the specific lesion or disorder, the disease process, and related management principles. The risk of hemodynamic decompensation is of special concern as the patient undergoes the stress imposed during labor, delivery, and the puerperium. Therefore, the nurse must integrate both obstetric and cardiac principles to provide a broader framework for care.

Before addressing the pathophysiology of specific disorders, normal cardiac anatomy and physiology are reviewed (Figure 11-1). Atria are low pressure chambers that serve as reservoirs of blood for the ventricles. The right atrium receives venous blood via the superior and inferior vena cavae and coronary sinus from the systemic bed. The left atrium receives oxygenated blood returning to the heart from the pulmonary bed via the four pulmonary veins. Approximately 70% of blood flows from the atria to the ventricles during early ventricular diastole, known as protodiastole. The ventricles serve as pumps to expel

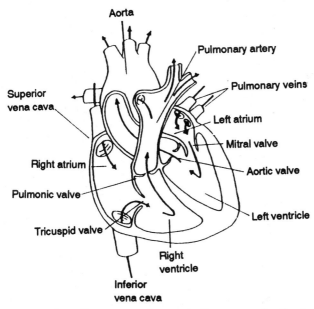

Figure 11-1. Normal cardiac anatomy (arrows indicate normal path of circulation).

blood. The right ventricle pumps deoxygenated blood into the pulmonary circulation via the pulmonary artery. The left ventricle pumps oxygenated blood into the systemic circulation via the aorta. The left side of the heart functions as a higher pressure system than does the right side.

Atrioventricular valves consist of the tricuspid valve on the right and mitral valve on the left. During diastole, valve leaflets open allowing unidirectional blood flow into the respective ventricle. As ventricular pressure increases during systole, valve leaflets close preventing retrograde flow. Semilunar valves consist of the pulmonic valve on the right and aortic on the left. Open during ventricular systole, each of these valves allows unidirectional blood flow to the respective arterial outflow tract. Following systole as arterial pressures increase, each valve closes to prevent retrograde flow during diastole.

Cardiac output, the amount of blood ejected from the left ventricle, is determined by the interaction of four variables: preload, afterload, contractility, and heart rate. *Preload* refers to the initial myocardial muscle fiber length and is determined by intraventricular volume and pressure. As preload increases in a normal heart, cardiac output increases. A higher preload than is normal is required to maintain adequate cardiac output in a failing heart. *Afterload* refers to ventricular wall tension during systole and is dependent primarily on pulmonary and systemic vascular resistance. In a normal heart, there is an inverse relationship between afterload and cardiac output. *Contractility,* or the inotropic state of the heart, is considered the force and velocity of ventricular contractions when preload and afterload remain constant. Finally, *heart rate* also directly influences cardiac output. Review of the pathophysiology for selected congenital, acquired, and ischemic cardiac disorders facilitates identification and understanding of appropriate methods to promote optimal hemodynamic function.

Congenital cardiac disorders may generally be subdivided into those involving the presence of an intracardiac shunt or ventricular outflow obstruction. An intracardiac shunt may result from a septal defect, patent ductus arteriosus, or tetralogy of Fallot. As a group, septal defects are the most common form of congenital cardiac anomaly. Many either close spontaneously or are corrected surgically in early childhood. The primary hemodynamic alteration in uncorrected septal defects is development of a left-to-right shunt. Pregnancy may exacerbate this condition by creating a large shunt whereby pulmonary vascular resistance increases, which then creates secondary pulmonary hypertension, shunt reversal, and cyanosis. This condition is known as Eisenmenger's syndrome. Two significant potential complications include arrhythmias and heart failure. In general, these women tolerate pregnancy well, especially in the absence of either a large left-to-right shunt or secondary pulmonary hypertension. Patent ductus arteriosus is characterized by open communication between the pulmonary artery and aorta. The primary hemodynamic alteration is development of a left-to-right shunt. As with septal defects, an uncorrected large patent ductus arteriosus with a concomitant large shunt and pulmonary hypertension carries significant risk of heart failure. In the absence of a large shunt, pregnancy is generally well tolerated. Tetralogy of Fallot refers to the cyanotic complex of ventricular septal defect, overriding aorta, right ventricular hypertrophy, and pulmonary stenosis. Most cases are corrected during early childhood with subsequent pregnancies generally tolerated well. The major pathophysiologic effect in uncorrected cases is right-to-left shunting secondary to the large ventricular septal defect and pulmonary artery stenosis resulting in cyanosis. Decline in systemic vascular resistance and venous return that may accompany pregnancy, labor, and delivery exacerbate this phenomenon. Risk is related to the degree of shunting and cyanosis.

Ventricular outflow obstruction may result from aortic stenosis, aortic coarctation, pulmonic stenosis, or idiopathic hypertrophic subaortic stenosis. Though rheumatic cardiac disease is probably the most common cause of aortic valvular disease, a congenital bicuspid aortic valve may lead to significant aortic stenosis. The primary defect involves noncompliant valvular leaflets that increase left ventricular volume during systole. The end result is left ventricular failure. Coarctation or gradual narrowing of the aorta most commonly occurs at the origin of the left subclavian artery. Other associated anomalies include a ventricular septal defect, patent ductus arteriosus, and intracranial aneurysm. Most women with uncomplicated aortic coarctation tolerate pregnancy well. However, risks include rupture of associated berry aneurysms, endocarditis, and death from aortic rupture or dissection.[26] Obstruction from pulmonic stenosis may be valvular, supravalvular, or subvalvular.[18] Degree of obstruction is the primary determinant of clinical function. With severe stenosis, right ventricular failure may occur. Idiopathic hypertrophic subaortic stenosis is accompanied by varying degrees of septal hypertrophy with resultant aortic stenosis or mitral regurgitation.

In addition to these, Marfan's syndrome, characterized by generalized weakness of connective tissue, is significant. The increased risk to the pregnant woman is caused by aortic root and wall involvement resulting in aneurysm formation, rupture, or aortic dissection.

Acquired rheumatic valvular diseases include mitral stenosis, pulmonic or tricuspid lesions, and aortic stenosis. Mitral stenosis, the most common rheumatic disorder in pregnancy, involves obstruction of blood flow from the left atrium to the left ventricle produced by a narrowed valve orifice. If the orifice is reduced to less than one half of normal, blood can flow to the left ventricle only with abnormally elevated atrial-to-ventricular pressure gradients. Adequate time for left ventricular filling is also crucial to maintain adequate cardiac output. Hemodynamically significant mitral insufficiency most commonly occurs in conjunction with other valvular lesions, with pregnancy generally well tolerated. Risks include development of atrial enlargement and fibrillation. Mitral valve prolapse, congenital rather than rheumatic in origin, is generally asymptomatic and well tolerated during pregnancy. Pulmonic and tricuspid lesions are unlikely to be symptomatic, and pregnancy, labor, and delivery are tolerated well. The primary risk is of right ventricular failure due to fluid overload. Aortic stenosis, though occasionally congenital in nature, is most commonly of rheumatic origin. It generally does not become hemodynamically significant until the orifice has diminished to one third or less of normal. The principal concern is maintenance of cardiac output. Pregnancy is usually well tolerated, yet with severe disease may be associated with fixed cardiac output. Risks include angina, myo-cardial infarction, syncope, or sudden death.

Myocardial ischemia occurs when local myocardial oxygen demands exceed oxygen delivery. Oxygen delivery is dependent on hemoglobin content of blood and amount of flow to the myocardium. Oxygen consumption parallels increases in heart rate, contractility, and afterload. If imbalance is prolonged, myocardial cell death or infarction occurs. Most infarctions involve the left ventricle.

Several methods may be identified to promote normal cardiac function. Cardiac output may be altered through manipulation of preload, afterload, contractility, and heart rate. When muscle fibers reach a point of stretch beyond which contraction is not enhanced, stroke volume decreases resulting in heart failure. Factors affecting preload follow:[32]

Increase in Preload	**Decrease in Preload**
Mitral insufficiency	Mitral stenosis
Left ventricular damage	Decreased circulating fluids
Vasoconstricting agents	Vasodilating agents
Increased circulatory fluids	Conduction anesthesia
Patient position	Patient position

When afterload becomes excessive, left ventricular stroke work increases, thereby increasing myocardial oxygen consumption, which results in left ventricular failure. The following are factors affecting afterload:[33]

Increase in Afterload	**Decrease in Afterload**
Aortic valvular stenosis	Vasodilating agents
Peripheral arterial vasoconstriction	Hemorrhage
Hypertension	Conduction anesthesia
Polycythemia	Patient position
Vasoconstricting agents	
Patient position	

Myocardial contractility may be manipulated via administration of inotropic cardiac drugs, which are shown in the following list:[33]

Positive Effect	**Negative Effect**
Digitalis	Quinidine
Isoproterenol	Barbiturates
Calcium	Propranolol
Catecholamines	
Norepinephrine	
Epinephrine	
Dopamine	
Dobutamine	

Sustained tachycardia may lead to heart failure because of decreased diastolic filling and shortened systolic ejection times. Conversely, cardiac output may also be compromised if the heart rate is too slow, as with heart block. Additional strategies include prevention of thromboembolism, infection, and anemia.

Assessment

Initial clinical assessment of the patient with cardiac disease begins with a thorough history. The patient's chief complaint should be determined and documented. History of her present cardiac disease should be elicited and include review of the specific lesion or disorder, functional classification, and current medications. The patient should be questioned regarding presence of symptoms such as chest pain, dyspnea, cyanosis, fatigue, palpitations, or skin changes. Complaints of pain require further evaluation including onset, duration, character, location, radiation, alleviating factors, aggravating factors, and accompanying signs or symptoms. Past medical history should also be reviewed including previous illnesses, surgical procedures, or hospitalizations. Family history should be evaluated including hereditary, familial diseases that pertain to the cardiovascular system. Assessment of social history includes smoking habits, alcohol consumption, chemical dependence, occupation, educational level, and support system.

General physical assessment involves use of inspection, palpation, percussion, and auscultation to determine the presence or absence of signs and symptoms associated with cardiac disease. Additional noninvasive assessment parameters include level of consciousness, blood pressure, hemoglobin oxygen saturation, electrocardiographic findings, and urinary output.

Invasive monitoring may be indicated for selected patients in order to more accurately assess hemodynamic function and adequacy of cardiac output. In such cases, the nurse is responsible for gathering and preparing appropriate equipment, assisting the physician during insertion, and supporting the patient. (See "Procedure for Assisting with Invasive Hemodynamic Monitoring in Obstetrics," page 317) In addition, thorough understanding of the principles of hemodynamic monitoring enables the nurse to interpret patient data, plan care, and initiate appropriate interventions.

Invasive hemodynamic monitoring may be accomplished via use of a central venous pressure or pulmonary artery catheter. The description, assessment capabilities, and associated complications for each follow.

The central venous pressure catheter is a single or multiple lumen catheter advanced through a peripheral or central vein until the tip is in the proximal superior vena cava (Figure 11-2). The internal jugular vein is used most often for central venous access because of the increased risk of pneumothorax with subclavian attempts during pregnancy. Use of this catheter permits evaluation of right preload, expressed in mmHg as central venous pressure, as well as access for administration of fluid or medications. The primary limitation is that right ventricular function may not accurately reflect left ventricular function, especial-

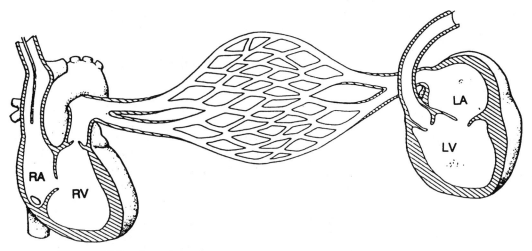

Figure 11-2. Central venous pressure catheter location. From Darovic, GO. *Hemodynamic monitoring: Invasive and noninvasive clinical application.* Philadelphia, WB Saunders, 1987. Reproduced with permission.

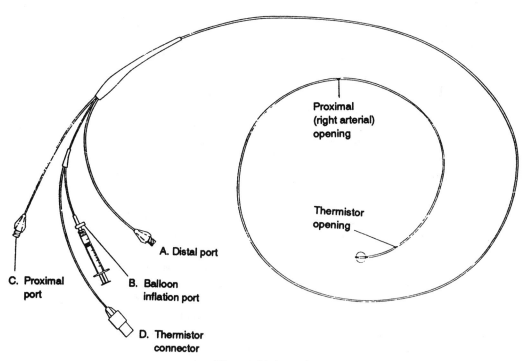

Figure 11-3. Pulmonary artery catheter.

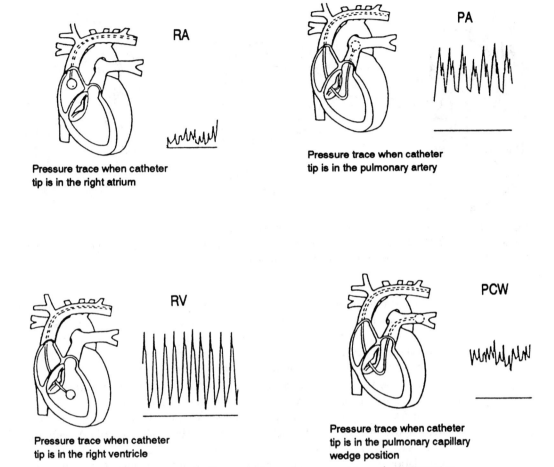

RA

Pressure trace when catheter
tip is in the right atrium

PA

Pressure trace when catheter
tip is in the pulmonary artery

RV

Pressure trace when catheter
tip is in the right ventricle

PCW

Pressure trace when catheter
tip is in the pulmonary capillary
wedge position

Figure 11-4. Waveforms during pulmonary artery catheter insertion.

ly in the patient with cardiac disease. Complications include trauma during establishment of venous access and infection related to the duration of invasive monitoring.

The pulmonary artery, or Swan-Ganz, catheter is a balloon-tipped, flow-directed, multiple lumen catheter (Figure 11-3). It is introduced through a central vein into the pulmonary artery. Characteristic waveforms may be visualized as the catheter tip passes through various cardiac structures (Figure 11-4). Following insertion, the catheter rests in the pulmonary artery with the balloon tip deflated. Use of this catheter permits continuous evaluation of pressures of the central vein and pulmonary artery. Intermittent inflation of the balloon permits evaluation of pulmonary capillary wedge pressure. This provides information regarding left preload by simulating closure of the pulmonic valve (Figure 11-5). Intermittent evaluation of cardiac output may also be conducted utilizing ther-

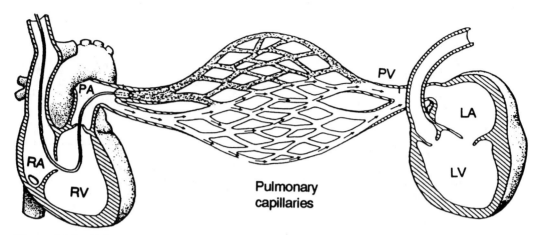

Figure 11-5. Pulmonary artery catheter location during assessment of pulmonary capillary wedge pressure. From Darovic, GO. *Hemodynamic monitoring: Invasive and noninvasive clinical application.* Philadelphia, WB Saunders, 1987. Reproduced with permission.

modilution technology. Other hemodynamic data may be derived through calculations based on the preceding basic parameters. Normal hemodynamic values during pregnancy are presented in Table 11-2.[34] Complications include trauma during establishment of venous access, infection related to the duration of monitoring, and arrhythmias during insertion as the catheter tip passes through the right ventricle. Rare complications include catheter knotting, pulmonary artery rupture, thromboembolism, and balloon rupture.

Cardiac disease in pregnancy is classified as a high-risk condition, thus including all the special psychosocial problems previously described with these groups of patients (see Chapter 4). In addition, fear, anxiety, and pain associated with labor and delivery may further compromise hemodynamic status via re-

TABLE 11-2
Normal Hemodynamic Values in Pregnancy

Parameter	Value and Standard Deviation
Cardiac output (liter/minute)	6.2 ± 1.0
Systemic vascular resistance (dyne/sec/cm^{-5})	1210 ± 266
Pulmonary vascular resistance (dyne/sec/cm^{-5})	78 ± 22
Mean pulmonary artery pressure (mmHg)	13 ± 2
Pulmonary capillary wedge pressure (mmHg)	7.5 ± 1.8
Central venous pressure (mmHg)	3.6 ± 2.5
Left ventricular stroke work index (g/m/m^{-2})	48 ± 6

lease and circulation of catecholamines. Psychosocial assessment includes evaluation of maternal anxiety level and availability of support resources.

Nursing Diagnoses

Identification of actual or potential diagnoses facilitates planning of appropriate nursing care. The following may be useful when caring for the pregnant woman with cardiac disease:

- Potential for congestive heart failure and pulmonary edema related to:
  Increased preload
  Increased afterload
- Potential for altered cardiac output: decreased, related to:
  Mechanical or structural factors
  Arrhythmias
  Congestive heart failure and pulmonary edema
- Potential for thromboembolism related to:
  Valvular defects
  Decreased venous return
  Hypercoagulability of pregnancy
- Potential for impaired gas exchange related to:
  Pulmonary venous congestion
  Pulmonary edema
  Thromboembolism
- Potential for increased oxygen demands and cardiac workload related to:
  Pain
  Anxiety and fear
  Infection
- Potential for infection related to:
  Pulmonary congestion
  Invasive hemodynamic monitoring
  Valvular disease
- Potential for spontaneous or iatrogenic preterm labor and delivery related to:
  Maternal hypoxemia
  Worsening maternal condition
- Altered comfort level and anxiety
- Potential for fetal hypoxia

Theoretical Basis for the Plan of Nursing Care and Intervention

The primary goal of nursing care for the patient with cardiac disease is promotion of adequate cardiac output to meet maternal and fetal demands. General issues that must be addressed in planning intrapartum care include route of delivery, use of anesthesia, hemodynamic monitoring, and antibiotic prophylaxis.

Vaginal delivery is preferable for most patients with cardiac disease, with cesarean section reserved for obstetric indications. Induction of labor at term may be preferable in order to promote a controlled course of labor and delivery, as well as coordinate medical and nursing regimes. In such instances, the patient may be admitted a day prior to induction to optimize hemodynamic function.

Conduction anesthesia, appropriate for most patients with cardiac disease, blunts changes in heart rate and cardiac output associated with pain. It also decreases preload secondary to peripheral vasodilation. Care must be exercised to avoid hypotension and subsequent reduction in preload, which may adversely influence cardiac output.

Invasive hemodynamic monitoring is indicated for patients with NYHA class III or IV disease. Pulmonary artery catheterization is most frequently the preferred method of surveillance (Figure 11-6). Hemodynamic alterations associated with labor, delivery, and the immediate postpartum period should be considered when interpreting data (Table 11-3). The nurse should frequently evaluate the patient for signs and symptoms of complications related to invasive monitoring and implement measures to reduce such risks. (See "Procedure for Assisting with Invasive Hemodynamic Monitoring in Obstetrics," page 317.)

Antibiotic prophylaxis is administered because patients with known cardiac defects may develop endocarditis during invasive procedures predisposing to

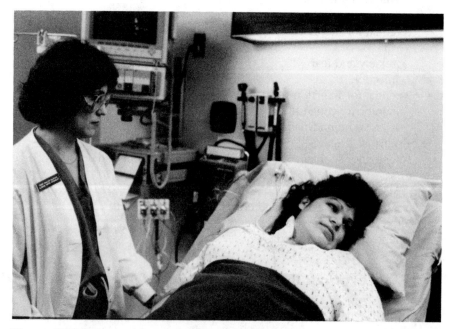

Figure 11-6. Intrapartum invasive hemodynamic monitoring with the pulmonary artery catheter.

TABLE 11-3
Cardiac Output during Normal Labor and Delivery

Stage of Labor	Cardiac Output (%)
Early first*	15
Late first*	30
Second*	45
Postpartum—5 minutes	65
Postpartum—60 minutes	40

*An additional 15% increase accompanies each uterine contraction.

bacteremia. Positive blood cultures have been reported to occur in up to 5% of uncomplicated vaginal deliveries.[35–37] Bacteremia may be more frequent following cesarean section depending on circumstances and indications of operative delivery. Despite the American Hospital Association's opinion that prophylaxis is not necessary for patients with valvular heart disease undergoing vaginal delivery, many physicians prefer to order prophylaxis in light of the risk–benefit ratio. Current recommendations for prophylaxis are presented in Table 11-4.[38]

Additional nursing issues may be identified when providing care for intrapartum patients with cardiac disease. These include the following:

- Single room care if possible
- Sufficient space to accommodate specialized procedures and equipment
- Proper positioning of patient to optimize cardiac output
- Administration of drugs as ordered to optimize hemodynamic function
- Regulation of all intravenous fluids with infusion pump
- Frequent assessments of intake and output
- Avoidance of hypotension
- Investigation of cause of tachycardia
- Anticipation of autotransfusion following delivery
- Avoidance of the lithotomy position during the second stage of labor

Patients with mitral stenosis require sufficient preload and diastolic filling times in order to maintain adequate cardiac output. Therefore, lateral position-

TABLE 11-4
Recommendations for Bacterial Endocarditis Prophylaxis

Ampicillin 2 g intravenously and Gentamicin 1.5 mg/kg/intravenously OR	30 Minutes prior to delivery
Vancomycin 1 g intravenously and Gentamicin 1.5 mg/kg/intravenously	30 Minutes to 1 hour prior to delivery Every 8 hours for 3 dosages

ing during labor should be encouraged. Left preload values, expressed as pulmonary capillary wedge pressures, are generally maintained between 12 and 14 mmHg and the heart rate kept below 100 beats per minute. Propranolol may be ordered for sustained maternal tachycardia. Epidural anesthesia is often utilized, and hypotension is avoided. Due to postpartum autotransfusion and the concomitant increased risk of left ventricular overload and pulmonary edema, lithotomy positioning for delivery should be undertaken with caution.

Patients with hemodynamically significant aortic stenosis, in order to maintain adequate cardiac output, must have a margin of safety in left ventricular end diastolic volume and avoid hypotension. Any event leading to decreased venous return may result in cardiovascular decompensation. Lateral patient positioning for labor should be encouraged. It is common for these women to have associated ischemic heart disease; therefore electrocardiographic monitoring may be ordered. Left preload (wedge pressure) is usually maintained in the range of 16 to 18 mmHg to help protect against the results of unexpected blood loss.

Pulmonary hypertension represents a unique nursing challenge as maternal risks are significant. Induction under controlled circumstances is usually undertaken. Systemic hypotension leads to decreased right ventricular filling pressures that may be inadequate to perfuse the pulmonary arterial bed. Profound hypoxemia and death may result. It is therefore crucial to maintain adequate right preload and to include a margin of safety. Epidural anesthesia is administered with caution as a result of the risks of hypotension.

Expected Outcomes

During the intrapartum period, the patient with cardiac disease will do the following:

1. Maintain adequate cardiac output to meet maternal demand
2. Maintain optimal hemodynamic parameters
3. Maintain adequate gas exchange and tissue perfusion
4. Exhibit normal electrocardiographic findings
5. Exhibit no signs or symptoms of thromboembolism
6. Exhibit no signs or symptoms of infection
7. Maintain reassuring fetal heart rate responses

References

1. Cunningham FG, MacDonald PC, Gant NF: *Williams' Obstetrics* (18th ed.). Norwalk, CT, Appleton & Lange, 1989, p. 779.
2. Oakley CM: Pregnancy and heart disease: Pre-existing heart disease. *Cardiovas Clin* 19:57, 1989.
3. Gilstrap LC: Heart disease during pregnancy. *Clin Obstet Gynecol* 32:1, 1989.
4. Metcalfe J, McAnulty JH, Ueland K: *Burwell and Metcalfe's Heart Disease and Pregnancy: Physiology and Management* (2nd ed.). Boston, Little, Brown, 1986, p. 116.

5. Mitchell SC, Korones SB, Berendes HW: Congenital heart disease in 56,109 births: Incidence and natural history. *Circulation* 43:323, 1971.

6. Ullery JC: Management of pregnancy complicated by heart disease. *Am J Obstet Gynecol* 67:834, 1954.

7. Ueland K: Cardiovascular diseases complicating pregnancy. *Clin Obstet Gynecol* 21:429, 1978.

8. Shime J, Mocarski EJM, Hastings D, et al: Congenital heart disease in pregnancy: Short- and long-term implications. *Am J Obstet Gynecol* 156:313, 1987.

9. Elkayam U, Cobb T, Gleicher N: Congenital heart disease and pregnancy, in Elkayam U, Gleicher N (eds.): *Cardiac Problems in Pregnancy: Diagnosis and Management of Maternal and Fetal Disease* (2nd ed.). New York, Alan Liss, 1990, p. 73.

10. Veasy LG, Wiedmeier SE, Orsmond GS, et al: Resurgence of acute rheumatic fever in the intermountain area of the United States. *N Engl J Med* 316:421, 1987.

11. Szekely P, Turner R, Smith L: Pregnancy and the changing pattern of rheumatic heart disease. *Br Heart J* 35:1293, 1973.

12. Ginz B: Myocardial infarction in pregnancy. *J Obstet Gynecol Br Commonw* 77:610, 1970.

13. Hankins GDV, Wendel GD, Leveno KJ, et al: Myocardial infarction in pregnancy: A review. *Obstet Gynecol* 65:139, 1985.

14. Homans DC: Peripartum cardiomyopathy. *N Engl J Med* 312:1432, 1985.

15. Sanderson JE, Andesanya CD, Anjorin FI, et al: Postpartum cardiac failure: Heart failure due to volume overload? *Am Heart J* 97:613, 1979.

16. Pyeritz RE, McKusick VA: The Marfan syndrome, diagnosis and management. *N Engl J Med* 300:772, 1979.

17. Gianopoulos JG: Cardiac disease in pregnancy. *Med Clin N America* 73:639, 1989.

18. Clark SL: Structural cardiac disease in pregnancy, in Clark SL, Hankins GDV, Cotton DB, Phelan JP (eds.): *Critical Care Obstetrics* (2nd ed). Boston, Blackwell 1991.

19. Criteria Committee of the New York Heart Association: *Nomenclature and Criteria for Diagnosis of Diseases of the Heart and Great Vessels* (8th ed.). New York, New York Heart Association, 1979.

20. Selzer, A: Risks of pregnancy in women with cardiac disease. *JAMA* 238:892, 1977.

21. Sobrevilla LA, Cassinelli MT, Carcelen A, et al: Human fetal and maternal oxygen tension and acid-base status during delivery at high altitude. *Am J Obstet Gynecol* 111:1111, 1971.

22. Whittemore R, Hobbins JC, Engle MA: Pregnancy and its outcome in women with and without surgical treatment of congenital disease. *Am J Cardiol* 50:641, 1982.

23. Brady K, Duff P: Rheumatic heart disease in pregnancy. *Clin Obstet Gynecol* 32:21, 1989.

24. McAnulty JH, Morton MJ, Ueland K: The heart and pregnancy. *Curr Prob Cardiol* 13:589, 1988.

25. Kumar A, Eklayam U: Hypertrophic cardiomyopathy in pregnancy, in Elkayam U, Gleicher N (eds.): *Cardiac Problems in Pregnancy: Diagnosis and Management of Maternal and Fetal Disease* (2nd ed.). New York, Alan Liss, 1990, pp. 129–136.

26. Ramin SM, Maberry MC, Gilstrap LC: Congenital heart disease. *Clin Obstet Gynecol* 32:41, 1989.

27. Nora JJ, Nora AH, Wexler P: Hereditary and environmental aspects as they affect the fetus and newborn. *Clin Obstet Gynecol* 24:851, 1981.

28. Coburn AF, Young DC: The Epidemiology of Hemolytic Streptococcus During World War II in the United States Navy. Baltimore, Williams & Wilkins, 1949, p. 170.

29. Stetson CA: The relation of antibody response to rheumatic fever, in McCarty M (ed.): *Streptococcal Infections*. New York, Columbia University Press, 1954, p. 208.

30. Taranta A, Spagnuolo M, Feinstein AR: Chronic rheumatic fever. *Ann Intern Med* 56:367, 1962.

31. Goldman ME, Meller J: Coronary artery disease in pregnancy, in Elkayam U, Gleicher N (eds.): *Cardiac Problems in Pregnancy: Diagnosis and Management of Maternal and Fetal Disease* (2nd ed.). New York, Alan Liss, 1990, pp. 153–165.

32. Nolan TE, Hankins GDV: Myocardial infarction in pregnancy. *Clin Obstet Gynecol* 32:68, 1989.

33. De Angelis R: The cardiovascular system, in Alspach JG, Williams SM (eds.): *Core Curriculum for Critical Care Nursing* (3rd ed.). Philadelphia, WB Saunders, 1985, pp. 101–118.

34. Clark SL, Cotton DB, Lee W, et al: Central hemodynamic assessment of normal term pregnancy. *Am J Obstet Gynecol* 161:1439, 1989.

35. Redleaf PD, Fadell EJ: Bacteremia during parturition. *JAMA* 169:1284, 1984.

36. McCormack WM, Rosner B, Lee YH, et al: Isolation of genital mycoplasmas from blood obtained shortly after vaginal delivery. *Lancet* 1:596, 1975.
37. Sugrue D, Blake S, Troy P, et al: Antibiotic prophylaxis against infective endocarditis after normal delivery: Is it necessary? *Br Heart J* 44:499, 1980.
38. Cox SM, Leveno KJ: Pregnancy complicated by bacterial endocarditis. *Clin Obstet Gynecol* 32:1, 1989.

12.

◆ ◆ ◆

Pulmonary Disorders in Pregnancy

Karen Dorman

Supportive Data

The incidence of primary pulmonary disorders in the pregnant population is rare. More commonly, they occur as a consequence of other disease processes and include disorders such as pulmonary edema, pulmonary embolisms, and adult respiratory distress syndrome (ARDS). Pneumonia of viral or bacterial etiology or as a result of gastric aspiration may also occur during pregnancy. However, it is difficult to accurately ascertain the incidence of each of these disorders since they often represent varying degrees of the same ongoing process. For example, amniotic fluid embolism often results in the development of pulmonary edema which may progress to ARDS. In addition, many pulmonary disorders have similar symptoms and may require invasive testing to confirm the diagnosis. Therefore, misdiagnosis and unconfirmed diagnosis also contribute to an underestimation of the true incidence.

The overall incidence of pulmonary edema in pregnancy is unclear. However, it has been reported that patients receiving intravenous betamimetic therapy for preterm labor have a 5% incidence of cardiogenic pulmonary edema due to sodium and water retention.[1] The incidence is as high as 50% for pregnancies of twins treated with betamimetics. Additionally, an increased incidence of noncardiogenic pulmonary edema has been reported when preterm labor was associated with maternal infection.[2] Bacterial pneumonia occurs in 0.04% to 1% of the pregnant population.[3] Deep vein thrombosis, the most common causative factor of pulmonary embolism, occurs with the same incidence in the antepartum period as in nonpregnant patients.[4] However, the incidence in the postpartum period increases by 3 to 8 times. The incidence of amniotic fluid embolism is reported to be 1 in 8000 to 80,000 deliveries.[5] Adult respiratory distress syndrome occurs in a small number of pregnant patients. However, its exact incidence is difficult to determine since it is not a primary process and actually represents the end point of many different pulmonary disorders.

Significance

Although relatively uncommon, pulmonary disorders during pregnancy may result in significant maternal morbidity and mortality. Cardiogenic pulmonary edema, when detected early, can be easily reversed. However, when pulmonary edema is due to cardiac failure or occurs in the presence of other complicating factors, reversal is much more difficult. Noncardiogenic pulmonary edema requires complex therapeutic intervention. Thus, severe cardiogenic and noncardiogenic pulmonary edema carry high morbidity. Pneumonia is a relatively common entity that carries moderately low morbidity and mortality since the introduction of antibiotics.[6] The clinical course of women in labor with pneumonia is dependent on many factors, such as the organism involved, the resistance of the host, prompt diagnosis, and treatment. Pneumonia resulting from aspiration of gastric contents has been reported as the cause of death in as many as 50% of maternal deaths in Great Britain.[7] The complications that arise as a result of gastric aspiration are dependent on the amount and the acidity of the gastric contents. The greater the amount and the greater the acidity, the more damage done. The clinical course may be apparent within minutes or may evolve over several hours. Noncardiogenic pulmonary edema, bronchospasm, atelectasis, decreased airway compliance, and, even, hypotension may occur.[8]

Two pulmonary disorders occurring during pregnancy, amniotic fluid embolism and ARDS, are associated with substantial morbidity and mortality. Mortality associated with amniotic fluid embolism is as high as 86%, the majority consisting of those dying within the first two hours after the incident.[9] If the patient survives the initial insult, disseminated intravascular coagulation occurs to some extent in up to 100% of patients with amniotic fluid embolism.[5,10] Pulmonary edema also occurs in a large percentage of these patients. The incidence of death in patients with ARDS has been reported as high as 67%.[11]

Significant maternal hypoxemia places the fetus at increased risk for morbidity or mortality. The placenta serves as the organ of respiration for the fetus with the exchange of oxygen and carbon dioxide occurring as a passive process. The oxygen supply available to the fetus is dependent on adequate maternal arterial oxygen content (Pao_2), placental perfusion, and fetal saturation of hemoglobin. Removal of carbon dioxide is dependent on fetal blood flow to the placenta, subsequent diffusion of carbon dioxide, and uptake by the maternal circulation. (Normal umbilical cord blood gases are listed in Table 12-1.)

Several mechanisms exist that facilitate fetal adaptation to brief periods of maternal hypoxemia. First, diffusion of oxygen to the fetus is enhanced due to elevation of maternal Pao_2 and reduction of arterial carbon dioxide concentration ($Paco_2$) associated with pregnancy. In addition, fetal hemoglobin has a stronger affinity for oxygen than does maternal hemoglobin and fetal hematocrit levels are higher than adult hematocrit levels. Finally, the fetus exhibits a com-

TABLE 12-1
Normal Umbilical Blood Gases Reported
as Average, Standard Deviation, and Ranges

	Umbilical Venous	Umbilical Arterial
*p*H	7.35 ± 0.05	7.28 ± 0.05
	(7.24 − 7.49)	(7.15 − 7.43)
P$_{CO_2}$ (mmHg)	38.2 ± 5.6	49.2 ± 8.4
	(23.2 − 49.2)	(31.1 − 74.3)
P$_{O_2}$ (mmHg)	29.2 ± 5.9	18.0 ± 6.2
	(15.4 − 48.2)	(3.8 − 33.8)
HCO$_3$ (mEq/liter)	20.4 ± 2.1	22.3 ± 2.5
	(15.9 − 24.7)	(13.3 − 27.5)

Source: From American College of Obstetricians and Gynecologists:
Assessment of fetal and newborn acid-base status. *ACOG Tech Bull* 127,
Apr. 1989.

pensatory mechanism that shunts blood flow to the brain and heart in the presence of hypoxic stress.

Chronic maternal hypoxemia, however, may result in failure of these compensatory responses and can lead to fetal hypoxia, acidosis, or death. Other complications include polycythemia and intrauterine growth retardation. Fetal hypoxia often results in the passage of meconium from the gastrointestinal tract, which if aspirated by the fetus during labor or delivery may cause respiratory distress syndrome.

Pulmonary edema is defined as an abnormal accumulation of water—more than may be drained by the lymphatic system—in the extravascular portions of the lung, which may involve both the interstitial and alveolar spaces.[12] Although not always clinically obvious until moderate in severity, it is frequently an early finding in the progression of many other disease processes.

Normally, the pulmonary capillaries are permeable to fluid, and there is constant movement of fluid across the capillary membrane into the interstitial spaces and back into the capillaries. The flow of fluid is regulated by the balance of two opposing forces. Pulmonary capillary hydrostatic pressure forces fluid out of the vessels, and plasma oncotic pressure pulls fluid into the vessels by the attraction of fluid to protein molecules in the blood. Pulmonary hydrostatic pressure is greater in the arterioles, and plasma oncotic pressure is greater in the venules. These two forces are usually balanced. The lymphatic system is also available to absorb any excess fluid that may accumulate in the interstitial space. This balanced system may be altered primarily by two mechanisms. An increase in capillary hydrostatic pressure results in cardiogenic pulmonary edema, and an increase in the permeability of the capillary membrane results in noncardiogenic pulmonary edema. Both mechanisms cause excess fluid accumulation

Etiology

in the extravascular compartment, the interstitial spaces, and the alveoli. Although the end result is the same, therapy is directed toward the causative factor. If inappropriately identified, treatment may be detrimental to the patient.

Cardiogenic, or hydrostatic, *pulmonary edema,* as the name implies, occurs as a result of heart dysfunction. The causes of ventricular failure in obstetrics include elevated preload, most frequently related to iatrogenic fluid overload; decreased contractility, secondary to myocardial infarction or cardiomyopathy; and elevated afterload, related to aortic stenosis or severe hypertension.[13,14] Regardless of the cause of left ventricular failure, the left ventricle becomes unable to empty efficiently and fluid accumulates, which results in an elevated pressure. As the ventricular failure continues, the left atrial pressure rises, which increases capillary hydrostatic pressure forcing excessive fluid into the extravascular spaces. The condition worsens as alveoli fill with fluid.

In contrast, noncardiogenic pulmonary edema is caused by increased pulmonary capillary permeability, does not involve heart dysfunction, and is referred to as *nonhydrostatic pulmonary edema.* It occurs as a result of physical or chemical damage of the pulmonary vascular membrane, which allows fluid as well as protein molecules to escape into the extravascular spaces. The causes of noncardiogenic pulmonary edema in obstetrics include aspiration of gastric contents, sepsis, blood transfusion reactions, disseminated intravascular coagulation, and amniotic fluid embolism.[14] The increased protein content in the extravascular spaces attracts additional fluid, which increases the pulmonary edema. This process results in a clinical picture similar to cardiogenic pulmonary edema.

Pneumonia in pregnancy may result from aspiration of gastric contents as well as viral or bacterial pathogens. In general, pneumonia is not tolerated as well by pregnant women as it is by nonpregnant women. Gastric aspiration occurs most commonly during intubation for general anesthesia but may also occur during eclamptic seizures. Pregnant women are at increased risk for aspiration due to the relaxation of the gastroesophogeal sphincter and displacement of the stomach by the uterus to a horizontal angle. In addition, there is an increase in gastric acid secretion and a decrease in gastric motility. Sedatives used in labor may decrease normal reflexes, thereby further increasing risk.

Bacterial pneumonia is rarely seen in patients with intact immune systems. The incidence increases if defense mechanisms are altered (*e.g.,* by a decrease in mechanical barriers from intubation, by decreased clearance of organisms due to poor cilial function as a result of smoking or certain viral infections, and by decreased immune response due to immunosuppressive drugs or chronic anemia).[3] The most common causative organism is *Streptococcus pneumoniae,* but other pathogens include *Haemophilus influenzae, Staphylococcus aureus,* and *Klebsiella pneumoniae. Mycoplasma pneumoniae* produces a slow-onset pneumonia, which is accompanied by low-grade fever that frequently abates without treatment. Viral pneumonia usually occurs as a complication of other diseases such as influenza, varicella, and measles.

Pulmonary embolism refers to the condition where a plug composed of a detached clot, bacteria, or other foreign body occludes a blood vessel in the pulmonary circulation. Two types reported during pregnancy are thromboembolism and amniotic fluid embolism. Deep vein thrombosis is the most common predisposing condition for pulmonary embolism and obstetric patients are at high risk for deep vein thrombosis because of increased venous stasis as well as the hypercoagulable state of pregnancy. Patients with documented deep venous thrombosis require heparin therapy until after delivery, with brief interruption of therapy around the delivery. Pulmonary thromboembolism results when a portion of a clot is dislodged from the venous circulation and migrates into the pulmonary vasculature where it occludes a pulmonary arteriole, preventing blood flow and infarcting the area beyond the clot.[15]

Though the exact mechanism remains unclear, amniotic fluid embolism results from escape of amniotic fluid into the maternal venous circulation. Several factors common to the majority of reported cases of amniotic fluid embolism include average maternal age of 32 years, multiparity, strong uterine contractions, significant amount of particulate matter in the amniotic fluid, larger than average fetus, stillbirths, and premature placental separation.[9] Detection of fetal squamous cells, hair, lanugo, and mucin in maternal blood is the cornerstone for diagnosis, with many cases diagnosed at autopsy. However, several clinicians have reported finding fetal squamous cells in blood aspirated from the pulmonary artery in patients without symptoms.[16,17] Many have suggested the primary finding is severe pulmonary arterial vasospasm as a result of amniotic fluid entering the lungs, followed by severe noncardiogenic pulmonary edema.[10,18,35] However, Clark and co-workers reexamined the findings of earlier clinicians and concluded that the elevation of pulmonary capillary wedge pressures and pulmonary arterial pressure were secondary to left ventricular dysfunction.[19]

Adult respiratory distress syndrome—previously referred to as shock lung, hemorrhagic pulmonary edema, and pump lung—was first described in 1967.[20] Diagnosis is made in patients with moderate-to-severe hypoxemia, bilateral diffuse infiltrates, no history of primary pulmonary disease, presence of a predisposing disease, and no increase in left atrial pressure. Other symptoms include cyanosis and decreased pulmonary compliance. Onset of the disease process becomes obvious several hours to several days following the initial insult. Predisposing factors include severe pulmonary edema, aspiration pneumonia, sepsis, pulmonary trauma, multiple transfusions, and pulmonary embolism.[21,22]

Framework for Accepted Therapy

Planning and provision of nursing care require an understanding first of normal respiratory function. *Ventilation* refers to the actual movement of air in and out of the lungs. *External respiration* refers to the oxygen exchange at the alveolar level, and *internal respiration* refers to the gas exchange at the cellular level. Although technically three separate entities, in reality it is difficult to separate these processes. The lungs have approximately 300 million alveoli that are composed of 90% type I alveolar epithelial cells and 10% type II alveolar epithelial cells. Type I cells are involved with the transfer of gas across the capillary membrane, are easily destroyed by injury, and do not regenerate. By contrast, type II alveolar cells produce and store surfactant, a phospholipid that prevents the collapse of the alveoli at end expiration and maintains elasticity of the lung. They can also regenerate and even become type I alveolar cells if there is a need. When surfactant is diminished, atelectasis occurs and diffusion is impaired. Sighing helps expand alveoli and spread surfactant into the distal areas of the lung not well ventilated with every breath.

Each alveolus is completely surrounded by a dense network of capillaries, each of which allows one red blood cell to pass at a time. As a red blood cell passes through the capillaries, it is exposed to approximately three alveoli in three fourths of a second. During this time, the oxygen saturation increases from 75% (normal mixed venous) to greater than 97% saturation (normal arterial blood). This saturation can occur in one fourth of a second in cases of tachycardia.[23] Oxygen and carbon dioxide diffuse easily across the alveolar capillary membrane; however, diffusion is decreased when the membrane is thickened as in ARDS and cardiogenic pulmonary edema.

Exchange of oxygen and carbon dioxide occurs by a process of diffusion, defined as movement from an area of high concentration to an area of low concentration to reach an equilibrium. The majority of oxygen is carried by the hemoglobin molecules (measured as oxygen saturation) with approximately 1–2% dissolved in plasma (measured as Pao_2).[24] As oxygen molecules dissolved in plasma diffuse into the tissue cells, more oxygen is released from hemoglobin molecules to be dissolved into plasma. Hemoglobin has a rather constant affinity for oxygen, though at a lower Pao_2 oxygen is more quickly released from hemoglobin to the tissues. At higher levels of Pao_2, the saturation of the hemoglobin molecules remains essentially constant. In conditions such as fever, increased $Paco_2$ (hypercarbia), and acidosis, hemoglobin dissociation is enhanced, which allows more oxygen to be released for use by the tissues. The opposite is true in conditions such as hypothermia, alkalemia, and hypocarbia. Oxygen delivery to the tissues is also affected by cardiac output and hemoglobin.

Another important aspect in ventilation is the movement of gas into and out of the alveoli. The diaphragm does approximately 80% of the work of ventilation during normal inhalation, and exhalation is a passive process. As the diaphragm contracts, the pleural cavity enlarges, creating a negative pressure that allows air to rush in. The pulmonary circuit is the largest vasculature of the body and generates a systolic and diastolic pressure far lower than those of the systemic circulation. The increase in plasma volume seen in pregnancy does not affect pulmonary pressure. Changes in intrathoracic pressure caused by maternal hyperventilation or positive pressure ventilation cause a profound variation in pulmonary pressure. This effect should be considered if invasive monitoring is to be used.

The pulmonary circuit is so intricate that hypoxemia can result from many different causes. The three most common categories are shunt, alveolar hypoventilation, and ventilation and perfusion inequality. The term *shunt* refers to a condition in which blood enters the arterial system without passing through ventilated parts of the lungs.[24] Shunts can be caused by congenital cardiac defects or arteriovenous fistulas. However, shunting can also be due to hypoventilation of a portion of the lung as occurs in atelectasis with alveolar collapse, pneumonia causing alveolar consolidation, and/or excessive mucous production as in chronic bronchitis. Hypoxemic patients with true shunts are not able to increase the Pao_2 to normal limits even with the administration of 100% oxygen. When the amount of oxygen available in the alveoli is less than required by the metabolic processes in the tissues, alveolar hypoventilation is the cause. In most cases this is also associated with an elevated $Paco_2$. Causes include reduced chest expansion, depressed central nervous system function, and lung expansion restriction. Oxygen therapy will benefit this condition; however, mechanical ventilation is often required.

Ventilation/perfusion (V/Q) inequality occurs when the alveoli are underventilated or underperfused. Common causes of V/Q mismatch are chronic obstructive lung disease, asthma, pneumonia, and pulmonary thromboembolism. Administration of oxygen is beneficial in these patients.[23]

Many of the shunts described here reflect impairment of gas exchange. The most common is fluid in the lungs as in cardiogenic and noncardiogenic pulmonary edema. Another problem with gas exchange occurs in ARDS when the interstitial membrane thickens and prevents the diffusion process from occurring. With these patients, perfusion is normal but ventilation is impaired. Thus, shunt also refers to the portion of the lung that is not able to oxygenate the blood.

The goal of treatment for specific pulmonary disorders in pregnancy is determined by the cause of the disorder and the severity of respiratory compromise. In patients with cardiogenic or hydrostatic pulmonary edema, insertion of a pulmonary artery catheter reveals an elevated pulmonary capillary wedge pressure, indicative of left ventricular failure, as well as increased pulmonary arterial pressures. The focus of treatment is improvement of left ventricular function and reduction of hydrostatic pressure with diuretics, inotropic medications, and afterload reduction with antihypertensives or possibly in combination, dependent on the primary problem. Patients with noncardiogenic pulmonary edema experience increased pulmonary capillary permeability. In contrast, insertion of a pulmonary artery catheter reveals normal-to-low pulmonary capillary wedge pressure. Since the permeability of the membrane cannot be manipulated, treatment is usually supportive in nature until membrane stabilization occurs.

Pneumonia in pregnancy resulting from gastric aspiration during intubation for general anesthesia may be prevented by the use of cricoid pressure during intubation (Sellick's maneuver). Administration of sodium citrate prior to intubation neutralizes the gastric acid present and may decrease the incidence of aspiration.[25,26] Anticholinergics, used to decrease gastric acid production, may take as long as 60 minutes to have the desired effect and are therefore not used.[27]

Once aspiration has occurred, treatment includes prompt suctioning and possibly bronchoscopy, if large particulate matter is involved. In the past, saline lavage was used but is contraindicated since it may actually spread aspirate throughout the lung. Though controversial, steroids and antibiotics are frequently given to stabilize the cellular membrane and prevent secondary bacterial infection. Prompt initiation of respiratory support including oxygen is imperative and, when necessary, mechanical ventilation is initiated. When the patient has bacterial pneumonia, broad spectrum antibiotic coverage pending sputum culture results and oxygen therapy are the mainstays of treatment.

Although pregnant women are not at great risk for contracting influenza, there is evidence that women in the third trimester are at increased risk for developing secondary viral pneumonia.[28] For high-risk patients such as those with cardiac or respiratory disease or a compromised immune system, vaccination is advisable since such infection may occasionally be fatal during pregnancy. Pneumonia generally occurs 2 to 3 days after infection with influenza and is treated with ribavirin. Patients are then carefully assessed for secondary bacterial infection. There is a 20% reported incidence of lung involvement in adults with varicella and in pregnant women this is associated with significant mortality.[29] Symptoms include dyspnea, cough, chest pain, and bloody sputum within 3 to 6 days of vesicular eruption. Acyclovir is the drug of choice for treatment of varicella pneumonia.

The treatment for pulmonary embolism includes heparin administration and supportive oxygen therapy as required. The most common symptoms of pulmonary embolism are tachypnea, dyspnea, chest discomfort, and apprehension. Since these symptoms are rather vague and indicative of many disease states, the presence of pulmonary embolism should be documented prior to instituting anticoagulant therapy. Diagnosis may be made with a V/Q scan, which reveals interruption of blood flow. If inconclusive, pulmonary angiography may be required.

Amniotic fluid embolism begins with such symptoms as severe dyspnea, chills, sweating, coughing, vomiting, and occasionally convulsions followed by cardiovascular and respiratory collapse. Initial treatment is aimed at restoring and maintaining cardiovascular and respiratory function and includes fluid and oxygen therapy, possibly mechanical ventilation, and administration of inotropic and vasoactive drugs.

Adult respiratory distress syndrome is characterized by severe pulmonary edema, pulmonary hemorrhage, formation of hyaline membranes, hyperplasia, and interstitial fibrosis.[22] Treatment is mainly supportive and includes mechanical ventilation, oxygen therapy with inspired oxygen concentration of 60% or less, and the use of positive end expiratory pressure to force fluid in the extravascular spaces back into the vessels and open collapsed alveoli.

Oxygen is the most frequently used and misused drug for patients with a pulmonary disorder, and it has both positive and detrimental effects. The goal of oxygen therapy is to achieve a Pao_2 of 70 to 100 mmHg with a hemoglobin saturation of at least 90%. The concentration required to treat patients is dependent on the total clinical picture including cardiac output and the amount and quality of hemoglobin. Once oxygen therapy is initiated, the patient is frequently assessed using arterial blood gases to decrease the oxygen concentration administered to the lowest therapeutic amount.

In addition to oxygen therapy, pharmacologic support may be administered to restore normal respiratory function. The drugs used in the treatment of pulmonary disorders vary according to the underlying problem. However, use of small amounts of sedation may be beneficial in most types of respiratory distress to quell the anxiety-triggered hyperventilation associated with air hunger. Morphine sulfate in small increments not only calms patients but has a relaxant effect on the pulmonary vasculature and slightly decreases venous return, which may be beneficial in disease states such as cardiogenic pulmonary edema. Care must be taken to monitor the effects as even mild overdosage could depress the respiratory center of the central nervous system thus decreasing the stimulus to breathe.

Another frequently used class of medication is steroids. Although use is often controversial, they are frequently used in the treatment of aspiration pneumonia, amniotic fluid embolism, and for many of the other precipitating causes of noncardiogenic pulmonary edema. The rationale for use of steroids is to decrease the local inflammatory response and stabilize the cellular membrane. They are usually instituted immediately after the initial insult and continued for several days afterward.

Antibiotic therapy is not routinely indicated for all pulmonary disorders. Many carry increased risk of infection either from the actual disease process as in bacterial or aspiration pneumonia or from manipulation of the airways permitting introduction of bacteria. In many pulmonary disorders, fluid and sputum accumulate in the alveoli, creating a facilitative medium for bacterial growth.

Assessment

Physical assessment of the patient with pulmonary complications should begin with a complete history. Symptoms such as shortness of breath, dyspnea, and chest pain, as well as explicit explanations of the severity and duration of these symptoms should be included. During an acute incident, the history remains important though relevant information should be gathered as quickly as possible from the patient or from another reliable source.

While gathering the patient's history, attention should be directed to general appearance, noting skin condition, ventilatory pattern, respiratory effort, and chest wall movement symmetry. Central cyanosis, if present, is a fairly late sign of hypoxia since it represents desaturation of greater than 5 gm/dl of blood in the capillaries.[30] This must be differentiated from peripheral cyanosis, which represents localized hypoxia.

Chest wall palpation may reveal tender areas and lumps. Assessment of tracheal position is important as deviation may signify a large pleural effusion, pneumothorax, or severe atelectasis. Presence of tactile fremitus, elicited via use of the palmar surface of the examiner's hands to evaluate vibrations caused by the patient's speech, may reveal pleural effusions or consolidation represented by increased and decreased vibrations, respectively. Respiratory excursion may be better evaluated using the examiner's hands placed on the patient's back to evaluate symmetry of movement. Pneumonia, pneumothorax, and splinting often cause asymmetrical movement.

Chest wall percussion is used to differentiate organ densities. The air-filled lung sounds resonant, whereas the stomach sounds tympanic and muscle sounds flat. Percussion should be performed especially on initial assessment, and abnormalities should be further investigated.

Auscultation of breath sounds is an important part of every physical examination. The quality and phases of respiration change throughout the lung fields as air moves from the trachea to the alveoli. The pattern of respiration as well as the presence or absence of adventitious sounds should be noted. The names of adventitious sounds have been simplified and are now referred to as *crackles, wheezes,* and *pleural friction rubs*. Crackles, previously referred to as rales, are caused by different pressures throughout the lung fields and opening of collapsed alveoli. They are only heard during inspiration. Wheezes are indicative of airway constriction and are heard throughout the respiratory cycle. Plural friction rubs are caused by irritated surfaces rubbing together causing a grating sound during inhalation and exhalation. Consolidation can best be detected by listening to the patient say, "*e,e,e*" or "ninety-nine," while listening to the posterior chest wall with a stethoscope. The sounds heard from a normal lung should be "*e,e,e*" and "*nin, nin*." If consolidation is present, the examiner would hear, "*a,a,a*" or "ninety-nine," clearly.

Evaluation of arterial blood gases is also an important step in the assessment of pulmonary disease. When interpreted correctly, they are helpful in determining the origin, chronicity, and severity of pulmonary dysfunction, as well as the patient's response to treatment. They should be obtained prior to initiation of therapy in order to establish a baseline. Patients requiring multiple arterial blood gases may benefit from an indwelling arterial catheter to reduce the risk of traumatic injury to the artery from repeated punctures. The Pao_2 value refers to the amount of oxygen dissolved in arterial blood. The normal range for adults on room air is 80 to 100 mmHg. The Pao_2 should be assessed first since, if low, oxygen supplementation is instituted immediately while the remainder of the values are assessed. The normal range of blood pH is 7.35 to 7.45. If less than 7.35, the patient is acidotic; if greater than 7.45, the patient is alkalotic. The next value examined is $Paco_2$ to determine respiratory acidosis, respiratory alkalosis, or normalcy. This value reflects the adequacy of ventilation; the normal range is 35 to 45 mmHg. The normal range for bicarbonate is 22 to 26 mEq/liter. A low bicarbonate level represents metabolic acidosis, and a high level is indicative of metabolic alkalosis. The blood gas values of the pregnant woman differ from those of a nonpregnant woman because of the normal change of hyperventilation of pregnancy; thus gases reflect a mild respiratory alkalosis.

Since many pulmonary disorders have vague or similar symptoms, additional tests are often required to differentiate the diagnoses. For the patient with pneumonia, sputum must be obtained for Gram's stain and culture, as well as a blood culture. Chest x-ray is one of the most commonly used tests, is easily performed, and can be done at the patient's bedside if necessary. X-rays make it possible to differentiate structures of different densities within the chest with bone being the most dense and air the least dense. Thus, bone and muscle appear white; blood and fluid, gray; and air, black. The presence and location of additional radiopaque items such as an endotracheal tube, pulmonary arterial catheter, and chest tubes can be documented with chest x-ray. The best view of the chest is the posteroanterior view, with patients standing and lungs fully expanded. This view is usually only available when the x-ray is taken in the radiology department. Portable film shows the anteroposterior view, with patients either upright or supine, and frequently not able to expand their lungs adequately. Thus the quality of film and clarity of structures are less than optimal and often inconclusive.

Ventilation/perfusion scans are most often used to diagnose pulmonary emboli. Hypothetically, in patients with normal pulmonary function, the ratio between ventilation and perfusion should be 1:1. However, due to normal physiological and anatomical shunting, there is always a mild mismatch. Patients with problems in either ventilation or perfusion would have a greater mismatch. The test is performed in two stages: first, perfusion and then ventilation. Radioactive dye is injected into the patient's vein, and the flow of dye through the pulmonary vasculature is reported through a cathode-ray tube, and photographs are taken. Obstructions to blood flow are usually representative of pulmonary embolism although tumors, pulmonary hypertension, arteriovenous fistulas, and vasculitis may also impede blood flow. Next the patient inhales a radioactive gas, and the distribution is carefully monitored. Ventilation abnormalities are suggestive of chronic obstructive pulmonary disease, pneumonia, severe pulmonary edema, cystic fibrosis, and airway obstruction. Portable V/Q scans are now available for critically ill patients.

Pulmonary function tests are used to quantify respiratory function, by actually measuring lung volume during normal and maximal ventilation. These tests are usually given to patients with known pulmonary disease or those who complain of dyspnea for baseline evaluation of lung mechanics to follow changes in respiratory function due to a chronic disease process. They are also performed for preoperative evaluation prior to surgery in patients with known pulmonary disease. The values routinely obtained are tidal volume, inspiratory reserve, inspiratory capacity, expiratory reserve volume, vital capacity, residual volume, functional reserve capacity, and total lung capacity. Patient understanding and cooperation are essential for measurement of many of these parameters.

An adjunct to the intermittent monitoring of arterial blood gases is continuous pulse oximetry. Hemoglobin saturated with oxygen absorbs more light than does unsaturated hemoglobin. Thus pulse oximetry introduces a beam of light into the capillary bed and measures the amount that is absorbed by the hemoglobin. The absorbed amount is indicative of the oxygen saturation of hemoglobin in the body. This value is not a substitute for arterial blood gases but can be used as additional information obtained on a continuous basis to monitor trends in the patient's condition.

Nursing Diagnoses

PULMONARY EDEMA (CARDIOGENIC)
- Ventilation and perfusion ratios, altered, related to excessive accumulation of fluid in alveoli
- Cardiac rhythm, altered, related to hypoxia, hypokalemia, medications or anxiety and concomitant disease
- Anxiety (acute), related to pain and discomfort, fear of suffocation
- Cardiac output, altered, related to left ventricular dysfunction
- Fluid and electrolyte imbalance, altered, related to diuretic therapy

ACUTE RESPIRATORY FAILURE (DUE TO AMNIOTIC FLUID EMBOLISM, PULMONARY EMBOLISM, ADULT RESPIRATORY DISTRESS SYNDROME)
- Anxiety related to dyspnea and fear of dying
- Airway clearance, ineffective, related to secretions, bronchial edema, bronchospasm, fibrosis, and parenchymal destruction
- Infection, related to retained secretions, use of respiratory equipment, impaired pulmonary defense system
- Impaired gas exchange, related to alveolar hypoventilation
- Tissue perfusion, altered: cardiopulmonary (decreased) related to embolism
- Gastrointestinal function, altered, related to ulcers and gastritis

MECHANICAL VENTILATION
- Anxiety related to disease process, diagnostic tests and procedures, therapy
  Mechanical ventilation
  Sensory deprivation (overload)
  Sleep deprivation
  Disorientation
  Inability to talk
- Breathing pattern, ineffective, related to ventilator malfunction, accidental extubation, barotrauma, pneumothorax
- Infection, potential for, related to bypass of normal filtering system
  Breach of aseptic technique for suctioning through tracheal tube
  Repeated traumatic or intrusive suctioning procedures
- Breathing pattern, ineffective, related to hyperventilation or hypoventilation

- Cardiac output, altered: decreased, related to increased intrathoracic pressures associated with mechanical ventilation (and, if used, positive end expiratory pressure)
- Gas exchange, impaired, related to oxygen toxicity secondary to high inspired oxygen concentrations
- Injury, potential for, related to pressure sores on side of mouth, nose, tracheostomy site, hyperplasia and inflammation, scarring and stenosis of trachea caused by trauma of endotracheal tube

Theoretical Basis for the Plan of Nursing Care and Intervention

Care of the woman in labor with pulmonary compromise is especially challenging since both mother and fetus are at risk for hypoxia. Adequate maternal oxygenation is important, however adequate cardiac output and placental perfusion are equally essential for fetal oxygenation. Oxygen should be administered in the required concentration via mask or cannula with patient comfort considered. The patient's respiratory status must be frequently assessed including rate, effort, skin color, and oxygen saturation via pulse oximetry. Arterial blood gases should be monitored if there is a change in respiratory status or therapy. Auscultation of breath sounds is required at least every 8 hours, more often if the patient's status changes. The fetus should be monitored closely for evidence of hypoxia, as reflected by abnormal fetal heart rate responses.

The method selected for oxygen delivery is dependent on the amount of oxygen required as well as patient comfort. It must be emphasized that the inspired concentration of oxygen is based on normal tidal volume and respiratory rate. Nasal cannulas are frequently used to deliver low concentrations of oxygen (*i.e.,* 1 to 5 liters/minute) or 24% to 44%. Cannulas are advantageous in that they are inexpensive, easy to use, and comfortable to wear. Higher flow rates should be avoided because of drying of the nasal mucosa. There have been concerns regarding the effectiveness of a nasal cannula with patients who predominantly breathe through their mouth, and studies have reported conflicting results.[31,32] In general, masks are less comfortable and many patients report a claustrophobic feeling. Simple masks are most commonly used for short-term oxygen therapy. They can deliver up to 60% oxygen, however actual concentration can be greater or more dilute as a result of the oxygen concentration of the exhaled air and rate of breathing. The mask may also be used for delivery of humidification or aerosol treatments.

The nonrebreathing mask has a reservoir and a one-way valve that prevent exhaled air from entering the reservoir bag. This mask requires a higher rate of flow (at least 8 liters/minute) to keep the reservoir bag inflated. A tightly fitting nonrebreathing mask can deliver 90% to 100% oxygen. However, due to loosely fitting masks and rapid respiratory rates, the concentration delivered is usually approximately 63%.[32] High-flow systems deliver all the air required by the patient, in addition to the proper concentration of oxygen from 24% to 100%. An advantage of this system is that respiratory rate and breathing pattern have no effect on the inspired oxygen concentration.

The Venturi mask is the most reliable mask for delivering exact oxygen concentrations, regardless of the patient's respiratory pattern. The mask delivers 100% oxygen at high velocity through an orifice the size of which can be adjusted to deliver different oxygen concentrations. The inspired oxygen concentration with various delivery devices are shown in Table 12-2.

Humidification of inspired air is necessary when the upper airway is bypassed as with intubation or when supplemental oxygen is required. It is important to prevent drying and irritation of the respiratory system, minimize fluid loss, and liquify secretions so they may be expectorated. Patients who already require ventilation are at greater risk for these complications. Humidification can be accomplished with warm or cold humidifiers, although cold humidifiers are only 50% effective.

Patients who have refractory hypoxemia or tissue hypoxia with supplemental oxygen therapy and are therefore unable to ventilate sufficiently require intubation and mechanical ventilation. The most commonly used ventilators are posi-

TABLE 12-2
Estimate of Delivered Oxygen Concentrations
with Low-Flow Oxygen Devices

100% O_2 Flow Rate (liter/minute)	Fi_{O_2}
Nasal Cannula	
1	0.24
2	0.28
3	0.32
4	0.36
5	0.40
6	0.44
O_2 Mask	
5–6	0.40
6–7	0.50
7–8	0.60
Mask with Reservoir Bag	
6	0.60
7	0.70
8	0.80
9	0.80+
10	0.80+

Note: Normal ventilatory patterns are assumed.
Source: From Shapiro BA, Harrison RA, Kacmarek RM, Cane RD: *Clinical Application of Respiratory Care*. Chicago, Year Book Medical Publishers, 1985.

tive pressure ventilators of which there are three types: volume cycled, pressure cycled, and time cycled. The volume-cycled ventilators are the most frequently used and work by delivering a preset volume of gas regardless of the patient's change in respiratory compliance. A pressure limit allows excess tidal volume to be shunted out through the tubing if pressure increases acutely.

Pressure-cycled ventilators are excellent for short-term use since they deliver gas until a preset pressure is reached. This ventilator is not used for patients requiring long-term therapy since pulmonary pressures are constantly changing with the patient's condition. Time-cycled ventilators are programmed to deliver gas during a preset time regardless of the patient's respiratory dynamics. Thus, they are indicated for short-term use, such as in the operating and recovery room.

Irrespective of the type of ventilator selected, several modes of ventilation are available. They include controlled; assist controlled; and intermittent mandatory, or synchronized intermittent mandatory ventilation. Controlled ventilation delivers a preset tidal volume at a preset per-minute rate during which the patient cannot trigger respirations. This mode is indicated for patients with respiratory paralysis or apnea secondary to central nervous system damage. Assist controlled ventilation features delivery of a preset tidal volume at a preset per-minute rate, but allows the patient to trigger extra breaths that are delivered by the machine at the preset tidal volume. This mode is suitable for patients who have respiratory failure or alveolar hypoventilation. The most frequently utilized mode is synchronized intermittent mandatory ventilation. This mode delivers a preset tidal volume at a preset rate; however the patient is able to breathe spontaneously at her own tidal volume. The synchronized setting prevents the machine from delivering a breath during exhalation of a spontaneous breath. This mode is indicated for weaning procedures and for patients with respiratory insufficiency who are spontaneously breathing.

Adding positive end expiratory pressure may be required in patients with decreased compliance or fluid-filled alveoli. This keeps the alveoli open in the expiratory phase and can force pulmonary fluid out of the alveoli toward the vasculature. Continuous positive airway pressure works on the same principle but is used when patients are not receiving intermittent positive pressure with a ventilator. Continuous positive airway pressure can be delivered by a tight-fitting mask, though an endotracheal tube is most often used.[33] Positive end expiratory pressure and continuous positive airway pressure must be carefully monitored, especially if the patient is hemodynamically unstable. Venous return and thus cardiac output are decreased with increased intrathoracic pressure. When high levels of positive end expiratory pressure are required, inotropic drugs or fluid therapy may be required to maintain cardiac output.[34] Use of positive end expiratory pressure in conjunction with mechanical ventilation may allow a reduction of Fio_2 to less toxic levels below 50%.

Nursing care of the patient requiring mechanical ventilation presents additional challenges. Though a lifesaving measure, mechanical ventilation can be quite frightening and introduces another set of possible complications to the already compromised patient. Care must be taken to assure that the ventilator is working properly prior to connection to the patient and that it continues to function for the duration of therapy. A qualified respiratory therapist must be readily available to troubleshoot ventilator problems. The nurse at the bedside must also be familiar with the ventilatory settings and alarms, must know how to detect common problems, and must be able to appropriately ventilate the patient with an Ambu bag until any problem is solved. All procedures and equipment should be explained thoroughly as this is the most effective way to allay fear and enhance patient cooperation. The patient must be able to communicate by writing on a pad or chalkboard, since speech is impossible and lip reading is difficult when orally intubated. Ventilatory settings must be validated according to hospital standards, and a complete patient assessment including breath sounds should be done at appropriate intervals. Suctioning is also an important therapy when the patient is being mechanically ventilated since she can no longer cough to clear secretions. Not a benign procedure, suctioning should be done only when necessary to clear the airway. Hyperoxygenation should be accomplished before and after suctioning. Suctioning should be rapid, using only intermittent suction during withdrawal of the catheter. If the patient requires positive end expiratory pressure, a special valve is available so that the positive pressure can be maintained if open suctioning is performed.

In the event of acute respiratory failure, priorities include attainment of a secure airway, ventilation with 100% oxygen if possible, and assessment and support of circulatory function. This must be maintained until further assistance is available. If the patient is breathing but experiencing difficulty, a mask delivering a high concentration of oxygen should be placed on the patient and a quick assessment performed to determine the cause of respiratory failure. If the patient has aspirated, rapid suctioning should be done prior to ventilation to prevent the gastric contents from being forced farther into the lungs. During the acute phase of respiratory failure, attention should be directed toward stabilization of the mother. Only after the mother has been stabilized should attention be directed toward the fetus. An important caveat to remember is if the mother is hypoxic, the fetus is also hypoxic and outcome will often be improved with *in utero* resuscitation. However, if the mother's condition includes absence of cortical activity or no chance of survival, cesarean section may be performed depending on fetal gestational age and condition.

It should be remembered that maternal hypoxia often triggers labor as a protective mechanism caused in part by decreased uteroplacental perfusion. Thus, the woman in labor with pulmonary complications should be assessed for uterine activity and rupture of membranes that may result from uterine contractions. If the patient is found to be in preterm labor and tocolytics are ordered, decisions regarding tocolysis require careful thought. For example, betamimetics may be indicated since they also cause bronchodilation. However, cardiovascular side effects could be devastating in the patient who is critically ill.

Expected Outcomes

During the intrapartum period, the patient with a pulmonary disorder will do the following:

1. Maintain adequate gas exchange and tissue perfusion
2. Maintain optimal hemodynamic parameters
3. Exhibit no signs or symptoms of infection
4. Maintain adequate cardiac output to meet maternal demand
5. Maintain reassuring fetal heart rate responses

References

1. Katz M, Robertson PA, Creasy RK: Cardiovascular complications associated with terbutaline treatment for preterm labor. *Am J Obstet Gynecol* 139:605, 1981.
2. Hatjis CG, Swain M: Systemic tocolysis for premature labor is associated with an increased incidence of pulmonary edema in the presence of maternal infection. *Am J Obstet Gynecol* 159:723, 1988.
3. Maccato J: Pneumonia in pregnancy, in Gilstrap LC, Faro S (eds.): *Infections in Pregnancy*. New York, Alan R Liss, 1990.
4. Villasanta U, Granados JL: Deep vein thrombophlebitis during pregnancy, in Zuspan FP, Christian CD (eds.): *Controversies in Obstetrics and Gynecology*. Philadelphia, Saunders, 1983.
5. Killam A: Amniotic fluid embolus. *Clin Obstet Gynecol* 28:32, 1985.
6. Benedetti TL, Valle R, Ledger WJ: Antepartum pneumonia in pregnancy. *Am J Obstet Gynecol* 144:413, 1982.
7. Crawford JS: Maternal mortality associated with anesthesia. *Lancet* 2:918, 1972.
8. Pritchard JA, McDonald PC, Gant NF: *Williams' Obstetrics* (17th ed.). Norwalk, CT, Appleton-Century-Crofts, 1985.
9. Mulder JI: Amniotic fluid embolism: An overview and case report. *Am J Obstet Gynecol* 152:430, 1985.
10. Courtney LD: Amniotic fluid embolus. *Obstet Gynecol Surv* 29:169, 1974.
11. Hankins GDV: Adult respiratory distress syndrome, in Clark SL, Hankins GDV, Cotton DB, Phelan JP (eds.): *Critical Care Obstetrics* (2nd ed). Boston, Blackwell, 1991.
12. Tranbaugh RF, Lewis FR: Mechanisms and etiologic factors of pulmonary edema. *Surg Gynecol Obstet* 158:193, 1984.
13. Benedetti TJ, Kates R, Williams V: Hemodynamic observations in severe preeclampsia complicated by pulmonary edema. *Am J Obstet Gynecol* 152:330, 1985.
14. Keefer JR, Strauss RG, Civetta JM, Burke T: Noncardiogenic pulmonary edema and invasive cardiovascular monitoring. *Obstet Gynecol* 58:47, 1981.
15. Roberts SL: Pulmonary tissue perfusion altered: Emboli. *Heart Lung* 16:128, 1987.
16. Kuhlman K, Hidvegi D, Tamma R: Is amniotic fluid material in the central circulation of peripartum patients pathologic? *Am J Perinatol* 2:295, 1985.
17. Lee W, Ginsburg KA, Cotton DB, Kaufman RE: Squamous and trophoblastic cells in the maternal pulmonary circulation identified by invasive hemodynamic monitoring during the peripartum period. *Am J Obstet Gynecol* 155:999, 1986.
18. Morgan M: Amniotic fluid embolism. *Anesth* 34:20, 1979.
19. Clark SL, Montz FJ, Phelan JP: Hemodynamic alterations associated with amniotic fluid embolism: A reappraisal. *Am J Obstet Gynecol* 151:617, 1986.

20. Ashbaugh DG, Bigelow DB, Petty TL, et al: Acute respiratory distress in adults. *Lancet* 2:319, 1967.
21. Bernard GR, Bradley RB: Adult respiratory distress syndrome: diagnosis and management. *Heart Lung,* 15:250, 1986.
22. Craig KC, Pierson DJ, Carrico CJ: The clinical application of positive end-expiratory pressure (PEEP) in the adult respiratory distress syndrome (ARDS). *Resp Care* 30:184, 1985.
23. West JB: *Respiratory Physiology: The Essentials* (3rd ed.). Baltimore, Williams & Wilkins, 1985.
24. Thelan LA, Davie JK, Urden LD: *Textbook of Critical Care Nursing: Diagnosis and Management.* St. Louis, Mosby, 1990.
25. Lahiri SK, Thomas TA, Hodgson RMH: Single-dose antacid therapy in the prevention of Mendelson's syndrome. *Br J Anaesth* 45:354, 1973.
26. Sellick BA: Cricoid pressure to control regurgitation of stomach contents during induction of anesthesia. *Lancet* 2:204, 1961.
27. Roberts RB, Shirley MA: Reducing the risks of acid aspiration during cesarean section. *Anesth Analg* 53:589, 1974.
28. Kort BA, Cefalo RX, Baker VV: Fatal influenza A pneumonia in pregnancy. *Am J Perinatol* 3:179, 1986.
29. Luby JP: Southwestern Internal Medicine Conference: Pneumonia in adults due to mycoplasma, chlamydia, and viruses. *Am J Med Sci* 294:45, 1987.
30. Hudak CM, Gallo BM, Lohr T: *Critical Care Nursing: A Holistic Approach.* Philadelphia, Lippincott, 1986.
31. Shapiro BA, Harrison RA, Kacmarek RM, Cane RD: *Clinical Application of Respiratory Care.* Chicago, Year Book Medical Publishers, 1985.
32. Spearman C, Sheldon R: *Egan's Fundamentals of Respiratory Therapy* (4th ed.). St. Louis, Mosby, 1982.
33. Domigan-Wenta J: CPAP mask. *AJN* 85:813, 1985.
34. Gallagher TJ, Civetta JM, Kirby RR: Terminology update: Optimal PEEP. *Crit Care Med* 6:323, 1978.
35. Clark SL, Cotton DB, Gonik B, et al: Central hemodynamic alterations in amniotic fluid embolism. *Am J Obstet Gynecol* 158:1124, 1988.

13
♦ ♦ ♦

Disseminated Intravascular Coagulation

Melissa Sisson

Supportive Data

Incidence

Disseminated intravascular coagulation (DIC) has been described since the 1950s, most notably in obstetric literature, presumably because of its propensity to accompany certain obstetric conditions. While not a separate clinical entity, DIC is an intermediary of other diseases. It represents a derangement of the balance between the precoagulant and fibrinolytic systems that occurs when normal regulatory mechanisms fail. As Weiner suggests, DIC is probably best viewed on a continuum along which clinical presentation and course may vary widely depending on the inciting mechanism.[1]

A consequence of this tendency toward clinical variation is difficulty in ascertaining the incidence of DIC in pregnancy. In the case of abruptio placentae accompanied by intrauterine fetal demise, the occurrence of DIC may be as high as 100%.[2] In contrast, DIC associated with intrauterine fetal demise without abruption is quite rare, except when products of conception are retained beyond 5 weeks. An insidious consumptive coagulopathy is more common in the obstetric patient than is an acute, fulminating DIC.[3] More imperative than defining actual incidence is the recognition that pregnant women may be predisposed to DIC, particularly when besieged by obstetric complications.[1]

Significance

The significance of DIC in pregnancy with regard to maternal–fetal morbidity and mortality is dependent on the precipitating event, its severity, and the ease with which it is eliminated. Most obstetric cases are amenable to correction of the underlying process and respond favorably to termination of the pregnancy. Morbidity and mortality are related to hemorrhage and end-organ damage secondary to ischemia. In the context of morbidity and mortality, placental abruption, preeclampsia–eclampsia, and amniotic fluid embolism have particular relevance and are described here.

Abruptio placentae, occurring in 1 : 250 deliveries, is generally considered the obstetric disorder most often associated with acute DIC.[4] Disseminated coagulopathy can be identified in 30% of those cases in which intrauterine fetal demise has occurred secondary to abruption.[4] Maternal mortality varies from 0% to 5.2%, while perinatal mortality is cited between 5% and 36.5%.[3] Abruption severe enough to result in intrauterine fetal demise and coagulopathy signals a serious danger to maternal well-being.

Preeclampsia–eclampsia is often associated with laboratory abnormalities consistent with coagulopathy, though symptomatic bleeding occurs only rarely. Some clinicians postulate that preeclampsia may actually represent a chronic low-grade DIC.[5]

Van Dam and co-workers reported DIC in 10 of 19 patients with hemolysis, elevated liver enzymes, and low platelets (HELLP syndrome) and found these patients most likely to develop more life-threatening complications at delivery.[6] Though many patients with preeclampsia–eclampsia demonstrate a subclinical coagulopathy, those experiencing compounding complications such as placental abruption or the HELLP syndrome are at significantly greater risk for mortality.

Fortunately a rare complication, amniotic fluid embolism has a maternal mortality of 80%. Should the initial cardiorespiratory insults be survived, 45% will develop DIC.[3] Amniotic fluid embolism is responsible for 10% of all maternal deaths, acquiring increasing significance as maternal mortality becomes less frequent.

Though acute coagulopathy during pregnancy is a rare event, it can have profound consequences for maternal–fetal well-being. Obstetric complications in isolation may carry significant risk for mother and fetus, but when compounded by disseminated coagulopathy, morbidity and mortality increase considerably. It is therefore incumbent upon all practitioners caring for pregnant women to be knowledgeable about DIC, thereby facilitating both early detection and improved outcome.

TABLE 13-1
Predisposing Conditions

General	Obstetric
Sepsis	Abruptio placentae
Metastatic carcinoma	Preeclampsia–eclampsia
Transfusion reactions	Retained intrauterine fetal demise
Hemolytic conditions	
Malignant hypertension	Saline abortion
Trauma	Amniotic fluid embolism
Snake bite	

As previously noted, DIC is a secondary complication arising from another disease process. Precipitating conditions include generalized vascular endothelial damage, such as those toxic, inflammatory, hypoxic, or immune in nature, or entrance of thromboplastic material into the circulation, for example cancer or leukemic cells.[7] A number of conditions have been associated with development of DIC and are presented in Table 13-1.

Etiology

Framework for Accepted Therapy

Central to any discussion of DIC is an understanding of normal coagulation. Hemostasis is the process by which blood is maintained in a liquid state within vessels, with loss of blood from damaged vessels prevented. Contributors to this process include the vascular endothelium, platelets, and circulating blood proteins. Disruption of the endothelium as a result of vascular damage sets into motion the first phase of hemostasis, which is formation of a temporary platelet plug. Exposure of subendothelial collagen results in platelet activation and adhesion. Release of histamine and serotonin promotes local vasoconstriction, whereby platelet cohesion occurs and a temporary plug is formed.

The second phase of hemostasis involves the local activation of the coagulation cascade resulting in thrombin production and eventual formation of a fibrin clot. Circulating blood proteins, the third component of hemostasis, include those of the coagulation system, the fibrinolytic system, the kinin system, and the complement system. These systems participate by providing a method of checks and balances that regulate clot formation.

The blood proteins in the coagulation system, traditionally referred to as clotting factors, can be functionally divided into enzymes and cofactors.[8] The enzymes (serine proteases) are activated clotting factors, and cofactors are substances that accelerate the rate of substrate activation by enzymes. The coagulation system is a series of self-amplifying substrate-to-enzyme interactions that is activated by three types of injuries: trauma to tissue, trauma to vascular endothelium, and trauma to red blood cells or platelets.

When one or more of these initiating injuries occur, thrombin is generated via the intrinsic pathway (contact system) or via the extrinsic pathway (tissue factor). The intrinsic pathway is activated when factor XII, or the Hageman factor, is exposed to collagen, phospholipid, or kallikrein or in conditions such as sepsis.[3] The extrinsic pathway is activated by tissue thromboplastin. The final stages of clot formation begin with the activation of factor X, the first step in a converging pathway that brings the intrinsic and extrinsic pathways together (see Figure 13-1).

The activation of factor X begins the final common pathway and leads to the conversion of circulating prothrombin to thrombin. Thrombin acts as a proteolytic enzyme cleaving fibrinopeptides A and B from fibrinogen, a large circulating plasma protein. Fibrin monomers are formed as a result of this cleavage, then are polymerized or joined by activated factor XIII and a stable clot is produced.[2]

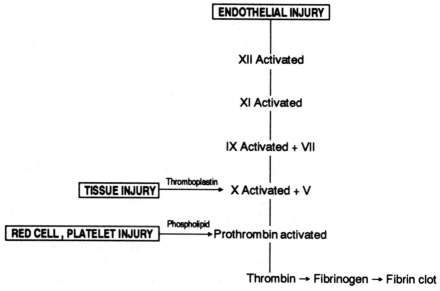

Figure 13-1. Summary of clotting sequence.

Three major regulatory mechanisms control coagulation: the fibrinolytic system, antithrombin III, and protein C. These systems, aided by rapid blood flow and removal of activated clotting factor by the reticuloendothelial system, serve to localize clot formation and to maintain the liquid state of blood.

The fibrinolytic system begins the breakdown of fibrin when the clot is formed (see Figure 13-2). Plasminogen is incorporated into the fibrin clot and, when activated, is converted to plasmin which systematically lyses fibrin. Four major fragments called fibrin degradation products, or fibrin-split products, are liberated: X, Y, D, and E. The fibrin degradation products have anticoagulant properties including disruption of fibrin polymerization, coating of platelets,

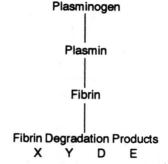

Figure 13-2. Summary of fibrinolysis.

and formation of soluble fibrin monomer complexes.[2] Fibrin degradation products exert their anticoagulant effect when they cannot be adequately cleared because of excess fibrin formation.

Antithrombin III is the central physiologic antagonist to coagulation. It is a glycoprotein that binds to activated factors XII, XI, IX, and X and slowly inactivates thrombin. When it combines with heparin, thrombin inactivation is accelerated and occurs rapidly.

Protein C is a vitamin-K-dependent proenzyme that is found in plasma. When activated by thrombin, protein C degrades activated cofactors V and VIII. It then exerts an anticoagulant effect by inhibiting a portion of the coagulation cascade.

Pregnancy has been referred to as a hypercoagulable state; the following list shows the hemostatic alterations in pregnancy:

> Increase in factors V, VII, VIII, IX, X, XII, and prothrombin time
> Increased fibrinogen
> Decrease in factors XI and XIII
> Decreased protein C
> Decreased fibrinolysis

There are elevations of all coagulation factors with the exception of factor XIII and possibly XI, which are believed to decrease.[3] In addition, fibrinolytic activity appears to be decreased during pregnancy with a speculated increase in plasminogen activator inhibitor. Levels of protein C are also decreased, while levels of antithrombin III remain unchanged. Alterations in the hemostatic mechanism occur in order to maintain the pregnancy and to protect the mother from blood loss at delivery.

Disseminated intravascular coagulation represents a failure of the normal regulatory mechanisms, so that fibrin generation is no longer confined to the area of injury. As a consequence of one or more precipitating events, there is massive consumption of the circulating clotting factors and activation of the fibrinolytic system. The result is (*a*) hemorrhage, (*b*) systemic production of fibrin monomers and polymers with fibrin thrombi producing end-organ ischemia and necrosis, (*c*) activation of the kinin system with resultant vascular permeability and hypotension, and (*d*) activation of the complement system with systemic manifestation.[3] The process is self-perpetuating, and the clinical picture is one of excessive thrombosis, depletion of circulating blood proteins necessary for normal coagulation, and lysis of existing fibrin, all resulting in hemorrhage and shock.

Disseminated intravascular coagulation is an intermediary of many primary disease processes, a number of them specific to the practice of obstetrics (see Table 13-1). In normal pregnancy, the coagulation and fibrinolytic systems appear to be in a hyperdynamic state with both increased production and turnover of many procoagulants.[9] It has therefore been suggested that pregnancy may represent a primed state in which there is an increased susceptibility to DIC. The intrapartum activation of coagulation, as evidenced by increases in fibrinopeptide A, activated Hageman factor, and soluble fibrin monomer complexes, and activation of fibrinolysis indicated by increased fibrin degradation products, implies that normal parturition may actually represent a low-grade DIC.[3] Hypothetically then, a pregnant woman exposed to an appropriate stimulus, such as release of tissue thromboplastin during placental abruption, may be at far greater risk to respond with an overt coagulopathy than her nonpregnant counterpart.

Therapy for DIC is predicated on the degree to which the underlying mechanism can be eliminated. Generally, pregnancy termination results in arrest of the process. Of equal importance is management of the systemic manifestations of DIC with volume replacement, blood product replacement, coagulation component replacement, cardiovascular support, and respiratory support.[3]

A chronic, subclinical DIC may be successfully managed by removing the underlying cause, often accomplished by pregnancy termination. Once the stimulus for coagulopathy is eliminated, serial monitoring of clotting studies, volume replacement as necessary, and periodic clinical evaluation are usually sufficient therapy.

An acute catastrophic DIC mandates a more aggressive approach. Therapy may involve correcting deficiencies in coagulation with blood component administration, vigorous volume replacement, and invasive support measures. The following list describes the principles of management.

> Eliminate underlying cause.
> Institute supportive measures to correct acidosis, hypotension, and hypoperfusion.
> Initiate vigorous volume replacement.
> Initiate blood component replacement.
> Consider pregnancy termination.

Antithrombin III concentrate is effective in the treatment of obstetric causes of DIC; however, it is also contained in fresh frozen plasma. There is no consensus that transfusion of antithrombin III concentrate is superior to conventional blood component therapy.[3]

Heparin does not seem to be generally accepted as useful therapy for obstetric causes of DIC. Heparin acts to neutralize thrombin by accelerating the activity of antithrombin III. However, if antithrombin III levels are depleted, as occurs in fulminating DIC, heparin therapy would not seem efficacious. Finley suggests limited low-dose heparin administration only in those patients with intact vascular systems, no evidence of bleeding diathesis, and a prolonged triggering mechanism.[3] Prevention of DIC hinges on successful identification of predisposing conditions. Once susceptibility is recognized, careful assessment enhances detection of initial signs and symptoms and promotion of early intervention.

Assessment

As outlined previously, the patient with DIC may have a diverse clinical picture. Signs and symptoms may be as innocuous as epistaxis or as disastrous as multiportal hemorrhage. Acute, fulminant DIC is most often associated with severe abruptio placentae and amniotic fluid embolism. However, chronic low-grade DIC is the more typical obstetric presentation and is associated with preeclampsia–eclampsia and retained intrauterine fetal demise. Patients with a compensated DIC are at great risk for the development of fulminant DIC.

Though hemorrhage is the initial sign of coagulopathy, it is always preceded by thrombosis, the signs of which vary with the organ affected. Seven percent of patients have clinical signs of thrombosis, which may include peripheral cyanosis, gangrene, renal impairment, drowsiness, confusion, coma, and cardiorespiratory failure.[9] Oozing may occur from venipunctures and other sites of trauma. Epistaxis, ecchymosis, purpura, petechiae, and other disruptions of the integument are common. Red blood cell lysis secondary to activation of the complement system is a potential occurrence.[3] Hypotension due to hemorrhage or activation of the kinin system almost always accompanies DIC.

In the patient with massive hemorrhage, the collection of laboratory data may prove academic, due to the obvious need for expedience. However, as a screening tool and guide for therapy, laboratory evaluation is essential. The following shows the barrage of laboratory tests that are available and the abnormalities that can result in DIC.

Platelet count: Decreased
Fibrinogen: Decreased
Prothrombin time: Prolonged
Partial thromboplastin time: Prolonged
Antithrombin III: Decreased activity
Fibrin degradation product: Greater than 40
Soluble fibrin monomer complexes: Increased

Antithrombin III levels are the most sensitive determinants of DIC, showing a decline in activity due to increased consumption.[1] Fibrin degradation products are nonspecific unless exceeding 40 mg and can be increased with the breakdown of an old clot. Fibrinopeptide A, since it has a half-life of 3 minutes, indicates excessive fibrin production and more accurately reflects current coagulation status.[3] The presence of soluble fibrin monomer complexes is also indicative of recent thrombin activity.[2]

The more common and most available tests for coagulation assessment include serum fibrinogen levels, prothrombin time, partial thromboplastin time, and platelet count. Prothrombin time, which reflects extrinsic coagulation, is prolonged in DIC as is partial thromboplastin time, which measures intrinsic coagulation. Generally, these tests are far less specific, but in the asymptomatic patient may be useful for screening. Of those patients with DIC, 50% have normal prothrombin and partial thromboplastin times, while most have a decreased fibrinogen, and 90% have thrombocytopenia.[1] Additional laboratory work should include hemoglobin level, hematocrit reading, and a peripheral smear.

In the patient who is actively bleeding with a living fetus, it may be necessary to immediately estimate the adequacy of hemostasis. In such a case, it is recommended that 5 to 10 ml of the patient's blood be drawn and placed in a non-heparinized tube and observed for clot formation at 37° centigrade every 30 seconds for 5 minutes; failure of clot formation suggests overt coagulopathy.[9]

Nursing Diagnoses

A number of nursing diagnoses pertain to the pregnant woman with DIC.[10] These include the following:

- Alteration in hemostasis
- Fluid volume deficit, actual or potential
- Gas exchange, impaired, maternal and fetal
- Alteration in health maintenance secondary to:
    Impaired cardiovascular function, actual or potential
    Impaired renal function, actual or potential
    Impaired liver function, actual or potential
    Impaired pulmonary function, actual or potential
    Impaired central nervous system function, actual or potential
- Anxiety
- Alteration in family process

Theoretical Basis for the Plan of Nursing Care and Intervention

The demands of caring for the patient with potential or manifest DIC vary from astute surveillance to active intervention. Initially, impact on the severity of the process can be maximized if the risk is recognized and coagulopathy is detected early. Assessment is also of paramount importance, and the attentive perinatal nurse who detects the subtle signs of bleeding may avert catastrophe.

The detection of an alteration in the hemostasis level, secondary to abnormal coagulation, requires assessment of both clinical and laboratory data. Patient screening includes assessment of baseline hemoglobin levels, hematocrit reading, serum fibrinogen levels, platelet count, prothrombin time, partial thromboplastin time, and fibrin degradation products. The frequency of collection of further laboratory data is determined by the detected abnormalities. Spurious results may be obtained if coagulation studies are drawn from an arterial line.[9]

TABLE 13-2
Blood Component Therapy

Component	Content	Volume	Goal
Packed red blood cells	Red cells: 1 U increases hematocrit 3%	200–225 ml	Hematocrit ≥ 30%
Fresh frozen plasma	Clotting factors: 1 U increases fibrinogen 10 mg/dl	180–200 ml	Replace clotting factors; fibrinogen greater than 100 mg/dl
Cryoprecipitate	Clotting factors: 1 U increases fibrinogen 10 mg/dl	15–20 ml	Replace clotting factors; fibrinogen greater than 100 mg/dl
Platelet concentrate	Platelets: 1 U increases count 5000 per μl	50 ml	Platelet count 50,000 per μl or greater

Physical assessment should be thorough and systematic with particular attention paid to discovery of petechiae, ecchymoses, hematoma formation, vaginal bleeding, gingival bleeding, hematuria, and hemorrhages in the conjunctiva. Trauma such as venipuncture or intramuscular injection should be avoided.

In the actively bleeding patient, blood loss should be quantified when possible. Blood component replacement is often necessary (see Table 13-2). The risks of blood administration include transfusion reaction, transmission of infectious disease, and circulatory overload.[11] Currently the risk of contracting Non A Non B hepatitis is 1:100, and that of contracting human immunodeficiency virus is 1:40,000 to 1:250,000 with transfusion.[12] The onset of transfusion reaction is characteristically rapid, and signs and symptoms may include fever, chills, nausea, paresthesia, muscle cramps, urticaria, shortness of breath, tachycardia, hypotension, convulsions, and cardiac arrest. If an adverse reaction occurs, the transfusion should be stopped immediately, the intravenous tubing flushed with normal saline, and the patient managed empirically. The risk of a fatal hemolytic anemia is approximately 1:100,000.[12] Rigid adherence to procedure for proper identification of blood components is critical.

Using blood components permits selection of the blood product most likely to provide maximum benefit to the patient. Packed red blood cells transfused with crystalloid for volume expansion have proved to be effective replacement for the patient in hemorrhagic shock.

Platelet transfusion is generally not recommended except as a prophylaxis in the clinically stable patient with a count of less than 10 to 20,000 or in the preoperative patient with a count of under 50,000.[12] Transfusion of fresh frozen plasma strictly for volume replacement is not indicated; however, it is advocated for replacement of clotting factors.[12] Cryoprecipitate provides an alternative to fresh frozen plasma for the volume-restricted patient since each unit is 15 to 20 ml. The disadvantage posed by cryoprecipitate is that it does not contain antithrombin III.

Fluid volume deficit accompanies hemorrhage. The need for fluid replacement may be assessed by measurement of urine specific gravity, hematocrit, central venous, pulmonary artery and pulmonary capillary wedge pressures, and intake and output. Circulating fluid volume can be restored with crystalloid or colloid solutions carefully quantified to replace estimated volume loss. Quantification of volume replacement is best achieved by monitoring central hemodynamic pressures.

Impaired fetal gas exchange may occur as a consequence of decreased uteroplacental perfusion due to maternal hemorrhage and shock. Continuous electronic fetal monitoring during the intrapartum period is beneficial for assessment of fetal well-being. Late decelerations, tachycardia, and loss of variability may be ominous and, pending maternal condition, may dictate expedient delivery. Additional interventions include lateral maternal positioning and administration of oxygen.

The systemic nature of DIC can precipitate impairment of cardiovascular, renal, liver, central nervous system, and pulmonary function, particularly when blood loss is great. Nursing care includes assessment of the patient's clinical condition and interpretation of laboratory data in order to ascertain compromise of major organ systems.

Blood pressure, pulse, and peripheral perfusion are monitored frequently with particular attention to the development of hypotension and tachycardia. Inotropic support may be necessary to maintain perfusion. Urine output should be measured and specific gravity determined. An output of greater than 25 ml/hour generally coincides with adequate perfusion of the kidneys. Serum creatinine and blood urea nitrogen levels are monitored closely for elevations consistent with renal involvement. Liver function tests are monitored serially with attention to elevation of SGOT, SGPT, and bilirubin. Nausea, vomiting, and right upper quadrant or shoulder pain suggest liver involvement. Continuous assessment of mental status is imperative since any alteration may be an early expression of cerebral hemorrhage. Pulmonary involvement may represent an iatrogenic complication resulting from fluid overload. Observation for dyspnea, tachypnea, cyanosis, and frequent auscultation of breath sounds assist in determining the presence of pulmonary edema. Pulse oximetry and measurement of arterial blood gases may also prove useful.

Emotional support is crucial for the patient and family experiencing such life-threatening complications as DIC. Anxiety is common, as is disruption in family process. Interventions include encouraging discussion, establishing trust, and offering explanations of procedures and equipment. The family should be encouraged to visit and, as possible, maternal–infant bonding facilitated by the perinatal nurse.

In summary, intensive surveillance is mandated in the intrapartum patient at risk for DIC. If the patient is acutely affected, many aspects of supportive care fall within the realm of nursing practice. The degree to which the patient responds to supportive measures, once the precipitating event is eliminated, determines outcome.

Expected Outcomes

If the initiating cause of DIC is successfully removed and the response to supportive therapy is positive, the following outcomes are possible:

1. Maintenance of hemostasis
2. Maintenance of adequate cardiac output and tissue perfusion
3. Prevention of fetal distress
4. Prevention of permanent renal dysfunction
5. Prevention of permanent liver dysfunction
6. Prevention of permanent pulmonary dysfunction
7. Prevention of permanent central nervous system dysfunction
8. Alleviation of anxiety
9. Diminished disruption of family process

References

1. Weiner CP: The obstetric patient and disseminated intravascular coagulopathy. *Clin Perinatol* 13:705, 1986.
2. Sher G, Statland BE: Abruptio placenta with coagulopathy: a rational basis for management. *Clin Obstet Gynecol* 28:15, 1985.
3. Finley BE: Acute coagulopathy in pregnancy. *Med Clin N America* 73:723, 1989.
4. Gilabert J, Estelles A, Aznan J, Galbis M: Abruptio placenta and disseminated intravascular coagulation. *Aeta Obstet Gynecol Scand* 64:35, 1985.
5. Kobayashi T, Terao T: Preeclampsia as chronic disseminated intravascular coagulation. *Gynecol Obstet Invest* 24:170, 1987.
6. Van Dam PA, Renier M, Backlandt M, et al: Disseminated intravascular coagulation and the syndrome of hemolysis, elevated liver enzymes and low platelets in severe preeclampsia. *Obstet Gynecol* 73:97, 1989.
7. Johansen, et al (eds.): *Standards of Critical Care* (3rd ed.). St. Louis, Mosby, 1988.
8. Brandt JT: Current concepts in coagulation. *Clin Obstet Gynecol* 28:3, 1985.
9. Hewitt P, Davies S: The current state of DIC. *Inten Care Med.* 9:249, 1983.
10. Doenges ME, Kenty JR, Moorhouse M: *Maternal Newborn Care Plans Guidelines for Client Care.* Philadelphia, FA Davis, 1988.
11. Committee on Technical Bulletin, American College of Obstetricians and Gynecologists: Blood component therapy. *ACOG Tech Bull* 78, 1984, pp. 1–4.
12. *FDA Drug Bulletin* 19:14, 1989.

14

Acquired Immune Deficiency Syndrome in Pregnancy

Abbe Bendell
JoNell Efantis-Potter

Supportive Data

Incidence

It has been estimated that one million people in the United States are infected with the human immunodeficiency viruses (HIV).[1] States are required to report all cases of acquired immune deficiency syndrome (AIDS) and, as of June 30, 1991, there was a total of 182,834 cases of AIDS among adults and adolescents.[2] Women accounted for 19,652 cases or 11% of the total and 78% of those cases were diagnosed between the ages of 25 to 39 years.[2] Although women make up only a minor percentage of all cases of AIDS, there has been a 1.5-fold annual increase in the incidence of AIDS in children, the majority of whom are infected via maternal–fetal transmission. The World Health Organization estimates that by the year 2000 there will be 10 million infected infants and children in the world. It is also estimated that mothers or both parents of more than 10 million children will have died from HIV infection/AIDS.[3]

Currently available statistics of HIV infection and AIDS among women are probably underestimated. Some people may be asymptomatic and unaware of their infection and are therefore not tested. Others may suspect infection but choose not to be tested. Still other women who may be aware of their infection may choose to withhold test results because they fear discrimination or because they deny their diagnosis.

Epidemiologic studies are currently underway to establish the incidence of HIV infection among childbearing women. At a large hospital in New York City, 2% of the women attending an antenatal clinic had positive results when screened for HIV.[4] In the same city, 1.5% of the female registrants seeking maternity services in all five of the city's boroughs were seropositive.[5] Using serum samples from newborns as an indicator of maternal serological status, the state of Massachusetts determined 2.1 per 1000 (0.2%) women giving birth tested positive with HIV antibodies.[6] In a study in New Jersey, 4.3% of the participants delivering at an inner city hospital that serves a high-risk population were seropositive.[7] All pregnant women who were born in Haiti and delivered a child at a hospital in Dade county, Florida, were screened for HIV; 3.6% of them were confirmed as HIV seropositive.[8] By the end of June 30, 1991, there were 3140 reported pediatric cases of AIDS.[2] Among these patients, there were 2645 (84%) in whom the probable mode of transmission was perinatal.[2] Among children 5 years old or younger, perinatal transmission accounts for 84% of the cases.[2]

Health care workers involved in care and treatment of HIV-positive patients must be aware of the potential occupational risk of caring for these patients. Several studies have been published addressing the occupational risk of contracting HIV among health care workers. Although over 3000 health care workers have been exposed to the virus, enrolled in studies, and tested for HIV, the risk for seroconversion is estimated to be less than 1%.[9]

Significance

In June 1979, a 32-year-old man went into a New York City hospital with symptoms now associated with *Pneumocystis carinii* pneumonia. He was treated for pneumonia and evaluated for an immune dysfunction which allows opportunistic infections to flourish. Although this was an unusual case, 15 additional cases were reported during medical meetings in New York City over the next few months. Review of the cases revealed that all of them involved young men who were either homosexuals or drug abusers. During the same time, Kaposi's sarcoma was initially seen among healthy young homosexual males, many of whom also developed fatal opportunistic infections. Since that time the incidence of these opportunistic infections and rare cancers has spread in epidemic proportions.

This was the beginning of a new disease process that eventually became known as AIDS. The Centers for Disease Control (CDC) began an active surveillance system to track this disease process and by June 1983, 1600 total cases had been recognized. Most of the cases comprised homosexual males. The virus believed to be the causative agent for AIDS, HIV, was identified in 1983 by a team of scientists in both France and America.[10] The virus was named LAV and HTLV III respectively, but in 1986 the International Committee on the Taxonomy of Viruses renamed it HIV for future consistency.[10]

When a person is diagnosed with HIV infection, the presence of the HIV antibody [as determined by the enzyme-linked immunosorbent assay (ELISA) test and confirmed by the Western Blot or other confirmatory testing techniques] indicates the body has been exposed to HIV and has developed antibodies to it. Antigen testing or viral culture is not routinely done as a diagnostic test.

Acquired immune deficiency syndrome is classified by progression of the infection. After exposure, there is a period of acute infection that is generally characterized by a transient illness. Referred to as acute retroviral infection, which is mononucleosis-like with fever, upper respiratory symptoms, and often diarrhea, patients at this stage are classified as group I. Antibody seroconversion is required as evidence of initial infection. Once the acute syndrome has resolved, patients are then reclassified into another group. Group II comprises those patients with asymptomatic infection. At this stage, there is a latent period between infection and development of the disease. These patients are HIV-antibody positive and are symptom free.

Persistent generalized lymphadenopathy occurs in those patients in group III. Patients are classified into this group if there is palpable lymphadenopathy in two or more extrainguinal sites persisting for more than 3 months. Group IV is characterized by other diseases and includes five subgroups. Subgroup A is constitutional disease that includes one or more of the following: fever persisting for more than 1 month, involuntary weight loss of greater than 10% of body weight, and diarrhea persisting for greater than 1 month. Subgroup B includes one or more of the following: dementia (HIV encephalopathies), myelopathy, and peripheral neuropathy. In 1987, subgroup C was revised and broadened by the CDC to include AIDS case definitions. Thus, diagnosis was allowed without laboratory evidence of HIV infection and with laboratory evidence of an opportunistic infection considered to be indicative of AIDS (see Table 14-1). Subgroup D includes patients with a diagnosis of one or more kinds of cancers associated with HIV infection, such as Kaposi's sarcoma and non-Hodgkin's lymphoma. Subgroup E includes patients with other conditions associated with HIV infection.[11]

In children, *HIV infection* is defined as the presence of the virus in the blood or tissues, confirmed by viral culture or other laboratory methods such as antigen detection. The presence of HIV antibody in an infant less than 15 months

TABLE 14-1
Opportunistic Infections

1. Candidiasis of the esophagus, trachea, bronchi, or lungs
2. Cryptococcosis, extrapulmonary
3. Cryptosporidiosis with diarrhea persisting >1 month
4. Cytomegalovirus disease of an organ other than liver, spleen, or lymph nodes in a patient >1 month of age
5. Herpes simplex virus infection causing a mucocutaneous ulcer that persists longer than 1 month; or bronchitis, pneumonitis, or esophagitis for any duration affecting a patient >1 month of age
6. Kaposi's sarcoma affecting a patient <60 years of age
7. Lymphoma of the brain (primary) affecting a patient <60 years
8. Lymphoid interstitial pneumonia and/or pulmonary lymphoid hyperplasis (LIP/PLH complex) affecting a child <13 years of age
9. *Mycobacterium avium* complex or *M. kansaii* disease, disseminated (at a site other than or in addition to lungs, skin, or cervical or hilar lymph nodes)
10. *Pneumocystis carinii* pneumonia
11. Progressive multifocal leukoencephalopathy
12. Toxoplasmosis of the brain affecting a patient >1 month of age

of age may not be indicative of actual HIV infection but may be due to passive maternal transmission. Maternal antibodies to the virus may be present for as long as 15 months in the neonate. Abnormal immunological levels indicating both humoral and cellular immunodeficiencies in the presence of HIV antibody, and/or identification of the virus in the blood or tissues, or confirmation of symptoms meeting the CDC case definition of AIDS define *infant infection.*

In children under the age of 13 years HIV infection has been classified into three major groups. Class P-0 refers to children with indeterminate infection. This includes infants and children up to 15 months old who were perinatally exposed and cannot be definitively diagnosed as infected but who have the HIV antibody.

Class P-1 includes those with asymptomatic infection. These patients test positive for HIV and have no signs or symptoms that would lead to classification in P-2.

Class P-2 includes those children with symptomatic infection and is subdivided into six subclasses. Subclass A includes two or more nonspecific findings persisting for greater than 2 months. The nonspecific findings include fever, failure to thrive or weight loss of 10% of baseline body weight, hepatomegaly, splenomegaly, generalized lymphadenopathy, parotitis, and diarrhea that is persistent or recurrent. Subclass B includes progressive neurologic disease. Subclass C includes lymphoid interstitial pneumonia and pneumonitis. Pneumonia

TABLE 14-2
Classification of Human Immunodeficiency Virus Infection in Children under 13 Years of Age

Class P-0. Indeterminate infection
Class P-1. Asymptomatic infection
  Subclass A. Normal immune function
  Subclass B. Abnormal immune function
  Subclass C. Immune function not tested
Class P-2. Symptomatic infection
  Subclass A. Nonspecific findings
  Subclass B. Progressive neurologic disease
  Subclass C. Lymphoid interstitial pneumonitis
  Subclass D. Secondary infectious diseases
    Category D-1. Specified secondary infectious diseases listed in the CDC surveillance definition for AIDS
    Category D-2. Recurrent serious bacterial infections
    Category D-3. Other specified secondary infectious diseases
  Subclass E. Secondary cancers
    Category E-1. Specified secondary cancers listed in the CDC surveillance definition for AIDS
    Category E-2. Other cancers possibly secondary to HIV infection
  Subclass F. Other diseases possibly due to HIV infection

Source: Adapted from Centers for Disease Control: Classification system for HIV infection in children under 13 years of age. *MMWR* 36:225–230, 1987.

and pneumonitis are accepted as indicative of AIDS in children but not in adults. Subclass D includes secondary infectious diseases indicative of AIDS as listed in the adult CDC definitions: recurrent serious bacterial infectious diseases persisting for greater than 2 months. Subclass E includes secondary cancers. The final subclass, F, includes other diseases possibly due to HIV infection (see Table 14-2).[12]

If current mortality trends continue, AIDS can soon be expected to become one of the five leading causes of death in women of reproductive age.[3] Women infected with HIV are the major source of infection among infants; thus trends in AIDS mortality among women forecast the impact of HIV on mortality among children as well.

Immunity is the body's specific response to an invading organism.[13] The body utilizes two types of immunity or immune responses in dealing with foreign organisms—natural and acquired. Natural immunity is present at birth and is general or nonspecific. It includes physical barriers such as intact skin and mucous membranes, which prevent entrance of foreign organisms into the body, as well as cilia, which clear pathogens from the upper respiratory tract.[13] Chemical barriers (*i.e.,* acid gastric juices) destroy invading organisms non-specifically. Blood cells and their responses (such as phagocytosis) are part of both natural and acquired immune responses. Acquired immune responses are developed during a person's lifetime as a result of contact with a disease or immunization. Acquired immunity includes both humoral and cell-mediated immunological responses and can last for long periods of time.[13]

Etiology

When a foreign organism invades the body, a phagocytic immune response occurs as the white blood cells engulf and destroy the foreign organisms. Humoral immune response then occurs with manufacture of antibodies produced by B lymphocytes, which are specific to the foreign organism. The B lymphocytes, macrophages, and special T lymphocytes all take part in the recognition phase of the foreign organism (antigen) and in antibody production.[13] The T cells carry the antigenic message back to the B cells so that antibodies are produced or are reactivated. Antibodies then bind with the antigen, and phagocytosis can occur.

Cell-mediated, or cellular, response then occurs involving T lymphocytes. The antigens bind with receptor sites on the T cells that in turn stimulate the production of killer cells. The function of killer cells is to secrete a chemical substance known as lymphokinase which also facilitates destruction and removal of the antigen with help from other cells.

Humoral and cellular immune responses work in conjunction. T helper cells (T_4 cells) improve B lymphocyte function and, therefore, antibody production, as well as differentiate killer cells. Suppressor cells (T_8 cells) stop the production of B cells and, therefore, the production of B antibodies. Once this process has been completed, the antibodies become inactive but retain the ability to be recalled if the antigen is presented again.

Human immunodeficiency virus is a member of a unique group of viruses called retroviruses. Unlike most cells, these viruses carry their genetic coding materials as ribonucleic acid instead of deoxyribonucleic acid (as in most cells). After HIV has entered the bloodstream, it bonds to receptors on the surface of the T_4 helper cell. In order for ribonucleic acid to be converted into deoxyribonucleic acid, the enzyme, reverse transcriptase, orders the host cells' genetic material to be reproduced as retroviruses. The number of active T_4 cells decreases, and the remaining T_4 cells no longer function to fight infection. Consequently, an individual becomes susceptible to develop opportunistic infections caused by other organisms that would not affect a person with a normal functioning immune system.[14] Human immunodeficiency virus has been isolated in plasma, semen, saliva, urine, tears, breast milk, cerebrospinal fluid, lymph nodes, the brain, bone marrow, and cervical and vaginal secretions. However, only blood, semen, vaginal secretions, and breast milk have been implicated in transmission of the virus. Transmission due to exposure to infected blood can occur as a result of blood transfusion, needle sharing, unintentional needle stick, or open-wound or mucous-membrane exposure. However, HIV is fundamentally a sexually transmitted disease that may be contracted by homosexual, bisexual, and heterosexual activity. The risk of acquiring HIV from one or more sexual encounters with an infected person is not known.[15]

Perinatal transmission (*i.e.,* from mother to fetus) accounts for 84% of pediatric AIDS cases.[2] The actual transmission rate during gestation is estimated as 20% to 50%.[8] The exact time of maternal-to-offspring transmission is not known,[16] although HIV has been isolated from aborted fetal tissues supporting a theory of early pregnancy transplacental transmission.[17] Mode of delivery (cesarean versus vaginal) does not alter the intrapartum HIV transmission rate.[18]

There are case reports of mothers who were infected during the postpartum period by blood transfusion and whose infants subsequently became infected, possibly by breast-feeding.[19] Because breast milk has been implicated as a source for perinatal transmission, breast-feeding is currently not recommended for mothers who are HIV seropositive.

The epidemiology of AIDS has identified specific groups of people whose behaviors place them at higher risk for infection. Human immunodeficiency virus was initially identified in young homosexual men and for many years was considered to be a gay man's disease. Intravenous drug abusers are at high risk due to contaminated needle sharing among addicts. The contamination occurs when infected blood from an addict remains in the needle and syringe and is then injected into another person.

Heterosexuals are at high risk if they engage in sexual encounters with multiple sex partners, drug abusers, bisexuals, infected hemophiliacs, transfusion recipients of HIV-infected blood, partners known to be infected, or persons born in countries where heterosexual transmission is thought to play a major role. Children are at high risk for pediatric AIDS if their mothers have or are at risk to contract HIV infection or if they were a recipient of an infected blood transfusion, blood components, or tissue prior to 1985.

Framework for Accepted Therapy

Literature regarding the effect of pregnancy on maternal HIV infection is meager. Although pregnant women who are HIV positive commonly have concerns about whether their disease will worsen during pregnancy, accurate information is not available about the role played by pregnancy in disease progression. One study suggested that when HIV-infected women become pregnant, the natural immunologic change of decreased cell-mediated immunity during the second and third trimesters accelerated HIV disease and hastened the onset of symptoms of AIDS.[20] Another study also suggested that the disease progressed more rapidly in women with HIV infection who went to term than it did in nonpregnant women with the infection.[21] These studies, however, were conducted with small populations and lacked control groups for comparisons. European studies concluded that pregnant and nonpregnant women observed over a period of approximately 3 years showed no statistically significant difference in the progression of HIV disease.[22]

Similarly, the effect of HIV on pregnancy is as yet unclear. Women who are seropositive may be at increased risk for certain complications, although the data are again controversial. Preliminary reports suggest there may be an increased risk of prematurity, premature rupture of membranes, low birth weight, and coexistent sexually transmitted disease.[21,23,24] The course of these complications may be more closely associated with drug addiction and low socioeconomic status than with HIV infection. Clarification of these findings must await the publication of matched-controlled studies currently underway.

During normal pregnancy, women experience a variety of immunologic changes, including decreased lymphocyte function, decreased levels of T_4 helper cell counts, and a decreased T_4:T_8 ratio—all evidence of depressed cell-mediated immunity. The altered immune state of pregnancy, when in the presence of HIV infection, may accelerate disease progression by increasing susceptibility to opportunistic infections. Among nonpregnant patients with AIDS, changes in absolute T_4 helper cell counts are used to evaluate the severity of immunocompromise, and depressed levels have been associated with the development of opportunistic infections. Similarly, opportunistic infections among pregnant AIDS patients are almost exclusively observed among women whose T_4 helper cell counts are significantly reduced.[25]

Antiretroviral therapy in adults has greatly reduced the short-term mortality and frequency of opportunistic infections. The first double-blind placebo-controlled trial demonstrating clinical efficacy of zidovudine was terminated when mortality was found to be significantly higher in the placebo groups.[26] In another study, retrovir significantly slowed the rate of progression of HIV infection in patients with depressed T_4 helper cell counts.[27]

Antiretroviral therapy is offered to pregnant women who are severely immunocompromised in an effort to prevent progression of disease. Phase I pharmokinetic studies of zidovudine are near completion in asymptomatic pregnant women to determine therapeutic dosage, as well as safety and efficacy of this therapy during pregnancy. What effect this drug has on neonatal outcome and perinatal transmission is yet to be determined. However, to date, no adverse fetal effects have been reported.

Pneumocystis carinii pneumonia is one of the most common opportunistic infections observed among AIDS patients. The standard treatment is sulfamethoxazole–trimethoprim, which readily crosses the placenta but does not appear to be teratogenic. Patients taking this regime should be observed for signs and symptoms of drug toxicity, which include rash, fever, nausea, neutropenia, and thrombocytopenia. Sulfonamides readily cross the placenta competing with bilirubin for binding to plasma albumin. There is increased risk, especially when administered close to delivery, for neonatal hyperbilirubinemia.

Pentamidine isethionate appears to be equally effective against *Pneumocystis carinii* pneumonia. However, experience with its use in pregnancy is lacking. After initial therapy for an acute episode of this pneumonia, aerosolized pentamidine may be administered as a form of prophylaxis; however, a potential complication is the development of systemic dissemination of *Pneumocystis carinii* pneumonia. If administered, patients must be monitored closely for potential side effects, which include upper airway irritation, mild cough, burning sensation in the throat, bronchospasm, and fatigue.[28,29]

Fungal infections caused by *Candida albicans* are common opportunistic infections seen in women with AIDS. *Candida esophagitis* is the most serious, and *Candida vaginitis* the most frequent.[30] Vaginal mucosal irritation and pruritus may cause severe discomfort, especially during labor and delivery. Although *Candida* infections respond well to therapy, recurrent episodes are common whenever antifungal medications are discontinued. Generally, patients continue medication after symptoms disappear because of the high rate of recurrence. Often topical therapy in combination with a systemic antifungal agent is necessary.

Herpes simplex virus infections are common among HIV-infected patients and can be severe, prolonged, persistent, and painful. Neonatal transmission following rupture of membranes is possible. In the nonpregnant state, acyclovir administration decreases the duration and severity of symptoms, as well as suppressing recurrent episodes.[31] The safety of acyclovir in pregnancy has not been demonstrated. However, after delivery, initiation of acyclovir prophylaxis should be considered for those patients with a history of herpes. Common side effects associated with the use of acyclovir include rash, hives, hypertension, headache, nausea and vomiting, and renal dysfunction.

Toxoplasmosis is caused by a protozoan found in feline feces or undercooked meat of infected animals, and its rate is increased among HIV-infected patients. Headache is the classic symptom, but other symptoms include fever, neurologic deficits, seizures, and coma. The drugs of treatment are pyrimethamine and sulfadiazine (which can be used in late pregnancy). The side effects of pyrimethamine include inhibition of folate metabolism resulting in leukopenia, thrombocytopenia, anemia, anorexia, nausea and vomiting, diarrhea, rash, headache, central nervous system effects, and photophobia. The side effects of sulfadiazine include anorexia, nausea and vomiting, diarrhea, rash, headache, elevated liver enzymes, drug fever, neuropathy, and decreased renal function. Clindamycin may also be added with potential side effects of nausea, vomiting, diarrhea, abdominal pain, rash, elevated liver enzymes, neutropenia, and jaundice.[14]

Other opportunistic infections associated with HIV infection that occur less frequently include cytomegalovirus, cryptococcosis, cryptosporidiosis, and *Mycobacterium avium intracellulare*. Cytomegalovirus can cause infection in the eyes, lungs, gastrointestinal tract, and central nervous system and can also have fetal effects. *Cryptococcus neoformans* is a fungus that manifests as a form of meningitis. Cryptosporidiosis, as a result of the protozoan parasite, usually causes diarrhea. *Mycobacterium avium intracellulare* may manifest itself as gastrointestinal symptoms or as tuberculosis.

Prior to the early 1980s, Kaposi's sarcoma was primarily seen in older males of Jewish or Mediterranean descent. Since AIDS has become more prevalent, Kaposi's sarcoma is now observed in both young men and women with immunodeficiency. Lesions are both internal and external and are seen as red, brown, or bluish nodules often on the face, in the mouth, or other body surfaces. Circulation may be impaired due to swelling in the extremities.

Assessment

A concise and comprehensive review of the medical history and current symptoms as well as thorough medication histories must be conducted. Particular attention is paid to symptoms such as chills, fever, fatigue, anorexia, vaginitis, or vaginal lesions, which may indicate signs of progressive disease. During the initial physical examination and throughout labor, the patient is assessed for signs of dehydration, maternal or fetal tachycardia, elevated temperature, abdominal tenderness, perineal lesions, and/or purulent discharge.

On admission, a complete blood count with differential leukocyte count, urinalysis, cervical and vaginal smear and cultures, and/or chest x-ray may be ordered to evaluate for HIV-related illness. A complete blood count and differential leukocyte count are performed because anemia and leukopenia and neutropenia are common in patients with HIV infection. A urinalysis is performed to evaluate for proteinuria, which may be seen in HIV nephropathy. T-cell subsets are ordered to evaluate immune status and are reported as percentage of T_4, percentage of T_8, and T_4:T_8 ratios. Absolute T_4 is most significant when establishing risk of opportunistic infections and progression of HIV infection.

Persons with $T_4 > 500$ have minimal risk of opportunistic infection; therefore, no prophylaxis is recommended. Zidovudine use is controversial in this group.

Opportunistic infections may occur in patients with T_4 between 200 and 500, but are not common. Reports have shown zidovudine to be of benefit to patients in this group. Persons with $T_4 < 200$ are at increased risk for opportunistic infections, and prophylaxis for *Pneumocystis carinii* pneumonia is usually provided.

Nursing Diagnoses

There are multiple nursing diagnoses that may be used to guide care for patients with HIV infection and AIDS. The following is a list of potential nursing diagnoses:

- Ineffective individual coping, related to:
    Depression in response to identifiable stressors
    Disease process
    Loss of income
    Loss of relationships
    Change of lifestyles
- Anticipatory grieving, related to:
    Knowledge of disease process
- Powerlessness, related to:
    Hospitalization
    Illness
- Disturbance in self-concept–body image, related to:
    Weight loss
    Appearance of skin lesions
    Fear of sexually transmitting the disease
- Social isolation, related to:
    Uncertain future
    Uncertain diagnosis
    Withdrawal from social contacts
    Loss of self-esteem
    Doubts about ability to survive
- Ineffective airway clearance, related to:
    Ineffective cough
    Inability to remove airway secretions
    Bronchospasm
    Food or fluid particles
    Trauma
- Alteration in nutritional status, related to:
    Increased metabolic needs
    Anorexia, nausea, and emesis
    Excessive diarrhea
    Stomatitis
    Medications

- Alteration in bowel elimination, related to:
  Viral disease process
  Food intolerance
  Untoward side effects of drugs
  Tube feeding
- Alteration in oral mucous membranes, related to:
  Trauma
  Ineffective oral hygiene
  Poor nutritional status
  Mouth breathing
  Stomatitis
- Alterations in thought process, related to;
  Inability to evaluate reality secondary to depression, anxiety, isolation, and physiologic process
- Alterations in sensory perception, related to:
  Sensory overload
  Inability to interpret incoming stimuli secondary to encephalitis, meningitis, and pneumonia
  Musculoskeletal changes
  Metabolic changes
  Impaired oxygen transport
- Alteration in comfort or pain, related to:
  Acute pain
  Chronic pain
  Secondary to infectious process
- Dysfunctional grieving, related to:
  Loss
  Perceived support system
  Unavailable support system
- Fluid volume deficit: actual or potential, related to:
  Excessive diarrhea
  Emesis
  Fever
  Night sweats
  Nasogastric suction
  Lung secretions
- Impairment of skin integrity: actual or potential, related to:
  Immobility
  Malnutrition
  Altered skin turgor
  Excretions and secretions
  Emaciation
  Secondary to viral process
- Impaired mobility: actual or potential, related to:
  Neoplasms

Immunoblastic sarcomas
Peripheral neuropathy
- Alteration in peripheral tissue perfusion: actual or potential, related to:
  Multiple venipunctures
  Multiple arterial punctures
  Toxic and viscous medications
  Increased volume of fluids
  Decreased patient movement
- Potential further opportunistic infection, related to:
  Abnormal white blood cell ratio
  Dehydration
  Skin breakdown
  Nutritional deficit
  General debilitation
- Alteration in actual activity tolerance, related to:
  Shortness of breath
  Decreased nutritional status

Theoretical Basis for the Plan of Nursing Care and Intervention

As this epidemic continues to grow, more and more nurses are becoming involved in patient counseling prior to and following HIV testing. Nurses involved in such counseling should be aware of the need for completeness, consistency, and strict confidentiality. Most states have legislation that mandates confidentiality and informed consent and regulates partner notification practices. Nurses must be familiar with the legislation specific to the state in which they practice.

With regard to universal practices, nursing care for identified intrapartum patients with HIV infection does not differ from that for noninfected patients. Because seroprevalence studies have revealed increasing numbers of women with HIV infection, many of whom are unaware of their disease, and because it is not possible to identify all patients who are HIV positive, the practice of strict adherence to universal precautions during the antepartum, intrapartum, and postpartum period is essential for all patients.

Although HIV has been isolated from a number of body fluids, blood is the only body fluid implicated in transmission of HIV to health care workers. Blood is the single most important source of HIV in the occupational setting, particularly in the labor and delivery suite. Infection control precautions must focus on the prevention of exposure to blood. Although vaginal secretions have been implicated in the sexual transmission of HIV, they have not been implicated in the occupational transmission from patient to health care worker.

Universal precautions were recommended by the CDC for use with all patients in 1987.[32] These recommendations have implications for practice in obstetrics and, specifically, the labor and delivery suite. Specific policies and procedures for implementing universal precautions are necessary to ensure that all health care professionals are following appropriate guidelines. With the advent of universal precautions in the care of all patients, concern regarding exposure to infectious patients should be minimized. Gloves, masks, goggles, and protective aprons should now be a part of routine labor and delivery attire.

Gloves should be worn when in contact with blood, amniotic fluid, nonintact skin and mucous membranes, and initial handling of the neonate until bathed. Water-resistant gowns or aprons as well as foot covers should be worn when there is potential for clothing to be splashed or saturated with blood or body fluids. Goggles, safety glasses, or face shields should also be worn when splashing of blood or body fluids is possible Masks should also be worn as a part of normal aseptic technique and if there is possibility of facial splashing or if patients require respiratory precautions. Instruments in labor and delivery should be washed and then either sterilized or disinfected by high-level disinfectant, such as an EPA approved glutaraldehyde solution, as appropriate. Special care should be taken when disposing of syringes and needles so that unintentional needlestick injuries do not occur. All linen and garbage or waste should be considered and treated as contaminated.

The use of mouth suction devices places the health care professional at risk because of the potential for exposure to blood-contaminated secretions of neonates. Therefore, wall or bulb suction should always be used to clear secretions from the neonate's oropharynx.[33]

In general, nursing care should be directed toward the system affected. Patients with AIDS have increased incidence of multisystem compromise including skin irritations and gastrointestinal, respiratory, and neurologic disorders. Skin irritations commonly affect the perineum, and nursing measures are thus palliative. Sitz baths or warm wet compresses can be applied. Topical analgesia is often indicated as well.

For patients with gastrointestinal complications, accurate intake and output are essential, and laboratory values are monitored for electrolyte imbalance. Skin turgor is assessed for signs of dehydration, and rehydration as appropriate is accomplished. Hyperalimentation may become necessary. Diarrhea and emesis may require medication and skin care of the perianal area. Gastrointestinal problems may contribute to a fragile nutritional state, thus patients are assessed for complications such as changes in oral mucosa. Special attention should be paid to mouth care. Patients may not be able to tolerate large meals but may require small frequent feedings when allowed to eat.

Since changes in respiratory status are common, an emphasis should be placed on the respiratory system and its care. Respiratory status is assessed and treatment initiated if gas exchange and airway are impaired. Effective airway clearance is of prime importance. Patients with *Pneumocystis carinii* pneumonia commonly require respiratory support in the form of respiratory treatments, oxygen, and/or ventilatory support. Nursing care aimed at improved gas exchange includes encouraging coughing to keep the airway clear and suctioning if necessary. Anxiety and stress are decreased by explaining the details of care to patients. Patients are taught pursed-lip breathing, deep breathing, and coughing. The head of the bed is elevated. Fluids may be increased to help thin secretions. Blood gas monitoring is often required, and physicians are notified if acute distress or worsening conditions occur.

Another challenge for labor and delivery nurses is evaluating the neurologic status of patients which may be impaired due to HIV illness or other obstetric or medical conditions such as preeclampsia, eclampsia, or stroke. If there is an alteration in mental status, nursing actions should include assessment of mental status and behavior changes that may require assistance from partners or families. Patients are also assessed for thought processes and judgment capabilities and may need to be oriented to person, place, and/or time. Often the environment must be modified for safety, which may include restriction of activity. All tests, procedures, and events should be carefully explained, and repetition of information may be required. The effect of stimulation is evaluated, and restriction or minimization accomplished if needed.

If a seizure occurs, the time and duration of the seizure should be noted. Protection from injury with padded side rails, and antiseizure medication is usually ordered. Following the seizure, neurologic status should be monitored and patients reoriented to their surroundings. Once patients are able to respond verbally, nurses must determine if they experienced a preseizure aura and note its qualities. Patients must then be instructed to immediately report if they experience the aura again.

Patients with HIV infection or AIDS may also use intravenous drugs and will therefore have the increased incidence of associated complications. Adequate pain management is most important for these patients, and analgesia and anesthesia should not be withheld or diminished. (See Chapter 8.)

It is not unusual for patients in an acute stage of AIDS to require hemodynamic monitoring and/or ventilatory support. Nurses skilled in critical care monitoring become an essential component in the provision of obstetric care for patients with HIV infection or AIDS. Each hospital should have a preestablished plan regarding where patients will be admitted and who will participate in their care.

Psychosocial support and counseling are of primary importance and a vital component to intrapartum nursing care. Women with HIV infection may experience periods of intense anxiety along with feelings of anger, guilt, self-pity, and confusion. Nurses must use their skills to offer supportive counseling, which is a continuous process particularly for this patient population. Once patients feel they are in a trusting, nurturing, and safe environment, compliance with medical regimens necessary during labor and delivery will be enhanced. It is essential that health professionals working with these women understand the complex issues they face and assist them in coping. It is important to recognize that many patients with AIDS and HIV infection are afraid for their future and are very sensitive to the reactions of others to them and their disease.

Caring for terminally ill obstetric patients in the labor and delivery unit is a rare event. Usually, obstetric care is delivered to primarily healthy women or women with chronic disease. The nursing staff may exhibit concern and/or unease in dealing with these patients. Nurses need to come to terms with their own feelings and then, through their exposure to perinatal bereavement counseling techniques, work with patients who are in the grieving process during labor and delivery. Families may also be part of the grieving process and require bereavement counseling. Therefore, patients with HIV infection and AIDS and their families require extensive psychologic support and counseling through labor, delivery, and the recovery process, which increase care requirements.

Specific issues that need to be addressed by terminally ill pregnant women and new mothers are childbearing and future child custody—issues that include adoption or legal guardianship. There is a very real possibility that pregnant AIDS patients may die either during the pregnancy or shortly thereafter. Pregnant women are often worried they may become too ill to care for their children. If arrangements have not been made, labor and delivery nurses may be instrumental in obtaining the necessary resources to complete these arrangements or to refer the family to appropriate resources.

Intrapartum nurses need to be cognizant of the potential need for bereavement counseling for patients with HIV infection and AIDS, which may be further complicated by the way in which women regard their own bereavement; whether they have had a previous child die or have one currently dying of AIDS; and the dying or death of their male partner or spouse. As women with HIV infection and AIDS enter into the labor and delivery suite, their thoughts may not be about the ideal baby they are going to deliver. Instead they may be wondering whether their babies will have the HIV infection and whether they may die. Or, perhaps, they may be concerned about other problems concerning the newborn. So, instead of entering labor and delivery in a mode of happy anticipation, these patients may be depressed, fearful, and have a high degree of anxiety. Bereavement counseling should be aimed at letting patients discuss their thoughts, fears, and concerns; helping them mobilize their resources; and making referrals as needed.

Following delivery, decisions regarding placement should be made if patients are no longer able to care for themselves. Some options for care include staying in the acute care facility,[14] home care with hospice or other support services such as a visiting nurse, a residential hospice facility, or a skilled nursing facility. Referrals to community resources including volunteer networks and organizations need to be completed.

Expected Outcomes

The patient will do the following:

1. Maintain vital signs within normal ranges (if not terminal or end stage)
2. Avoid vena cava compression and hypotension by maintaining appropriate maternal positioning

3. Maintain adequate hydration and acid–base balance
4. Maintain a stable neurologic status by the absence of seizure activity and no change in mental status
5. Maintain normal gastrointestinal activity
6. Maintain adequate pulmonary function via a patent airway, normal ventilation, and normal blood gas values
7. Verbalize decreased fear and increased understanding of risks to the fetus and self
8. Verbalize understanding of how she will be cared for while in the labor and delivery unit
9. Demonstrate maternal–infant bonding
10. Verbalize issues related to grief regarding herself, her baby, or her family

The fetus will do the following:

1. Maintain fetal heart rate between 110 and 160 beats per minute
2. Maintain a reassuring fetal heart rate pattern on the electronic fetal heart rate monitor as evidenced by:
   a. Absence of fetal heart rate decelerations and
   b. Presence of accelerations (as appropriate for gestational age)
   c. Minimal or greater fetal heart rate variability (as appropriate for gestational age and monitoring method)
3. Exhibit intrauterine activity

References

1. Centers for Disease Control. HIV prevalence and AIDS case projections for the United States: Report based on a workshop. *MMWR* 39:30, 1990.
2. Centers for Disease Control. HIV/AIDS surveillance report. July 1991.
3. Centers for Disease Control. The HIV/AIDS epidemic: The first 10 years. *MMWR* 22:357, 1991.
4. Landesman S, Minkoff H, Holman S, et al.: Immunodeficiency virus infections in parturients: Implications for HIV testing programs of pregnant women. *JAMA* 253(3)363–366, 1987.
5. Weisfuse I, Back S, O'Hare D, et al.: The seroprevalence of HIV-I infection among women attending maternal infant care clinics in New York City. *IV International AIDS Conference, Montreal, Canada.* Abstract 4038, 1988.
6. Hoff R, Berardi V, Weiblen J, et al.: Seroprevalence of human immunodeficiency virus among childbearing women. *N Engl J Med* 319(9):525–530, 1988.
7. Conner K, Goode L, Morrison J, et al.: Seroprevalence of HIV of parturients at University Hospital, Newark, NJ. *IV International AIDS Conference, Montreal, Canada.* Abstract 6085, 1988.
8. Scott G, Hutto C, Mastrucci M, et al.: Probability of perinatal infections in infants of HIV-I positive mothers. *IV International AIDS Conference, Montreal, Canada.* Abstract 6583, 1988.
9. Centers for Disease Control. Recommendations for prevention of HIV transmission in health care settings. *MMWR* 36:285–289, 1987.
10. Sinclair B: Epidemiology and transmission of infection by human immunodeficiency virus. *NAACOG's Clinical Issues in Perinatal Women's Health Nursing* 1(1):1, 1990.
11. Centers for Disease Control. Revisions of the CDC surveillance case definitions for AIDS. *MMWR* Suppl 36:3S–15S, 1987.

12. Centers for Disease Control. Classification system for HIV infection in children under 13 years of age. *MMWR* 36:225–230, 1987.
13. Brunner L, Suddarth D: *Textbook of Medical Surgical Nursing,* 6th ed., Chapter 45, pp. 1176–1193. Philadelphia, PA, J.B. Lippincott, 1988.
14. Lewis A: *Nursing Care of the Person with AIDS/ARC.* Rockville, MD, Aspen, 1988.
15. Friedland G, Klein R: Transmission of HIV. *N Engl J Med* 317:1125–1133, 1987.
16. Hauer L, Dattel B: Management of the pregnant woman infected with HIV. *J Perinatol B* 8:256–262, 1988.
17. LaPointe N, Michaud J, Pekovik D, et al.: Transplacental transmission of HTLVIII virus. *N Engl J Med* 312:1325, 1985.
18. Efantis J: In-patient maternity care for the HIV-positive woman and her newborn. *NAACOG's Clinical Issues in Perinatal and Women's Health Nursing* 1(1):50, 1990.
19. Weinbeck P, Loustand V, Denis F, et al.: Breastfeeding and HIV-I transmission. *IV International AIDS Conference, Montreal, Canada.* Abstract 5102, 1988.
20. Peckham CS, Senturia YD, Ades AE: Obstetric and perinatal consequences of human immunodeficiency virus (HIV) infection: A review. *Br J Obstet Gynaecol* 94:403–407, 1987.
21. Minkoff H, Nada D, Mendez R, et al.: Pregnancies resulting in infants with AIDS or AIDS-related complex. *Obstet Gynecol* 87:288–291, 1987.
22. Berrebi A, Kobuch W, Puel J, et al.: Effects of HIV infection on pregnancy. *International Conference on AIDS in Women and Children, Paris, France.* Abstract B17, 1989.
23. Gloeb DJ, O'Sullivan MJ, Efantis J: Human immunodeficiency virus infection in woman: I. The effects of human immunodeficiency virus on pregnancy. *Am J Obstet Gynecol* 159:756, 1988.
24. Berrebi A, Puel J, Tricoire J, et al.: The influence of pregnancy in the influence of HIV infection. *Fourth International Conference on AIDS, Stockholm, Sweden.* Abstract 4041, 1988.
25. Minkoff H, Feinkind L: Management of pregnancies of HIV-infected women. *Clin Obstet Gynecol* 32:467–476, 1989.
26. Fischl MA, Richmann DD, Grieco MH, et al.: The efficacy of Azidothymidine (AZT) in the treatment of patients with AIDS and AIDS-related complex: A double blind, placebo controlled trial. *N Engl J Med* 317;185, 1987.
27. Volberding P, Lagakos S, Koch M, et al.: Safety and efficacy of zidovudine in asymptomatic HIV-infected individuals with less than 500 CD4+ cells/mm.^{3} *N Engl J Med* 320: 1990.
28. Birdsall C, Uretsky S: How do you give pentamidine aerosol for PCP? *Am J Nurs* 88:1126–1127, 1988.
29. Haley C: Pentamidine in *Pneumocystis carinii* pneumonia. *Microlink Update* 3:1–4, 1987.
30. Carpenter C, Majer K, Fisher A: Natural history of acquired immunodeficiency syndrome in women in Rhode Island. *Am J Med* 86:771–775, 1989.
31. Minkoff HL: Care of pregnant women infected with human immunodeficiency virus. *JAMA* 258:2714–2717, 1988.
32. Centers for Disease Control. Recommendations for prevention of HIV transmission in healthcare settings. *MMWR* Suppl 37:3S-17S, 1987.
33. Sinclair B: Management of the parturient who is HIV positive. *NAACOG Newsletter* 15:12, 1988.

15
◆ ◆ ◆

Trauma in Pregnancy

Jane B. Daddario
Gayle Johnson

Supportive Data

Incidence

Trauma occurs with alarming frequency and has had a significant impact on our society, not only in terms of human loss but economic cost as well. It is the leading cause of death and disability among individuals under age 40 and, following heart disease, cancer, and stroke, the fourth leading cause of death among all age groups.

The magnitude of this problem has also been felt within the obstetric community. Trauma is responsible for 22% of nonobstetric-related deaths of pregnant women.[1,2] It has been estimated that accidental injury occurs in 7% of all pregnancies, with the distribution of reported cases increasing as pregnancy progresses.[3,4] Approximately 10% of injuries occur during the first trimester, about 40% in the second, and the remaining 50% in the third trimester of pregnancy.[5]

Several causes of traumatic injury may be readily identified. Motor vehicle accidents, responsible for 48,700 deaths in 1987 alone, have greatly increased mortality in the general population.[6] Though often associated with minor injuries, motor vehicle accidents cause death nearly 10 times more frequently than other sources of trauma and represent the most common cause of injury during pregnancy. Domestic violence is also a significant problem. Research demonstrates that 15% to 20% of all pregnant women are battered.[7] Therefore, until ruled out, battery should be considered a possible cause of trauma in female patients who do not have clear histories.[8,9] Other sources of trauma during pregnancy include falls, burns, and firearm injuries.

Significance   Although most traumatic injuries during pregnancy are minor in nature, significant morbidity and mortality may be encountered. An understanding of the impact of trauma on the mother and fetus facilitates nursing assessment and development of an appropriate plan of care. Foreknowledge of not only typical traumatic injuries but also associated complications allows few surprises for the nurse who encounters a pregnant trauma victim.

MATERNAL MORTALITY

Maternal mortality is most often due to injuries sustained from motor vehicle accidents, specifically head injuries followed by multiple internal injuries, which lead to hypovolemic shock and exsanguination.[10] These injuries tend to worsen if the victim is ejected from the vehicle. Studies have demonstrated that mortality would decrease if a properly placed lap belt in conjunction with a shoulder harness were worn by the mother (see Figure 15-1 for proper belt placement).[11] Other life-threatening injuries that may be encountered in the multiple trauma victim include dissection of major thoracic and abdominal vessels, pleural space intrusion, liver and splenic lacerations, bowel perforation, multiple extremity fractures, and pelvic hematomas or fractures.

Certain injuries and associated complications are unique to the pregnant trauma victim and include uterine damage, placental abruption, and amniotic fluid embolism. Disseminated intravascular coagulation may also develop in the

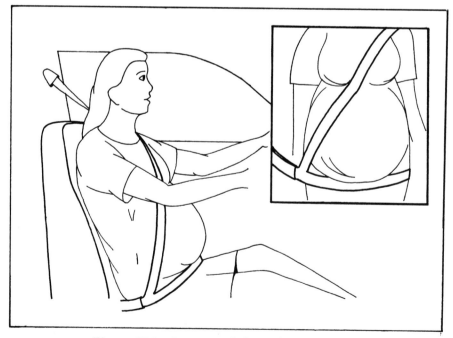

Figure 15-1. Proper seat belt use during pregnancy.

presence of a large placental abruption, significant hemorrhage, or intrauterine fetal demise. It is not uncommon following blunt or penetrating abdominal trauma for a transplacental fetal–maternal hemorrhage to occur. In a study of 32 pregnant trauma patients, the incidence of fetal–maternal hemorrhage was 28%, with a mean blood loss of 16 cc and a range from 5 to 40 cc.[12,13] Uterine rupture has been reported in association with accidents involving deceleration forces that tear the uterus away from its fixation point, cases where pregnant women were run over by moving vehicles causing extreme compression of the abdomen, and, rarely, other motor vehicle accidents.[11,14] However, placental abruption is much more likely to occur than is uterine rupture and has been reported as late as 5 days following the initial injury.[15,16] Though no statistics are available regarding the incidence of preterm labor and premature rupture of membranes secondary to trauma, any injury resulting in hypoxic insults may increase such risk.

A review of significant trauma statistics in the general population also helps anticipate the concomitant impact on maternal outcome. Direct cerebral and high spinal cord injuries account for approximately 50% of all trauma deaths.[17] Most head and spinal injuries occur as a result of falls or direct blows. Head injuries range from mild concussion to intracranial hemorrhage or herniation and occur in 70% of all traffic accidents, whereas 10% of motor vehicle accidents result in spinal injuries.[18]

Thoracic trauma is the primary cause of death in 25% of all fatal accidents and is a concurrent injury in 50%.[19] Blunt trauma accounted for the majority of these injuries and is most often due to the impact of a steering wheel or dashboard during a motor vehicle accident. Pregnant drivers who wear improperly placed seat belts or none at all are susceptible to such complications as pneumothorax, flail chest, pericardial tamponade, hemothorax, ruptured diaphragm, tension pneumothorax, great vessel dissection, and pulmonary or myocardial contusions. Penetrating trauma, however, is becoming more and more common, especially in urban areas. The extent of tissue damage depends largely on the kinetic energy involved; for example, low-velocity missiles or knives generally produce less significant bleeding and tissue destruction than high-velocity weapons.[19] Associated injuries include open pneumothorax, pericardial tamponade, hemothorax, and great vessel dissection. Intraabdominal organs may also be affected if the path taken by the penetrating object transects the diaphragm.

Abdominal trauma may result from either blunt or penetrating sources. Blunt injuries, in addition to uteroplacental damage discussed previously, may include genitourinary trauma such as bladder rupture, urethral lacerations, and renal contusion or avulsion. Penetrating abdominal wounds may be produced by a variety of objects yet are most often caused by bullets.[19] The uterus often serves as a protective shield to other organs though the fetus may be placed in a position of greater susceptibility. Maternal mortality from bullet wounds was low in 77 cases reported, whereas fetal mortality ranged from 41% to 71% and was dependent on gestational age.[20] Stab wounds are the second most frequent type of penetrating abdominal injury and are generally less severe than bullet wounds since the bowel is likely to slide away from the penetrating object. The extent of injury is greater with multiple wounds, especially those to the bowel. Patterns of injury may be predicted by following the path of the instrument involved. Perinatal mortality for all intrauterine wounds approximates 40%.[20]

Pelvic fractures continue to cause significant morbidity and mortality and remain the third most common injury in motor vehicle accidents.[21] There is an increased incidence of extensive retroperitoneal hemorrhage due to engorged pelvic veins. The pelvis usually fractures in two places due to the bony ring structure. Such injury does not necessarily preclude vaginal delivery.

Pregnant women may sustain burn trauma, though case reports are rare. Less than 0.1% of gravid burn patients suffer a thermal injury severe enough to warrant hospital admission.[4,21,22] Injury may be due to contact with hot objects, electric currents, or exposure to chemicals. Inhalation injury and carbon monoxide intoxication may complicate the clinical picture if there was prolonged exposure to flames, heated gases, or smoke. In the absence of inhalation injury, maternal survival depends on the extent and depth of the burn.[23] Those sustained as a result of an explosion may also be accompanied by significant blunt or penetrating trauma. Although thermal injury may result in superficial destruction of the skin and underlying tissue, alteration of virtually every organ system may occur. The pregnant burn victim is especially vulnerable to intravascular volume deficit and hypoxia.[4,11,23,24]

FETAL MORTALITY

The most common cause of fetal death in cases of trauma is maternal death. The second leading cause is placental abruption.[25,26] It has been documented that placental laceration, although rare, has always been associated with fetal loss.[27] Rapid compression and expansion of the uterus produce shearing forces that tear an essentially rigid placenta from the flexible uterine wall. Maternal and fetal bleeding ensue and fetal death results from exsanguination of the fetal blood volume into the uterine cavity.[26]

Perinatal mortality secondary to noncatastrophic trauma does not greatly increase if the fetus is healthy prior to the insult.[28] The frequency of direct fetal injury following trauma is unknown. Though it is uncommon to have a serious fetal injury in the absence of maternal injury, studies demonstrate that fetal injuries may be diagnosed with the uterus intact.[29]

Amniotic fluid provides a cushioning effect and in cases of minor blunt trauma the fetus usually survives intact. As the uterus rises out of the pelvis, the fetus becomes more vulnerable. The most common direct fetal injuries are skull fracture and intracranial hemorrhage.[27,29] Fetal skull fractures are most often associated with motor vehicle accidents and result from fetal impact against the sacral prominence of the symphysis pubis, as well as from forward flexion of the torso over the gravid uterus. Other reported fetal fractures include the mandible, clavicle, vertebrae, and long bones.[30]

As previously noted, trauma may result in rupture of the amniotic membranes.

If a rupture occurs and the fetus is preterm or not engaged in the maternal pelvis, a cord prolapse may occur resulting in compression and fetal compromise. Maternal hypovolemia or hypotension may result in significant reduction in uteroplacental perfusion, thus contributing to fetal hypoxia or acidemia. Abdominal trauma secondary to battering has been reported to cause significant fetal heart rate abnormalities. Regardless of the severity of maternal injury, fetal heart rate abnormalities may serve as predictors of fetal head trauma.[12]

The fetus, if injured but alive and beyond 24 weeks, is potentially salvageable. Gestational age has a significant impact on decision making with regard to timing of delivery. Regarding route of delivery, vaginal birth is preferable to cesarean section in most instances.

Etiology

Many social issues contribute to the overall high incidence of trauma. Drunk driving, nonuse of vehicle restraints or helmets, prevalence of handguns, and violent crime associated with drugs are just a few (see Chapter 8). Factors that have led to the high incidence of maternal injuries include increased societal mobility, presence of women in the workplace throughout pregnancy, entrance of women into jobs previously held by men, and exposure to violent behavior.[31]

Traumatic injuries result from mechanical, electrical, or thermal injuries to organs or tissues.[32] Mechanical or kinetic energy is responsible for the vast majority of injuries. Certain patterns of injury may be expected to occur depending on the mechanism of the event. Knowledge of these injury patterns will guide the nursing assessment and encourage a high index of suspicion for possible injuries that may not be immediately visible. An accident in which the body is subjected to a significant amount of kinetic energy is likely to produce serious or critical injuries. The following are some mechanisms that involve significant energy absorption:[33]

1. Falls of 20 ft or more
2. Motor vehicle accidents in which a change in speed of 20 mph has occurred, major vehicular damage is present, rollover is involved, passenger is ejected, or death of occupant within either car occurs
3. Pedestrian hit at speeds of 20 mph or more

Framework for Accepted Therapy

The mechanism of injury, gestational age of the fetus, and associated complications determine the maternal–fetal response to trauma. Certain physiologic and anatomic changes of pregnancy may significantly mask injury and influence patterns of injury and patient responses. For these reasons, such changes should be considered in planning care for the pregnant trauma patient (see Table 15-1).

Obstructions and reductions in blood flow from trauma are poorly tolerated by the mother and fetus since pregnancy is considered a high-flow, low-

TABLE 15-1
Changes to Consider in Planning Care for Pregnant Trauma Patients

Physioanatomic Changes during Pregnancy	Clinical Impact
CARDIOVASCULAR	
Blood volume increases by 50%	May lose 30–35% of blood volume before shock is evident
Plasma volume increased more than red blood cells; heart rate increases 15–20 beats per minute	Physiologic anemia
Decreased systemic vascular resistance; cardiac output increased by 50%	May not develop cool, clammy skin
RESPIRATORY	
Respiratory rate increased; tidal volume increased 30–40%; functional residual capacity decreased 25%	Compensated respiratory alkalosis
Metabolic rate and oxygen consumption increased	Reduced oxygen reserve; less tolerant of hypoxia
Chest wall broadened and diaphragm elevated	Thoracostomy performed above the normal site
Peripheral edema, dyspnea, and third heart sound present	May clinically mimic congestive ventricular failure
Abdominal viscera displaced and compressed; stretched abdominal musculature; decreased bowel sounds	Increased risk of liver or splenic rupture; abdominal injury may be masked or mimicked by pregnancy; altered patterns of referred pain; rebound tenderness may be present or absent
Decreased gastric motility; prolonged gastric emptying time; incompetent esophageal sphincter	Increased risk of aspiration
Pelvic venous congestion	Increased risk of hemorrhage
Protruding uterus and/or bladder	Increased risk of injury
HEMATOLOGIC	
Increased clotting factors VII, VIII, IX, and X; increased fibrinogen level	Hypercoagulability

resistance cardiovascular state. Hemorrhage may go unnoticed because the increased blood volume may mask hypotension. The pregnant woman may lose up to 35% of her circulating blood volume before signs of shock are evident and, for this reason, does not have the same ability to compensate for blood loss.[1] Therefore, correcting hypovolemia is a priority.

The difference in the ratio of plasma to red blood cells results in a decrease in hematocrit and albumin concentration. Due to decreased colloid osmotic pressure, the pregnant woman is vulnerable to leakage of plasma into the extravascular compartment. Thus, vigorous fluid resuscitation may increase the likelihood of pulmonary edema. However, the risk of volume overload should not prevent intravascular volume replacement but rather promote careful calculation in order to decrease capillary leakage. If the pregnant trauma patient requires immediate surgery under conduction anesthesia, additional fluid administration may be required in order to stabilize the blood pressure because of blood sequestered in the dilated vascular beds.

Oxygen reserve is decreased as a result of increased metabolic rate, thus enhancing the risk of maternal and fetal hypoxia. The chronic compensated respiratory alkalosis of pregnancy also decreases blood-buffering capacity. Associated alterations in arterial blood gas values should be considered when caring for these women. For example, the pregnant trauma patient with a Pco_2 of 40 mmHg may indeed have respiratory acidemia. Therefore, hypoventilation should be considered even though such a value in the nonpregnant woman would be normal.

The uterine vasculature has both alpha and beta receptors, but, due to the vasodilatory state of pregnancy, there is no uteroplacental vasoconstriction to impede blood flow. Perfusion pressure determines blood flow to the uterus since the uteroplacental vascular bed functions as a dilated, passive, low-resistance system.[34] Every 8 to 11 minutes the total circulating blood volume flows through the uterus, thus making the potential for bleeding a major consideration. Because of stretching of the abdominal wall and displacement of intra-abdominal organs, diminished response to peritoneal irritation may be observed complicating patient assessment.

Administration of oxygen and vasopressors alone will not improve blood flow to the uterus and placenta during hemorrhage or hypotensive episodes. Blood flow will be enhanced only through restoration and maintenance of circulating blood volume.[34] Once the pregnant woman experiences hypovolemic shock, compensatory mechanisms become activated. The uterus is then treated as a nonvital organ with blood shunted away to the brain, heart, kidney, and lungs. Fetal hypoxemia, metabolic acidemia, and death may ensue.[16]

Assessment

There is high risk for the pregnant patient with trauma because the normal anatomic and physiologic changes that have occurred as a result of her pregnancy will frequently mask serious derangements in maternal physical integrity and homeostasis. The trauma victim's initial contact with medical and nursing personnel often occurs in the emergency department setting, where lack of familiarity with obstetric principles and normal changes associated with pregnancy are not uncommon. Conversely, medical and nursing obstetric specialists may be unfamiliar with the principles of trauma stabilization and management. Therefore, the most effective strategy in providing the highest quality of care for the pregnant trauma victim requires collaboration between the emergency trauma and obstetric specialists. The nurse, well-grounded in both obstetric and trauma care, is invaluable in assuring coordination of care for this patient population.

An organized and systematic approach in assessing the trauma patient will ensure that priorities of management and stabilization are met. Assessment begins

Maternal Assessment

immediately upon encountering the patient and should follow a strict sequence, allowing life-threatening injuries to be corrected before more obvious, but non-life-threatening, injuries are managed.

The trauma assessment may be conceived as a "two-tier" system, more generally known as primary and secondary surveys. Initial emphasis is placed on the primary survey, in which life-threatening conditions are identified and resuscitation of vital signs is undertaken. Upon stabilization of vital signs, a secondary survey is performed. This includes a detailed head-to-toe examination, management of non-life-threatening injuries, and continual reassessment of the patient's condition.

The ABCs of initial trauma management are encompassed in the primary survey, which may be accomplished within minutes when performed efficiently and with a directed approach. Correctly applied, the primary survey includes *simultaneous* assessment and intervention when significant, immediately life-threatening injuries are present. Assessment and treatment priorities for the trauma patient should follow these steps:

1. Airway maintenance (and concurrent control of the cervical spine)
2. Assessment of breathing and circulation
3. Control of hemorrhage and treatment of shock

Assessment of the airway includes the basics: look, listen, and feel for movement of air. For the conscious patient, airway assessment can be accomplished at a glance; that is, the talking or shouting patient obviously has an open airway. An unconscious patient requires a closer assessment and may need assistance in gaining an airway. Opening a trauma patient's airway requires a modified jaw

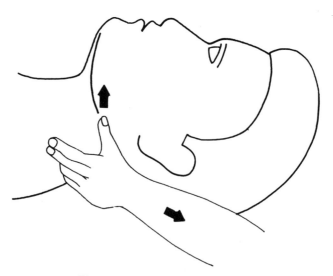

Figure 15-2. Modified jaw thrust.

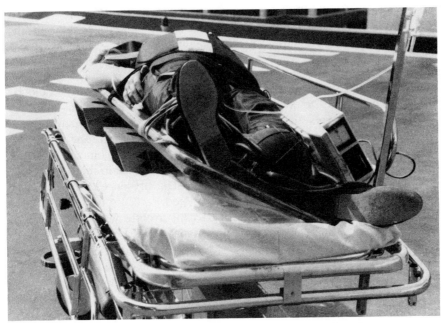

Figure 15-3. Tilting pregnant woman on spine board.

thrust without extension of the neck, rather than the head tilt–chin lift method (see Figure 15-2).

Clearing the airway of vomitus, blood, teeth, or foreign matter may be accomplished with suction and/or forceps. In no instance should the trauma victim's head be turned while clearing the airway, since cervical spine injuries can be exacerbated and can result in iatrogenic cord injury. An important axiom in airway management for the trauma patient is to assume cervical spine injury until proved otherwise by radiographic exam of all cervical vertebrae, including the superior surface of the first thoracic vertebra.

If turning a patient to the side is necessary in order to gain an adequate airway, this may be accomplished by turning her as a "whole-body" unit. Log-rolling, while manually maintaining cervical alignment or tilting a patient who is fully secured to a spine board, will accomplish this objective (see Figure 15-3). The cervical spine may be immobilized at this point by application of a cervical collar or other stabilization device, if this has not already been accomplished by prehospital care personnel.

Breathing and circulation may be assessed simultaneously since attention is directed to the neck and chest during this step of the primary survey. After establishing an adequate airway, assessing respiratory function by evaluating its rate and quality follows. Indications of distress include tachypnea, bradypnea, use of accessory muscles, shallow or painful respirations, asymmetric chest excursion, dyspnea, and inability to move air despite an open airway. Any of these symptoms should trigger suspicion of such chest injuries as pneumo- or hemothorax, tension pneumothorax, rib fracture or flail chest, and open sucking chest wounds. High-flow oxygen should be administered at this point, even in the absence of respiratory distress, since the pregnant patient's oxygen requirement is 10% to 20% greater than normal.[35]

Following assessment of respiratory rate and quality, attention should be directed to the neck. The trachea must be inspected and its position—whether or not it is midline—noted. Deviation of the trachea to either side may indicate the presence of tension pneumothorax or massive hemothorax. The neck veins must be assessed for flatness or distention. The former will accompany hypotension secondary to hypovolemia, while the latter may occur in the presence of tension pneumothorax or cardiac tamponade. The presence of edema, subcutaneous air, or discoloration must also be noted.

Assessment of circulation is performed concurrently with assessment of breathing in the primary survey. It is important to note that time-consuming blood pressure measurement need not be performed during the primary survey in order to diagnose shock. Palpation of the pulse of the carotid artery indicates a systolic pressure of at least 60 mmHg. The pulse of the femoral artery may be palpated if systolic pressure is at least 70 mmHg. Palpation of the pulse of the radial artery, indicating a systolic pressure of at least 80 mmHg, can be performed while visually inspecting the thorax.[10]

The chest is assessed for contusions, asymmetric excursion, paradoxical breathing, deformities, or open sucking wounds. The thorax is then palpated, and the presence of pain, rib instability, or subcutaneous emphysema is noted. Breath sounds must be auscultated; if decreased or absent on one side, percussion may indicate pneumothorax (hyperresonance) or hemothorax (dullness). Heart sounds should be *briefly* assessed to ascertain if they are distant or muffled. Pericardial tamponade will muffle heart sounds. Several life-threatening thoracic injuries should be detected during the primary survey. All demand immediate intervention to avoid catastrophe. Table 15-2 briefly describes each injury and its suggested initial management.

Circulatory assessment is completed by observing the patient's skin color and temperature, determining her mental status, and measuring capillary refill through a nail blanch test. Poor circulatory status is reflected in the patient who is cool, pale, agitated, and has prolonged capillary refill.

The third step of the primary survey should already have been initiated by other members of the trauma team by the time the first two steps have been assessed. Direct pressure and pressure bandages control most sources of peripheral bleeding; vessel ligature or tourniquets are rarely necessary. Military AntiShock Trousers, whose primary mechanism of action involves an increase in peripheral vascular resistance, may have already been placed by prehospital personnel in an effort to control hemorrhage, stabilize fractures, or treat shock (see Figure 15-4).[10,36] The abdominal compartment of the trousers should not be inflated for the gravid patient, since increased intraabdominal pressure may exacerbate compression of the vena cava.[1,10] Definitive surgical intervention will usually be required to achieve hemostasis for internal hemorrhage.

TABLE 15-2
Life-Threatening Thoracic Injuries

Type of Injury	Clinical Manifestations	Interventions
Airway obstruction	1. Profound shock 2. Cyanosis 3. No air movement	If attempts to clear airway with finger sweep, modified jaw thrust, suction, or laryngoscopy fail, perform immediate surgical cricothyrotomy.
Tension pneumothorax	1. Cyanosis and acute respiratory distress 2. Profound shock 3. Trachea deviated away from affected side 4. Jugular vein distention 5. Breath sounds absent and decreased on affected side 6. Hyperresonance on affected side	Immediately relieve tension by inserting 14 gauge needle into fifth intercostal space, midaxillary line, on affected side; use chest tube for long-term management.
Flail chest	1. Respiratory distress 2. Multiple unstable rib fractures 3. Paradoxical respirations 4. Poor air movement despite open airway	Internally stabilize rib fractures by immediate intubation with positive pressure ventilation.
Open pneumothorax	1. Respiratory distress 2. Open sucking chest wound 3. Subcutaneous emphysema	Cover immediately with petrolatum gauze or any airtight dressing; use chest tube for long-term mangement, and observe closely for development of tension pneumothorax.
Pericardial tamponade	1. Profound shock 2. Tightly distended jugular veins 3. Muffled heart sounds	Perform immediate pericardiocentesis or prompt thoracotomy with pericardial decompression and repair of myocardial injury.
Massive hemothorax	1. Profound shock 2. Respiratory distress 3. Breath sounds decreased or absent on affected side 4. Dullness to percussion on affected side	Immediately use chest tube with aggressive blood volume replacement, autotransfusion.

It is particularly important to pay close attention to the gravid patient's hemodynamic status. As previously noted, significant hemorrhage may be masked by the hypervolemic state of pregnancy, and the fetus may be placed at extreme risk of hypoxic injury even in the face of apparent maternal stability. One retrospective study of pregnant trauma victims associated an 80% fetal mortality with maternal shock.[37] Astute assessment and timely intervention will avoid increased

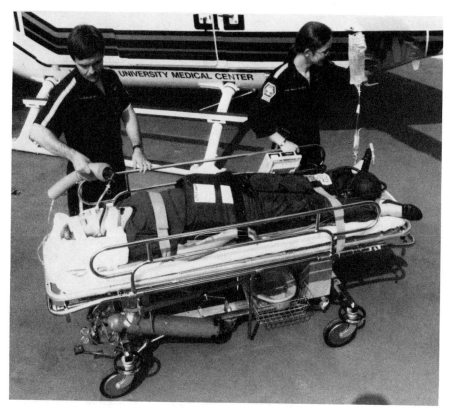

Figure 15-4. Pregnant woman in Military AntiShock Trousers.

morbidity. Treatment for shock or suspected hemorrhage must begin immediately. Placement of at least two large-bore intravenous catheters (14 or 16 gauge) with generous crystalloid and blood product administration should be initiated. Lactated Ringer's solution is the crystalloid of choice with a 3:1 replacement ratio (*i.e.,* 3 cc lactated Ringer's solution per 1 cc of estimated blood loss); it provides a base from which to begin fluid resuscitation.[1,10,38] If maternal shock has not been reversed after a bolus of 3 to 4 liters of lactated Ringer's solution, or if the patient arrives in profound shock secondary to catastrophic hemorrhage, transfusion with O-negative packed red blood cells should be immediately begun, followed by type-specific or cross-matched blood as soon as it is available.

Additional measures to combat hemorrhagic shock include placement of Military AntiShock Trousers in the emergency department if this has not already been done, use of Trendelenburg's position if ventilation is not impeded, and maintenance of patient's warmth. Shock will be exacerbated in the pregnant trauma victim by the well-known supine hypotensive syndrome, which can be avoided by tilting the entire spine board 15° laterally with pillows, blankets, or commercial wedges. Finally, continuous manual lateral displacement of the uterus by attending personnel may also be required.[38]

As previously noted, the primary survey includes assessment of and intervention in immediately life-threatening injuries. After resuscitation measures have been initiated, the secondary survey is performed. For the gravid patient, this includes a thorough head-to-toe examination with special attention given to the abdominal and pelvic assessment.

A brief neurologic assessment will reveal level of consciousness and sensorimotor function. Use of the mnemonic *AVPU* aids in rapid determination of level of consciousness:

> **A** = **A**lert and oriented
> **V** = Responds to **v**erbal stimulus
> **P** = Responds only to **p**ain
> **U** = **U**nresponsive

Although this is a very basic method for evaluating a patient's level of consciousness, its simplicity will promote clear communication about the patient's neurologic status among all caregivers. Descriptive labels such as lethargic, obtunded, or vegetative are subjective and are often interpreted differently by personnel involved in patient care. This method relies solely on objective assessment and enhances continuity. Early assessment is important, since establishing a baseline will assist in recognizing signs of deterioration.

After determining level of consciousness, examine the head for contusions, lacerations, and bony deformities. Basilar skull fractures are often accompanied by bleeding from the ear or nose, postauricular swelling and discoloration (Battle's sign), and periorbital edema and ecchymosis ("raccoon eyes"). The pupils must be evaluated for equality, reactivity to light, and accommodation. A portable cross-table lateral x-ray of the cervical spine, the radiograph of choice for initial evaluation of the cervical vertebrae, should be taken at this time.

Sensorimotor function may be easily evaluated in the conscious patient. If the patient is unconscious, how she responds to painful stimuli will indicate function. Withdrawal from or localization of pain indicates an intact sensorimotor system. Decorticate or decerebrate posturing accompanies deep cerebral hemispheric or upper brainstem injury. Spinal cord injury will produce flaccid paralysis below the level of the lesion.

The Glasgow Coma Scale is a common method for evaluating and monitoring neurologic status (Table 15-3). It has been shown to be a valid tool in predicting final outcome for head-injured victims.[35] Scores are derived by selecting the numerical value for the *best* response in three components of the evaluation and by calculating a total. An initial score of 8 or higher predicts a 94% favorable outcome, and scores of 3 or 4 predict only a 10% favorable outcome.[35]

The secondary survey should be continued by moving down the body. A thorough reassessment of the chest and circulation is performed, including a portable anteroposterior radiograph of the thorax. This is followed by an abdominal and pelvic exam. Abdominal pain, tenderness, or distention may not be observed in the pregnant patient, and peritoneal signs may be confusing or

TABLE 15-3
Glascow Coma Scale

Eye opening	Spontaneously	4
	To verbal command	3
	To pain	2
	None	1
Best verbal response	Oriented	5
	Confused	4
	Inappropriate words	3
	Incomprehensible sounds	2
	None	1
Best motor response	Follows commands	6
	Localizes pain	5
	Withdraws from pain	4
	Flexor posturing (decorticate)	3
	Extensor posturing (decerebrate)	2
	None	1
Total		3–15

unreliable, even in the presence of significant organ injury. If intraabdominal hemorrhage is suspected, the most reliable assessment tool in the trauma room is the diagnostic peritoneal lavage.[2,38,39] Although pregnancy was once considered a contraindication to this procedure, it has been shown that lavage has greater benefit than risk. It is 96% to 100% accurate in detecting intraperitoneal bleeding and is helpful in preventing undiagnosed hemorrhage.[2] Results are positive for intraperitoneal bleeding if the returned fluid is bloody. The fluid may also be examined microscopically. The following are criteria for a positive result:

1. More than 100,000 red blood cells per millimeter
2. More than 500 white blood cells per millimeter
3. Presence of bile, intestinal contents, or bacteria
4. Amylase level greater than 1.5 times the patient's serum amylase level[38,40]

Culdocentesis may be the individual physician's method of choice in evaluating intraperitoneal fluid, but should only be performed by someone thoroughly experienced with this procedure.

Abdominal and pelvic assessment assumes greater significance for the pregnant trauma victim. By this point in the secondary survey, maternal stabilization should be underway, if not already accomplished. Assessment of the uterus, fetus, and pelvis will provide some indication of fetal viability and well-being, and it is at this juncture that collaboration between trauma and obstetric specialists provides a critical enhancement of patient outcome.

A uterine assessment pertinent to the trauma victim includes measurement of fundal height to provide an estimate of gestational age; palpation of the uterus for tenderness and contraction frequency, intensity, duration, and resting tone;

assessment of fetal heart rate; and performance of a vaginal exam to assess cervical status noting vaginal bleeding or amniotic fluid leakage. Fetal assessment will be discussed in greater detail later in the chapter.

Pelvic bony structures should be evaluated clinically and radiographically. Significant, comminuted pelvic fractures may be obviously unstable when anteroposterior or medial pressure is manually applied at the iliac crests and pubic symphysis. An anteroposterior radiograph of the pelvis will reveal less obvious fractures and should be performed as part of the secondary survey. Blunt trauma forceful enough to produce fractures will usually result in at least two disruptions of the pelvic ring, with a potential loss of 6 to 8 U of blood.[41] Assessment of the urethral meatus for obvious tissue damage or bleeding must be made; if these are absent, a urinary catheter should be inserted to monitor urine output and to rule out hematuria. Hip fractures or dislocations may be clinically evident if the lower extremity on the affected side appears shorter or longer and is rotated medially or laterally.

An assessment of the extremities for soft tissue or skeletal injury completes the secondary survey. Injuries of the musculoskeletal system may appear dramatic, but rarely pose an immediate threat to life. Significant hemorrhage from femur fractures or any open fracture may occur, however, and hemostasis can usually be achieved through the use of pressure bandages and splinting. Assessment of the neurovascular function of an affected extremity includes evaluation of sensation, movement, color, capillary refill, swelling, and distal pulses.

Finally, optimal care of the pregnant trauma victim is promoted by a psychosocial assessment and the provision of emotional support for her and her family. Although an acute trauma resuscitation phase demands strict attention to the patient's physical condition, as much time as possible should be spent in determining her emotional status and extended support system and in reassuring her that aggressive care offers the fetus the best chance for survival. Extreme physical stress and fear have been shown to influence physiologic function during pregnancy and have been correlated with increased uterine activity and termination of pregnancy.[5] The pregnant patient and her family should be kept informed of her progress and the status of her baby and should be allowed to express their fear and anxiety within a supportive milieu. Family members should also be allowed to stay with the patient whenever appropriate.

FETAL ASSESSMENT

During initial maternal stabilization efforts, fetal assessment should address estimation of gestational age and evidence of well-being. More thorough assessment modalities may be implemented as maternal response permits. Medical and nursing personnel with expertise in obstetrics should be actively involved in this process as soon as possible.

The last menstrual period, fundal height, and biometric evaluation by ultrasonography may be used to assess the gestational age of the fetus. Due to the degree of injury, many trauma victims may be unable to provide precise dates for their last menstrual period, thus making this method unreliable. Fundal height measurement and ultrasound assessments are more practical, and accuracy of ultrasound is enhanced by early and serial sonograms.

Evidence of well-being and identification of stressors may be elicited by assessment of fetal heart rate responses. Examination by real time ultrasonography confirms the presence or absence of fetal heart activity and serves as an immediate indicator of fetal status.

Further assessment of fetal heart rate responses may be via auscultation or electronic fetal monitoring. Auscultation permits calculation of a baseline rate in beats per minute and may allow detection of marked changes in rate. By approximately 8 to 12 weeks gestation, fetal heart tones should be audible by Doppler and by a fetoscope by 16 to 19 weeks of gestation. However, auscultation with a fetoscope following blunt abdominal trauma may be difficult. Electronic fetal monitoring permits evaluation of baseline rate, variability, and periodic patterns.

A marked sinusoidal pattern has been identified frequently in fetuses who are severely anemic.[42] It has been observed that sinusoidal oscillations of more than 25 beats per minute are closely associated with poor fetal/neonatal outcome.[42] Other characteristics that indicate compromise include repetitive late, variable, or prolonged decelerations; absent variability; and tachycardia or bradycardia. In a hypovolemic patient, classic late decelerations may be alleviated by prompt volume replacement or repositioning. It should be remembered that placental abruption—a common cause of uteroplacental insufficiency in the obstetric trauma patient—though usually occurring within 48 hours of the injury, has been reported as late as 5 days.[1,27,42] Other tests that may be utilized to assess fetal status include ultrasonography, computerized tomography, magnetic resonanic imaging, and percutaneous umbilical blood sampling.

Continuous fetal heart rate monitoring is of benefit in the early diagnosis of traumatic fetal head injury; however, sequential ultrasound examinations may be necessary to confirm intracranial bleeding. Massive acute intracerebral hematomas have been readily diagnosed by ultrasound in the antepartum period.[43] It is important to realize, however, that slowly developing intracranial hemorrhages may require serial ultrasound over 3 to 5 days.[44]

Computed tomography scanning may be helpful in assessing direct fetal injury, as well as maternal intraabdominal bleeding, following blunt trauma. It has been used in place of peritoneal lavage, in some institutions, for the diagnosis of internal hemorrhage. A concern expressed about computed tomography is radiation dosage. The estimated absorbed dose of 2 mGy (0.2 rad) is about half that of standard pelvimetry.[26] To date, in animal and human data, exposure between 5 and 10 rad has not indicated an increase in gross congenital anomalies or intrauterine growth retardation.[45] Radiation exposure may be decreased by shielding the patient as much as possible and limiting the actual number of films for each individual view. Because of radiation exposure of the fetus, there is some question as to the use of computed tomography in early pregnancy for screening purposes. Yet in the near-term fetus with suspected trauma, the role is still emerging. It can be employed as an important diagnostic tool.

Magnetic resonance imaging is a noninvasive technology used for imaging of structural fetal defects as well as fetal function since it has the ability to detect some enzyme defects. Its major advantage over ultrasound is its ability to define soft tissue structures in the maternal pelvis. Magnetic resonance imaging has an important role in assessing the pregnant trauma victim, because maternal abdominal and pelvic structures can be more easily visualized than they are with ultrasound, which can be complicated by obesity and gas. Despite its clinical use in obstetrics, it is important to remember that its safety in human pregnancy remains undefined.[46]

Percutaneous umbilical blood sampling may be used to diagnose fetal coagulopathies, hemoglobinopathies, hemophilias, and congenital infections and may be used for rapid fetal karyotyping.[47] Since this procedure allows access to fetal circulation, the physician may use it to obtain a blood sample to help determine the severity of fetal injury as well as plan management.[47]

The interval between maternal death and delivery directly influences the survival rate of the infant. Studies indicate that surviving infants will be healthy if they are delivered within 5 minutes of maternal death.[34] Uncertainty about the time of the mother's death is not a contraindication to cesarean section. Neonatal outcome is critically affected by the elapsed time after the mother's death and gestational age of the fetus. An interval of less than 10 minutes between maternal death and delivery correlates with good neonatal survival.[48] Beyond 2 to 4 minutes, the chances of successful resuscitation of the mother diminishes. The obstetric nurse has approximately 4 minutes to restore hemodynamic stability.[34] The cardiopulmonary resuscitation team must ensure that there are pauses to determine the presence and status of the fetal heart beat. It is recommended that the fetus be delivered, regardless of gestational age, if the mother does not respond to open- or closed-chest massage within 15 minutes.

Nursing Diagnoses

Nursing diagnosis is an essential component of the nursing process, and formulation of appropriate diagnoses as they relate to the pregnant trauma patient will guide nursing intervention and assist evaluation of patient outcomes. These diagnoses may be categorized according to expected outcomes relating to maternal hemodynamic stability, adequate maternal pulmonary function, fetal well-being, and maternal psychosocial well-being. The following are examples of nursing diagnoses relating to the pregnant trauma patient:[49]

MATERNAL HEMODYNAMIC STABILITY
- Potential for maternal hemorrhagic shock secondary to traumatic injury
- Potential for maternal hemorrhage and shock secondary to uterine damage
- Potential for maternal hemorrhage and shock secondary to placental abruption

- Potential for maternal hemorrhage and shock secondary to bladder rupture
- Potential for maternal hemorrhage and shock secondary to penetrating trauma
- Potential for decreased cardiac output related to vena cava compression by the enlarged uterus

ADEQUATE MATERNAL PULMONARY FUNCTION

- Potential for venous stasis and pulmonary emboli related to coagulation alterations and immobility
- Potential inadequate airway related to obstruction
- Potential for impaired gas exchange related to pulmonary contusion
- Alteration in ventilation related to pleural space injuries
- Alteration in ventilation related to bony thorax fractures

FETAL WELL-BEING

- Potential for fetal hypoxia secondary to maternal shock
- Potential for fetal hypoxia secondary to uterine damage
- Potential for fetal hypoxia secondary to placental abruption
- Potential for premature rupture of membranes
- Potential for onset of preterm labor
- Potential for direct fetal injury secondary to maternal trauma
- Potential for fetal injury secondary to penetrating trauma
- Potential for emergency delivery secondary to fetal compromise and/or uterine or placental injuries
- Potential for alteration in uteroplacental perfusion related to cardiovascular compromise secondary to maternal positioning

PSYCHOSOCIAL WELL-BEING

- Potential for maternal and family anxiety related to sudden hospitalization during pregnancy
- Potential for maternal and family anxiety related to pending surgical procedures and possible fetal injury or death
- Alteration in maternal–infant bonding related to patient's condition and fetal outcome
- Alteration in maternal–infant bonding related to maternal injuries and clinical condition
- Alteration in grieving process related to maternal injuries and clinical condition

Theoretical Basis for the Plan of Nursing Care and Intervention

In addition to the management principles discussed earlier, the following general axioms and specific recommendations are presented in an effort to gain an overall view of initial stabilization of the pregnant trauma patient. Protection of the airway is of utmost importance. The conscious patient who has suffered minimal damage to the face and neck will usually have no difficulty in maintaining an airway. If airway patency is in doubt, several methods may be utilized to assure this is achieved. A simple device such as a nasopharyngeal or an oropharyngeal airway may be all that is necessary. However, complete control of the airway may be required, necessitating endotracheal intubation. Nasal intubation should be avoided in the pregnant patient, since increased vascularity in the upper airway passages predisposes her to significant bleeding during this sometimes traumatic procedure. If endotracheal intubation is elected, care must be taken to manually stabilize and prevent extension of the cervical spine. A more drastic measure, surgical cricothyrotomy may be required in rare cases to gain an adequate airway. Finally, pregnant women are at increased risk of aspiration. Insertion of a nasogastric tube and gastric decompression, along with vigilant assessment and rapid intervention in the event of vomiting, will decrease the incidence of this serious complication.

Aggressive ventilatory support is often demanded by the traumatized patient. Such a patient who is pregnant demands even greater attention to ventilation and oxygenation if fetal hypoxia is to be avoided. Oxygen should never be withheld from any patient who is short of breath, has a head injury, or is in shock; high-flow oxygen (12 liters/minute) should be administered via a nonrebreather face mask, the method of choice for the patient with an adequate airway. Trauma victims with a respiratory rate of less than 12 or greater than 25 breaths/minute may need additional assistance. Mechanical ventilation should be guided by arterial blood gases, with an awareness that the pregnant woman is normally in a state of compensated respiratory alkalosis. Acidosis should not be exacerbated by allowing her Pco_2 to rise above 35 to 40 mmHg.

When cardiopulmonary resuscitation is necessary, several issues associated with pregnancy should be considered. First, the thorax is less compliant, making mouth-to-mouth ventilation and chest compressions more difficult and less effective. Such alterations impede the success of standard closed-chest cardiopulmonary resuscitation.[50] Before 24 weeks gestation, the objective of cardiopulmonary resuscitation is maternal conservation. After 24 weeks gestation, fetal well-being may influence decision making. Prompt emergent delivery may enhance maternal resuscitation efforts. The limit for successful resuscitation in the presence of apnea and asystole of adults is 5 to 6 minutes.[34] Unless the pregnant woman shows a favorable response to resuscitation efforts within 4 minutes, bedside cesarean section or open-chest massage is recommended.[34,51] Postmortem cesarean section dates to when the procedure was performed as much for religious reasons as for medical benefit. It was only with improvement in surgical technique during the nineteenth century that postmortem cesarean section increased in numbers. Survival still remained less than 5%.[34]

Circulatory support is also critical for the pregnant trauma patient. Early resuscitation from hypovolemic or neurogenic shock will promote maternal well-being and adequate uteroplacental perfusion. Blood pressure should not be supported with vasopressor agents, since they do not specifically address the cause of the problem and they place the fetus at extreme risk for uteroplacental vasoconstriction.[2,5,31,52,53] The single exception to this axiom is neurogenic shock, which occasionally results from high spinal cord transection or injury. Sympathetic tone is lost in this circumstance, and diffuse vasodilation causes venous pooling of the blood. Such a clinical picture includes profound hypotension accompanied by bradycardia rather than tachycardia. If no source of hemorrhage is found, neurogenic shock may be reversed through fluid bolus and low-dose dopamine infusion.

Finally, circulatory assessment and further support may be accomplished via invasive hemodynamic monitoring devices (*e.g.,* intraarterial central venous, or pulmonary artery catheters). These adjuncts are useful especially for long-term management but are sometimes employed quite early in the resuscitative phase. Early insertion of a urinary catheter will also aid in monitoring circulatory status, since renal perfusion is a function of blood flow and decreased urinary output is one of the earliest signs of shock.[54,55]

The potential risks of medications given during pregnancy must be weighed against expected therapeutic benefits. In the presence of cardiopulmonary arrest, the full range of cardiotonic and vasopressor agents may be utilized in an effort to resuscitate the mother. Under less urgent circumstances, care should be exercised in the selection and administration of medications. Tetanus toxoid or human tetanus immunoglobulin should be administered following any break in skin integrity if the patient has not been immunized in the last 10 years.[10,36] Antibiotics are commonly required for trauma victims with open injuries. With the notable exceptions of tetracycline and sulfa drugs, there is a wide variety of antibiotics that are considered relatively safe to administer during pregnancy. These include the penicillins (*i.e.,* ampicillin, methicillin, and oxacillin), the cephalosporins (*i.e.,* cephalothin, cefoxitin, and maxalactasm), erythromycin, and clindamycin. Aminoglycosides (*i.e.,* kanamycin, gentamicin, tobramycin, and amikacin) should be used with caution since childhood otologic and renal sequelae may result.[56] The use of chloramphenicol is contraindicated in the third trimester, especially near term.[56] Diuretics and antihypertensives may decrease uterine blood flow and should, therefore, be used with caution. When anticoagulation therapy is necessary, heparin is the drug of choice, since coumadin crosses the placenta.[36]

Many trauma victims require surgical intervention. If general anesthesia is required, avoidance of maternal hypotension and hypoxia is more important than the specific agents used. Succinylcholine chloride may not be employed, however, since the risk of hyperkalemia is increased. Instead, nondepolarizing agents such as pancuronium bromide and vecuronium are preferred.[23] Other medications (*e.g.,* mannitol, dexamethasone, and naloxone), sometimes crucial to trauma resuscitation, have not been established as safe to use during pregnancy.[52] As noted previously, vasopressors should be employed as a last resort in the setting of trauma care and generally should be restricted to cardiopulmonary resuscitation efforts. A significant difference exists between such agents, relative to their effect on uterine blood flow. Peripheral vasoconstrictors will increase maternal mean arterial pressure, but decrease uterine blood flow. Central vasoconstrictors, however, will concomitantly increase uterine blood flow and mean arterial pressure.[3] Table 15-4 provides examples.

TABLE 15-4
Differences Associated with Vasopressors

Vasopressor		Mean Arterial Pressure	Uterine Blood Flow
Norepinephrine		↑	↓
Dopamine	5 µg/kg/minute	↑	↔
	10 µg/kg/minute	↑	↓
Ephedrine		↑	↑

Blood should be drawn while venous access for fluid resuscitation is accomplished. The most significant laboratory studies to be obtained are complete blood count with hemoglobin and hematocrit levels, white blood count with the differential, platelet count, fibrinogen level, prothrombin and partial thromboplastin time, fibrin degradation products, and type and cross-match. Clotting studies are indicated to provide a baseline in the event that disseminated intravascular coagulation occurs. The fibrinogen level and factors VII, VIII, IX, and X are increased during pregnancy; this coupled with a decrease in circulating plasminogen activator will provide some benefit if hemorrhage occurs.[2,36,54] Conversely, these hematologic alterations will increase the risk of thromboembolic disease if prolonged immobilization secondary to trauma is enforced.[2]

Additional blood should be obtained for levels of electrolytes, glucose, blood urea nitrogen, creatinine, amylase, arterial blood gases, SGOT, SGPT, alkaline phosphatase, lactic acid dehydrogenase, and calcium. The Kleihauer-Betke test, which diagnoses fetomaternal hemorrhage by detecting fetal erythrocytes in the maternal circulation, is also important, along with the indirect Coomb's test, which detects maternal Rh sensitization.[2,38] Blood and urine samples should be obtained to screen for toxic substances, and simple urinalysis should be performed. It is not useful to collect blood and body fluids for culture and sensitivity during the initial resuscitation period unless the patient has a known history of an infectious process or sepsis.

Immediate assessment and treatment priorities for the pregnant woman with burn trauma remain the same as for any other traumatic injury, with particular attention paid to airway patency if inhalation injury is suspected. Estimation of the severity of the burn occurs during the secondary survey and is based on the depth of the burn, the total body surface area involved, the patient's age, the severity of associated injuries, and the victim's preinjury state of health.[57] The primary goals of initial stabilization and ongoing management are to maintain a normal intravascular volume and provide maximum oxygenation, since the fetus is especially vulnerable to maternal shock and hypoxia.[4,11,23]

Uterine blood flow may be sustained by adequate fluid resuscitation. Use of the Parkland formula will provide a guide for fluid administration.[58] Based on this formula, 4 ml of crystalloid solution per kilogram of maternal body weight per percent of body surface burn is administered over the first 24 hours postburn, with one half of this total infused during the first 8 hours. The Parkland formula may be written as follows:

4 ml × Body weight (kg) × Percent body surface area (BSA) burned.

with one-half of the total given over the first 8 hours and the remainder infused over the next 16 hours. For example, consider a 70-kg female with a 60% BSA second-degree burn. Calculate the Parkland formula as follows:

$$4 \times 70 \times 60 = 16,800 \text{ ml over } 24 \text{ hours.}$$

with 8400 ml infused over the first 8 hours and 8400 ml over the next 16 hours. It is important to remember that the calculation of the time begins at the moment of the injury rather than admission to the hospital. Therefore, the patient arriving 2 hours postburn would require the first 8400 ml of fluid over the next 6 hours postadmission. It is important to remember that this is only a guide. More vigorous fluid resuscitation may be required to maintain a urine output of at least 50 cc/hour, which is a more specific indicator of an adequate maternal intravascular volume.

Oxygen should be administered to the pregnant burn victim even in the absence of apparent hypoxia. The effects of decreased maternal oxygenation are magnified in the fetus, and fetal death may occur at Po_2 levels that are compatible with maternal survival.[11] Intubation and mechanical ventilation are warranted if hypoxemia persists following oxygen administration via a face mask. Carbon monoxide intoxication, a frequent result of prolonged exposure to enclosed fires or suicide attempts, may also be managed by hyperbaric oxygen therapy.

Expected Outcomes

MATERNAL HEMODYNAMIC STABILITY
The patient will do the following:

1. Maintain vital signs within normal ranges
2. Maintain a normovolemic state as evidenced by adequate hemodynamic parameters
3. Avoid vena cava compression and hypotension by maintaining a lateral position
4. Avoid coagulopathy by maintaining a normal coagulation profile

ADEQUATE MATERNAL PULMONARY FUNCTION
The patient will do the following:

1. Maintain a patent airway
2. Maintain adequate gas exchange as evidenced by normal arterial blood gases
3. Maintain adequate ventilation as evidenced by normal, nonlabored respirations

PSYCHOSOCIAL WELL-BEING

The patient will do the following:

1. Demonstrate initial expression related to grief
2. Verbalize decreased fear and increased understanding related to status of both herself and her fetus
3. Verbalize understanding of assessment and intervention processes
4. Demonstrate appropriate behaviors related to maternal–infant bonding

FETAL WELL-BEING

The fetus will do the following:

1. Maintain reassuring fetal heart rate responses as evidenced by:
   a. Fetal heart rate between 110 to 160 beats per minute
   b. Minimal or greater fetal heart rate variability (when applicable)
   c. Presence of reassuring accelerations
   d. Absence of fetal heart rate decelerations
2. Exhibit movement (appropriate for gestational age)

References

1. Bremer C, Cassata L: Trauma in pregnancy. *Nurs Clin N America* 21:705–716, 1986.
2. Baker DP: Trauma in the pregnant patient. *Surg Clin N America* 62(2):275–289, 1982.
3. Patterson RM: Trauma in pregnancy. *Clin Obstet Gynecol* 27(1):32–37, 1984.
4. Rozycki GS: Trauma in pregnancy, in Moore EE (ed.): *Early Care of the Injured Patient*. Philadelphia, BC Decker, 1990.
5. Buchsbaum HJ: Trauma in pregnancy. *ACOG Update* 12(4):1–10, 1986.
6. Trunkey DD: Trauma: A public health problem, in Moore EE (ed.): *Early Care of the Injured Patient*. Philadelphia, BC Decker, 1990.
7. Campbell JC, Sheridan DJ: Emergency nursing with battered women. *J Emerg Nurs* 15(1), 1989.
8. Helton A: Battering during pregnancy. *AJN* 86:910–913, 1986.
9. McLeer SV, Anwar RAH, Herman S, Maquiling K: Education is not enough: A systems failure in protecting battered women. *Ann Emerg Med* 18(6):651–653, 1989.
10. Schwab EW, Shaikh KA: Shock in the pregnant patient. *Emerg Care Quart* 1(2):47–57, 1985.
11. Crosby W: Traumatic injuries during pregnancy. *Clin Obstet Gynecol* 26(4):902–912, 1983.
12. Sokal MM, Katz M, Lell ME, et al: Neonatal survival after traumatic fetal subdural hematoma. *J Reprod Med* 24:131–133, 1980.
13. Boehm FH: Fetal distress, in Eden RD, Boehm FH (eds.): *Assessment and Care of the Fetus*. Norwalk, CT, Appleton & Lange, 1990.
14. Landers DF, Newland M, Penney LL: Multiple uterine rupture and crushing injury of the fetal skull after blunt maternal trauma. *J Reprod Med* 34(12):988–993, 1989.
15. Smith LH: Surgical and gynecological complications, in Niswander KR (ed.): *Manual of Obstetrics: Diagnosis and Therapy*. Boston, Little, Brown, 1987, pp. 200–202.
16. Dees G, Fuller M: Blunt trauma in the pregnant patient. *J Emerg Nurs* 15(6):495–499, 1989.
17. Lewis FR: Prehospital trauma care, in Trunkey DD, Lewis FR (eds.): *Current Therapy of Trauma*. Philadelphia, BD Decker, 1984.
18. Roberts JR: Pathophysiology, diagnosis and treatment of head trauma. *Top Emerg Med* 1(1):41–62, 1979.
19. Trunkey DD: Thoracic trauma, in Trunkey DD, Lewis FR (eds.): *Current Therapy of Trauma*. Philadelphia, BD Decker, 1984.

20. Sandy EA, Koerner M: Self-inflicted gunshot wound to the pregnant abdomen: Report of a case and review of the literature. *Am J Perinatol* 6(1):30–31, 1989.
21. Fox MA, Fabian TC: The pelvis, in Moore EE (ed.): *Early Care of the Injured Patient*. Philadelphia, BC Decker, 1990.
22. Lavin JP, Polsky SS: Abdominal trauma during pregnancy. *Clin Perinatol* 10:423–438, 1983.
23. Deitch EA, Rightmire DA, Clothier J, Blass N: Management of burns in pregnant women. *Surg Gynecol Obstet* 161(1):1–4, 1985.
24. Taylor JW, Plunkett GD, McManus WF, et al: Thermal injury during pregnancy. *Obstet Gynecol* 47:434–438, 1976.
25. Smith CV, Phelan JP: Trauma in pregnancy, in Clark SL, Hankins GDV, Cotton DB, Phelan JP (eds.): *Critical Care Obstetrics*. (2nd ed.). Boston, Blackwell, 1991.
26. Civil ID, Talucci MD, Schwab CW: Placental laceration and fetal death as a result of blunt abdominal trauma. *J Trauma* 28(5):708–710, 1988.
27. Stuart GCE, Harding PGR, Daires EM: Blunt abdominal trauma in pregnancy. *Can Med Assoc J* 122:901–905, 1980.
28. Frees M, Hankins G: DV: motor vehicle accident associated with minimal maternal trauma but subsequent fetal demise. *Ann Emerg Med* 18(3):301–304, 1989.
29. Agran PF, Dunkle DE, Win DG, et al: Fetal death in motor vehicle accidents. *Ann Emerg Med* 16:1355–1358, 1987.
30. Bowdler N, Faixd RG, Elkins T: Fetal skull fracture and brain injury after a maternal automobile accident: A case report. *J Reprod Med* 32:375, 1987.
31. Daddario JB: Trauma in pregnancy. *J Perinat Neonat Nurs* 3(2):14–22, 1989.
32. Halpern JS: Mechanisms and patterns of trauma. *J Emerg Nurs* 15(5):380–388, 1989.
33. Committee on Trauma of the American College of Surgeons: Hospital and prehospital resources for the optimal care of the injured patient. *Am College Surg Bull* 71:4–40, 1968.
34. Lee RV, Mezzadri FC: Cardiopulmonary resuscitation of pregnant women, in Elkayam U, Gleicher N (eds.): *Cardiac Problems in Pregnancy*. New Jersey, Alan R. Liss, 1990.
35. Campbell JE: *Basic Trauma Life Support: Advanced Prehospital Care*. Bowie, MD, Prentice-Hall, 1985.
36. Smith LG: The pregnant trauma patient, in Cardona VD, et al (eds.): *Trauma Nursing: From Resuscitation through Rehabilitation*. Philadelphia, WB Saunders, 1988.
37. Rothenberger D, Quanttlebaum FW, Perry JF, et al: Blunt maternal trauma: A review of 103 cases. *J Trauma* 18:173–179, 1978.
38. Higgins SD: Perinatal protocol: Trauma in pregnancy. *J Perinatol* 8(3):288–292, 1988.
39. Auerbach PS: Trauma in the pregnant patient. *Top Emerg Med* 1(1):133–137, 1979.
40. Cummings PH, Cummings SP: Abdominal trauma, in Parker JG (ed.): *Emergency Nursing: A Guide to Comprehensive Care*. New York, Wiley, 1984.
41. McQuillan K, Wiles CE, III: Initial management of traumatic shock, in Cardona VD, et al (eds.): *Trauma Nursing: From Resuscitation through Rehabilitation*. Philadelphia, WB Saunders, 1988.
42. Higgins SD, Garite TJ: Late abruptio placentae in trauma patients: Implications for monitoring. *Obstet Gynecol* 63(3):10S–12S, 1984.
43. Bondurant S, Boehm FH, Fleischer AC, et al: Antepartum diagnosis of fetal intracranial hemorrhage by ultrasound. *Obstet Gynecol* 63:25S–27S, 1984.
44. Donn SM, Barr M, McLeary RD: Massive intracerebral hemorrhage in utero: Sonographic appearance and pathologic correlation. *Obstet Gynecol* 63:28S–30S, 1984.
45. Esposito TJ, Gens DR, Smith LG, Scorpio R: Evaluation of blunt abdominal trauma occurring during pregnancy. *J Trauma* 29(12):1628–1632, 1989.
46. Mattison DR, Angtuaco T, Miller F, et al: Magnetic resonance imaging in maternal fetal medicine. *J Perinatol* 9(4):411–419, 1989.
47. Dunn PA, Stuart W, Ludomirski A: Percutaneous umbilical blood sampling. *JOGNN*, 17(5):308–313, 1988.
48. Katz VL, Dotters DJ, Droegemueller W: Perimortem cesarean delivery. *Obstet Gynecol* 68:571–576, 1986.

49. Strange JM: Abdominal trauma during pregnancy: Blunt and penetrating, in Strange JM (ed.): *Shock Trauma Care Plans*. Springhouse Corporation, 1987, pp. 99–106.
50. Marx GF: Cardiopulmonary resuscitation of late pregnant women. *Anesthesiology* 56:156, 1982.
51. *American Heart Association: Advanced Cardiac Life Support*. Dallas, AHA, 1987.
52. Stauffer DM: The trauma patient who is pregnant. *J Emerg Nurs* 12(2):89–93, 1986.
53. Vander Veer JB: Trauma during pregnancy. *Top Emerg Med* 5:72–77, 1984.
54. Bocka J, Courtney J, Pearlman M, et al: Trauma in pregnancy. *Ann Emerg Med* 17:829–834, 1988.
55. Troiano NH: Cardiopulmonary resuscitation of the pregnant woman. *J Perinat Neonat Nurse* 3(2):1–13, 1989.
56. Cesario TC: Antibiotic therapy in pregnancy, in Elkayam U, Gleicher N (eds.): *Cardiac Problems in Pregnancy*. New Jersey, Alan R. Liss, 1990.
57. Bunkis J, Walton RL: Burns, in Trunkey DD, Lewis FR (eds.): *Current Therapy of Trauma*. Philadelphia, BD Decker, 1984.
58. Shuck JM, Moncrief JA: Thermal, electrical and chemical injuries, in Schwartz GR, Safar P, Stone JH, et al (eds.): *Principles and Practice of Emergency Medicine* (2nd ed.). Philadelphia, WB Saunders, 1986.

III

NURSING CARE PROTOCOLS AND PROCEDURES

Linda K. Davis

Protocol for the Nursing Management of the Patient in Preterm Labor Requiring Intravenous Tocolytic Therapy

◆ ◆ ◆

PURPOSE

To outline nursing management of patients in preterm labor requiring tocolytic therapy.

LEVEL

Interdependent

SUPPORTIVE DATA

Preterm labor is defined as labor occurring prior to 36 completed weeks gestation. In addition to this definition both the presence of uterine contractions and cervical change must be documented.

The incidence of preterm births is approximately 8% to 10% of all births in the United States. The effects, however, are significant as preterm births account for 60% of all perinatal morbidity and mortality. Respiratory distress syndrome, intraventricular hemorrhage, necrotizing enterocolitis, and neurosensory impairment are serious complications that the neonate may face with preterm birth.

One goal of treatment is prevention of further cervical change by decreasing or stopping uterine activity. Intravenous tocolytic therapy is utilized for this purpose. Magnesium sulfate and ritodrine are the two most common drugs used in intravenous tocolytic therapy. Ritodrine is the only medication with approval from the Federal Drug Administration for use in tocolytic therapy. Neither medication is without serious risk for the patient.

Side effects of magnesium sulfate include nausea and vomiting, headache, visual blurring, and sensa-

tions of heat and burning. At toxic levels, respiratory and cardiac arrest may occur. Side effects of ritodrine include maternal and fetal tachycardia, electrocardiographic changes, and possible pulmonary edema.

Nursing management not only includes administration of medication and monitoring for effectiveness, but also assessment for side effects and intervention when potentially life-threatening outcomes occur.

CONTENT

Magnesium Sulfate Administration

1. Prepare magnesium sulfate infusion as specified in "Procedure for Intravenous Magnesium Sulfate Administration," page 313.
2. Usual loading dose for tocolysis is 4 to 6 g intravenously by infusion pump over 15 to 20 minutes.
3. Maintenance dosage for tocolysis is usually 2 to 3 g intravenously per hour by continuous infusion pump.

Nursing Assessment during Magnesium Sulfate Tocolysis

1. Assess pulse, respirations, and blood pressure:
   a. Every 15 minutes during loading dose or increases in dosage of maintenance infusion
   b. Hourly during maintenance infusion
   c. Every 15 minutes if vital signs become unstable
2. Assess deep tendon reflexes and level of consciousness hourly.
3. Assess for signs or symptoms of magnesium sulfate toxicity:

a. Absence of reflexes

b. Marked lethargy

c. Decreased level of consciousness

d. Hypotension

e. Decreased respirations of less than 10 per minute

4. Ensure antidote to Mg SO$_4$, calcium gluconate, is at bedside, 1 g of 5% or 10% solution for intravenous push administration.

5. Anticipate orders for serum magnesium levels to follow therapeutic levels.

Ritodrine Administration

1. Prepare ritodrine infusion as specified in "Procedure for Intravenous Ritodrine Administration," page 309.

2. A bolus of primary intravenous fluid of 300 cc over 15 minutes may be given prior to the initiation of ritodrine infusion.

3. A baseline electrocardiogram may be obtained prior to the initiation of ritodrine infusion. If obtained, check results.

4. Ritodrine infusion is usually initiated at 0.05 to 0.1 mg/minute (50–100 µg/minute).

5. Increase dosage by increments of 0.05 mg/minute every 20 minutes until desired response is obtained.

6. The maximum dosage of ritodrine is 0.35 mg/minute.

7. After desired response is achieved, maintain ritodrine infusion at constant dosage for 60 minutes.

8. If response continues after 60 minutes, begin decreasing ritodrine dosage in increments of 0.05 mg/minute every 30 minutes until lowest dosage with desired response is achieved. Continue this rate as per physician order or until desired response is no longer present.

9. Do not decrease dosage lower than 0.05 mg/minute.

10. If labor recurs, notify physician and increase infusion as outlined in Steps 4 to 8.

Nursing Assessment during Ritodrine Tocolysis

1. Assess maternal pulse, respirations, blood pressure, and fetal heart rate:

a. Every 15 minutes during dosage increases

b. Hourly during maintenance infusion

c. Every 15 minutes if vital signs become unstable

2. Assess urine for ketones hourly or every void if indwelling catheter is not inserted.

3. Assess breath sounds by auscultation every 2 hours during maintenance infusion.

4. Assess for cough, chest pain, or shortness of breath every 2 hours during maintenance infusion.

5. Ensure propranolol (1 mg), antidote to ritodrine, for intravenous push and cardiac monitor are at bedside.

Oral Tocolytic Regimen

1. After receiving physician's order to wean from intravenous tocolytic to oral maintenance dose, administer oral tocolytic as ordered.

a. 10 mg ritodrine orally **or**

b. 2.5 mg terbutaline orally are commonly ordered

2. Continue current intravenous tocolytic infusion:

a. Ritodrine—continue for 30 minutes

b. Magnesium sulfate—continue for 60 minutes

3. Once oral tocolytic is administered and current intravenous tocolytic infusion is completed as specified, assess the patient for the following:

a. Blood pressure, pulse, respirations, and temperature

b. Breath sounds

c. Uterine activity for contraction frequency, duration, and intensity

d. Fetal heart rate for baseline rate, periodic and nonperiodic changes, reassuring or nonreassuring characteristics

4. Discontinue intravenous infusion if patient remains stable.

5. Assess vital signs, breath sounds, fetal heart rate, and uterine activity every 30 minutes × 2.

6. Patient is then evaluated by the physician for transfer to antepartum unit or reinstitution of intravenous tocolytic therapy.

Nursing Interventions

1. Maintain bed rest in lateral recumbent position to increase uterine perfusion.
2. Maintain strict hourly intake and output.
3. Patient should have nothing by mouth except for ice chips, given sparingly.
4. Encourage patient to void every 2 to 3 hours. Anticipate need for indwelling catheter if patient is unable to void or if quantity is insufficient for measurement.
5. Initiate "Protocol for Fetal Heart Rate Monitoring," page 305, and evaluate fetal heart rate every hour during maintenance infusion for baseline rate, periodic and nonperiodic changes, and reassuring and nonreassuring characteristics.
6. Evaluate uterine activity every hour for frequency, intensity, and duration of contractions during maintenance infusion.
7. Initiate cardiac monitoring if dyspnea, chest pain, irregular heart rate, or maternal heart rate ≥120 beats per minute occur.
8. Notify physician for the following:
   a. Abnormal breath sounds
   b. Maternal pulse ≥120 beats per minute, a systolic pressure <90 mmHg, or a diastolic pressure <40 mmHg
   c. Maternal respirations >24 per minute or <12 per minute
   d. Decreasing deep tendon reflexes or level of consciousness
   e. Mild coughing and complaints of shortness of breath or dyspnea
   f. Increase in intensity or frequency of contractions
   g. Baseline fetal heart rate >160 beats per minute
   h. Nonreassuring fetal heart rate.
   i. Abnormal magnesium level (>8 mEq/liter)
   j. Electrocardiographic changes in rate or rhythm

Complications

1. Magnesium sulfate

   a. Discontinue infusion, and notify physician of signs or symptoms of magnesium sulfate toxicity or abnormal magnesium level.
   b. Obtain calcium gluconate for administration.
   c. Usual dose is 1 g of 5% or 10% solution given intravenous push over 1 to 2 minutes.
   d. Monitor blood pressure, pulse, respirations, deep tendon reflexes, and level of consciousness every 5 minutes until stable and then every 15 minutes until stable.
2. Ritodrine
   a. Discontinue infusion, and notify physician of signs or symptoms of ritodrine intolerance.
   b. Apply cardiac monitor if patient is not currently monitored.
   c. Obtain propranolol for administration.
   d. Usual dose is 1 mg intravenous push.
   e. Monitor blood pressure, pulse, and respirations every 5 minutes until stable and then every 15 minutes until stable.
   f. Continue cardiac monitoring for 12 to 24 hours after infusion is discontinued.
   g. Take strict hourly intake and output measurements and auscultate lung fields every 2 hours for 12 to 24 hours after infusion is discontinued.

PSYCHOSOCIAL ASSESSMENT AND INTERVENTIONS

1. Explain to patient and support persons reasons for "stopping" labor.
2. Explain all procedures, equipment, medications, and side effects and answer all questions.
3. Allow for expression of anxiety concerning infant's prematurity. Arranging for the staff of the neonatal intensive care unit to visit the patient to answer questions may be helpful.
4. Continually update patient and family on maternal and fetal status.
5. Begin patient education to increase knowledge and skills concerning preterm labor. Patient education is individualized but may include the following:

a. Medication administration, scheduling, and side effects
b. Abdominal palpation and timing of contractions
c. Importance of bed rest in lateral recumbent position
d. Subtle signs or symptoms of preterm labor and importance of immediately reporting symptoms
e. Adequate hydration

Documentation

1. Pertinent maternal and fetal assessments
2. Initiation of protocols used in patient care
3. All nursing and medical interventions and patient's response
4. Magnesium sulfate in grams per hour
5. Ritodrine in milligrams per minute

6. Initial and subsequent tocolytic dosages as well as times of dosage changes
7. Physician notification including indication and response.

REFERENCES

1. American College of Obstetricians and Gynecologists: Preterm labor. *ACOG Tech Bull* 133, 1989.
2. Aumann GM, Blake GD: Ritodrine hydrochloride in the control of preterm labor: Implications for use. *J Obstet Gynecol Neonat Nurs* Mar.–Apr.: 75–79, 1982.
3. NAACOG, The Organization for Obstetric, Gynecologic, and Neonatal Nurses: Labor and tocolytics. *OGN Nurs Prac Resource* 10, Sept., 1984.
4. NAACOG, The Organization for Obstetric, Gynecologic, and Neonatal Nurses: *Standards for the Nursing Care of Women and Newborns* (4th ed.). Washington, DC, NAACOG, 1991.

Protocol for the Nursing Management of the Patient Requiring Oxytocin for Induction and Augmentation of Labor

◆ ◆ ◆

PURPOSE

To outline the nursing management of patients requiring continuous oxytocin infusion for the induction and augmentation of labor.

LEVEL

Interdependent

SUPPORTIVE DATA

Induction is defined as the stimulation of labor by artificial methods. Oxytocin is the drug used in the medical induction of labor and is also used to augment existing contraction patterns that may not be adequate for progression of labor.

CONTENT

Oxytocin Administration

1. Prepare oxytocin infusion as specified in "Procedure for Intravenous Oxytocin Administration," page 311.
2. Induction of labor
   a. Begin infusion at 0.5 to 1.0 mU/minute.
   b. Dosage may be increased by 1 to 2-mU increments every 30 to 60 minutes.
3. Augmentation of labor
   a. Begin infusion at 0.5 mU/minute.
   b. Dosage may be increased by 1.0-mU increments every 30 to 60 minutes.
4. The infusion rate is increased until adequate uterine activity is achieved as evidenced by the following:
   a. Contraction duration of 40 to 90 seconds
   b. Contraction frequency of 2 to 3 minutes
   c. Moderate-to-strong contraction intensity by palpation or, if using an intrauterine pressure catheter, an average amplitude of 40 to 90 mmHg, or Montevideo units between 180 to 240. (Montevideo units are calculated as follows: intensity of contraction in mmHg minus uterine resting tone, expressed as a total in mmHg over 10 minutes.)
   d. Adequate uterine resting tone or ≤20 mmHg if using an intrauterine pressure catheter
5. Oxytocin dosage exceeding 20 mU/minute requires physician evaluation and order.

Nursing Assessment during Oxytocin Administration:

1. Assess maternal pulse, respirations, and blood pressure every 30 to 60 minutes depending on stage and phase of labor and presence of associated complications.
2. Assess maternal temperature every 4 hours if membranes are intact, or every 2 hours if membranes are ruptured.
3. Assess intake and output every hour.
4. Assess fetal heart rate every 15 minutes for the following:
   a. Baseline rate
   b. Variability (if appropriate)
   c. Periodic and nonperiodic changes
   d. Reassuring and nonreassuring characteristics
   Note: "Protocol for Fetal Heart Rate Monitoring" (page 305), should be initiated in conjunction with this protocol.

5. Assess uterine activity every 15 minutes for the following:
   a. Uterine resting tone
   b. Frequency, intensity, and duration of contractions
6. Assess for signs and symptoms of uterine rupture
   a. Uterine hypertonus
   b. Uterine hyperstimulation
   c. Abdominal rigidity and pain
   d. Hypotension
   e. Tachycardia
   f. Vaginal bleeding
7. Assess for signs and symptoms of water intoxication
   a. Headache
   b. Nausea and vomiting
   c. "Feeling" sick and mental confusion
   d. Decreased urinary output
   e. Hypotension
   f. Tachycardia
   g. Cardiac arrhythmias

Complications

The following are complications that may occur when using oxytocin for induction and augmentation of labor:
1. Uterine hypertonus
2. Uterine hyperstimulation
3. Uterine rupture
4. Fetal hypoxia
5. Water intoxication
6. Prolapsed cord
7. Precipitous labor

Nursing Interventions

1. Oxytocin infusion should be discontinued for the following:
   a. Nonreassuring fetal heart rate response
   b. Uterine hypertonus or hyperstimulation
   c. Suspected uterine rupture
   d. Suspected water intoxication

2. If oxytocin is discontinued due to complications:
   a. Position patient on side and administer oxygen via face mask at 8 to 10 liters/minute.
   b. Increase primary intravenous rate except in case of water intoxication when primary intravenous rate should be decreased to the rate that keeps the vein open.
   c. Notify physician of suspected complications and subsequent nursing interventions.
   d. Anticipate emergency preparations if surgical intervention becomes necessary for prolapsed cord or nonreassuring fetal heart rate responses.
   e. Oxytocin infusion may be restarted with physician's order at the initial dosage and titrated as specified under (page 287) **Oxytocin Administration** (page 287).

Documentation

1. Pertinent maternal and fetal assessments
2. Initiation of protocols used in patient care
3. All nursing and medical interventions and patient's responses
4. Oxytocin dosage in milliunits per minute
5. Initial and subsequent dosages, as well as times of dosage changes
6. Physician notification including indication and response

REFERENCES

1. American College of Obstetricians and Gynecologists: *ACOG Standards for Obstetric Gynecologic Services* (6th ed.). Washington, DC, ACOG, 1985.
2. American College of Obstetricians and Gynecologists: Induction and augmentation of labor. *ACOG Tech Bull* 157, 1991.
3. NAACOG, The Organization for Obstetric, Gynecologic, and Neonatal Nurses: *Practice Competencies and Educational Guidelines for Nurse Providers of Intrapartum Care.* Washington, DC, NAACOG, 1988.
4. NAACOG, The Organization for Obstetric, Gynecologic, and Neonatal Nurses: The Nurse's role in the induction/augmentation of labor. *OGN Nurs Prac Resource.* 1988.

Protocol for the Nursing Management of the Patient with Pregnancy-Induced Hypertension

◆ ◆ ◆

PURPOSE

To outline nursing management of the intrapartum patient with pregnancy-induced hypertension.

LEVEL

Interdependent

SUPPORTIVE DATA

Pregnancy-induced hypertension is defined as blood pressure ≥140/90 or a 30-mmHg rise in systolic pressure or 15 mmHg rise in diastolic pressure above baseline accompanied by proteinuria and edema after the twentieth week of pregnancy. The etiology of pregnancy-induced hypertension is unknown, however, the goals of therapy are to treat symptoms and minimize complications that may affect multiple organ systems. Eclampsia refers to seizure activity not associated with neurologic disease. Intravenous magnesium sulfate ($MgSO_4$) decreases the uptake of acetylcholine at the myoneural junction and is given to prevent or control seizure activity.

CONTENT

Drug Administration

1. Prepare and administer $MgSO_4$ as specified in the "Procedure for Intravenous Magnesium Sulfate Administration," page 313.
2. Usual loading dose is 4 to 6 g intravenously by infusion pump over 15 to 20 minutes.
3. Maintenance dosage is usually 1 to 2 g intravenously per hour by infusion pump.
4. Monitor serum $MgSO_4$ levels as ordered.
5. Observe for signs or symptoms of $MgSO_4$ toxicity including:
   a. Respiratory rate of ≤ 12 per minute
   b. Decreased level of consciousness
   c. Absent deep tendon reflexes

Nursing Assessments

1. Check blood pressure, pulse, and respirations every 30 minutes; notify physician of systolic and/or diastolic blood pressure ≥160/110.
2. Assess temperature every 4 hours unless otherwise indicated.
3. Assess for signs or symptoms of disease progression.
   a. Headache
   b. Blurred vision or scotomata
   c. Nausea and vomiting
   d. Change in level of consciousness
   e. Epigastric pain
4. Assess deep tendon reflexes and clonus hourly.

Fluid Balance Assessment

1. Insert indwelling urinary catheter to straight drainage.
2. Maintain strict hourly intake and output.
3. Assess hemodynamic parameters hourly if pulmonary artery catheterization is utilized, unless otherwise indicated.
4. Notify physician of urinary output <30 cc/hour.
5. Check urine hourly for protein and specific gravity.
6. Total hourly intake is usually limited to between 100 and 125 cc unless otherwise ordered.

7. Auscultate breath sounds every 2 hours.
8. Notify physician of signs or symptoms of pulmonary edema or abnormal invasive hemodynamic parameters.
   a. Tightness in chest
   b. Shortness of breath
   c. Shallow, rapid respirations
   d. Wheezing
   e. Cough, with or without frothy sputum
   f. Tachycardia
   g. Increased pulmonary capillary wedge pressure
   h. Increased pulmonary artery diastolic pressure

Fetal Monitoring

1. Initiate Protocol for Fetal Heart Rate Monitoring (page 305).
2. Encourage lateral recumbent position to increase uterine perfusion.
3. Observe closely for signs or symptoms of abruptio placentae and uteroplacental insufficiency.

Emergency Management of Seizure Activity

1. Turn patient to side, do not restrict movements.
2. Protect patient.
   a. Raise and pad side rails of bed.
   b. Remove constrictive clothing.
3. Insert airway if possible, do not force jaw open.
4. Notify physician and call for assistance.
5. Administer $MgSO_4$ as ordered to control seizure activity.
6. Once seizure activity stops:
   a. Administer O_2 at 10 liters/minute by tight face mask.
   b. Suction mouth as necessary

c. Assess blood pressure, pulse, respirations, and fetal heart rate every 5 minutes until stable.
d. Note characteristics of seizure:
   • Presence or absence of aura
   • Site of initial body movements and progression of movements
   • Duration of seizure
   • Tonic, clonic phases
   • Duration of postictal phase
   • Length of unconsciousness
   • Maternal and fetal responses
e. Assess for placental abruption and/or imminent delivery.
7. Provide support to patient and family.

Documentation

1. Pertinent maternal and fetal assessments
2. Initiation of all protocols used in patient care
3. All nursing and medical interventions and patient response
4. Physician notification including indication and response
5. Any seizure activity and subsequent fetal and maternal responses

REFERENCES

1. American College of Obstetricians and Gynecologists: *ACOG Standards for Obstetrical and Gynecological Services* (6th ed.). Washington, DC, ACOG, 1985.
2. American College of Obstetricians and Gynecologists: Management of preeclampsia. *ACOG Tech Bull* 91, 1986.
3. Alonso BK: Hypertensive disorders of pregnancy. *NAACOG Update Ser* 3(3), 1985.
4. Knuppel RA, Drukker JE: *High Risk Pregnancy: A Team Approach*. Philadelphia, Saunders, 1986.
5. NAACOG, The Organization for Obstetric, Gynecologic, and Neonatal Nurses: *Standards for the Nursing Care of Women and Newborns* (4th ed.). Washington, DC, NAACOG, 1991.

Protocol for the Nursing Management of the Intrapartum Patient with Insulin-Dependent Diabetes

◆ ◆ ◆ ────────────────────

PURPOSE

To outline the nursing priorities and care specific to the intrapartum patient with insulin-dependent diabetes.

LEVEL

Interdependent

SUPPORTIVE DATA

Maternal morbidity and mortality are increased in the presence of type I or type II diabetes mellitus. The fetus is at risk for congenital anomalies, intrauterine fetal demise, macrosomia, and hypoglycemia, and the mother with diabetes is at risk for infections, diabetic ketoacidosis, accelerated hypoglycemia, operative delivery, and postpartum hemorrhage. Achievement and maintenance of euglycemia during the intrapartum period may decrease fetal and maternal complications.

CONTENT

Insulin Administration

1. Induction of labor and scheduled cesarean section.
   a. Withhold usual insulin dosage and diet on the morning of the scheduled procedure.
   b. Intravenous solution of 5% dextrose to be infused at 125 cc/hour.
   c. Begin insulin infusion if blood glucose level is >120 mg/dl.

2. Spontaneous labor
   a. Withhold insulin dosage.
   b. Patient must not have anything orally.
   c. Intravenous solution of 5% dextrose infused at 125 cc/hour.
   d. Begin insulin infusion if blood glucose level is >120 mg/dl.
3. Prepare insulin infusion as specified in "Procedure for Intravenous Insulin Administration," page 315.
4. Intravenous insulin dosage is titrated to patient's blood glucose values.
5. Intravenous insulin infusion is discontinued prior to delivery to decrease the incidence of postpartum hypoglycemia.
6. Dextrose 50% is maintained at the bedside in the event of hypoglycemia.

Nursing Assessments

1. Assess maternal vital signs hourly unless condition or stage of labor indicate otherwise.
2. Assess temperature every 4 hours.
3. Maintain hourly intake and output.
4. Assess urine for ketones.
   a. Hourly if indwelling catheter is inserted
   b. At every void if indwelling catheter has not been inserted
5. Examine skin over insulin injection sites noting the following:
   a. Bruising
   b. Areas of hypertrophy
6. Examine feet noting the following:
   a. Lesions
   b. Ulcers
   c. Lower extremity pulses
7. Assess for signs and symptoms of urinary tract infection or upper respiratory infection.

Blood Glucose Monitoring

1. Assess blood glucose level on admission.
2. Review patient's home blood glucose monitoring record to assess baseline values and evaluate trends and individual responses.
3. When the patient has nothing orally, check blood glucose level every 2 hours.
4. When the patient is receiving intravenous insulin, check blood glucose level hourly.
5. Assess blood glucose level if signs and symptoms of hypoglycemia occur.

Fetal Monitoring

1. Initiate "Protocol for Fetal Heart Rate Monitoring," page 305.
2. Encourage lateral recumbent position to increase uterine perfusion

Complications

1. Monitor for signs and symptoms of hypoglycemia.
   a. Cold, clammy skin
   b. Shaking
   c. Sweating
   d. Mental confusion or anxiety
   e. Light-headedness
   f. Pallor
   g. Numbness of tongue or lips
2. Monitor for signs and symptoms of diabetic keto-acidosis.
   a. Blood glucose level >300 mg/dl
   b. Presence of ketonuria
   c. Altered level of consciousness
   d. Kussmaul's breathing
   e. Acetone breath

Nursing Interventions

Hypoglycemia

1. If the patient is symptomatic, obtain blood glucose value and notify physician.
2. If blood glucose value is <60 mg/dl, initiate treatment.

3. Treatment of hypoglycemia:
   a. For the conscious patient taking food by mouth:
      • Give 8 oz of skim milk or other snack (*e.g.,* a complex carbohydrate such as peanut butter and crackers).
      • If hypoglycemia occurs preceding a meal, serve meal immediately.
   b. For the conscious patient who must have nothing orally, but who is receiving 5% dextrose intravenously, do the following:
      • Administer 300 cc of 5% dextrose over 25 to 30 minutes.
      • Recheck blood glucose level after administering bolus.
   c. For the unconscious patient, do the following:
      • Notify physician.
      • Administer 10 cc of 50% dextrose over 5 minutes. Subsequent doses may be necessary.
      • Blood pressure, pulse, and respirations must be taken every 5 minutes until stable.
      • Recheck blood glucose level every 15 to 30 minutes until >80 mg/dl.
   d. For the patient receiving intravenous insulin, do the following:
      • Notify physician.
      • Discontinue insulin infusion immediately.
      • Increase primary line infusion of 5% dextrose to 125 cc/hour.

Diabetic Ketoacidosis

1. Obtain values of blood glucose and urine ketones and notify physician.
2. Establish clear airway.
   a. Administer O_2 at 8 to 10 liters/minute via tight face mask.
   b. Assess arterial blood gases
   c. Anticipate need for intubation and mechanical ventilation.
3. Insert indwelling catheter and obtain urine for culture and sensitivity.
4. Discontinue beta agonists if being administered.
5. Begin fluid resuscitation. The usual recommended schedule includes the following:
   a. Administer 1 to 2 liters of normal saline over 30 minutes as ordered per physician.

b. Decrease fluids to 200 to 250 cc/hour.
- If sodium level is <155 mEq/liter, use 5% normal saline.
- If blood glucose level is <200 mg/dl, use 5% dextrose.

c. Anticipate need for invasive hemodynamic monitoring.

d. Assess for signs or symptoms of pulmonary edema.
- Dyspnea
- Tachypnea
- Tachycardia
- Wheezing
- Cough (with or without frothy sputum)

e. Assess for hypovolemia.
- Decrease in blood pressure
- Increase in pulse rate.
- Urine output <30 cc/hour
- Slow capillary refill.
- Decrease in central venous pressure and pulmonary capillary wedge pressure if monitoring initiated

6. Begin intravenous insulin infusion concomitantly with fluid resuscitation per physician order. The usual recommended dose is the following:

a. 20 to 30 U regular insulin bolus intravenously.

b. Follow with 12 U/hour infusion.

c. If blood glucose level is <200 mg/dl, decrease insulin dose.

d. Intravenous insulin dosage is titrated to blood glucose level.

e. Monitor blood glucose level every 15 to 20 minutes.

f. Monitor for signs and symptoms of hypoglycemia.

g. Monitor for signs and symptoms of cerebral edema (especially if blood glucose level has decreased at a rate >75 to 100 mg/dl/hour).
- Headache
- Vomiting
- Deteriorating mental status
- Widening of pulse pressure due to rise in intracranial pressure
- Bradycardia
- Sluggish pupillary light reflex

h. Notify physician of signs and symptoms of cerebral edema or hypoglycemia immediately.

7. Apply cardiac monitor and assess for the following:

a. ST-segment depression

b. Inverted T waves

c. Appearance of U waves after T waves

8. Monitor serum potassium levels.

a. Anticipate need for potassium replacement if potassium is <3.0 mEq/liter.

b. Potassium replacement is discontinued if urinary output is <40 cc/hour.

9. Monitor serum bicarbonate levels.

a. Anticipate need for intravenous bicarbonate if *p*H is <7.10.

b. The usual recommended dosage is 44 mEq sodium bicarbonate over 1 to 2 hours.

10. Obtain blood and/or sputum cultures as ordered.

11. Administer antibiotics as ordered.

12. Ensure that resuscitation equipment is immediately available.

Documentation

1. Pertinent maternal and fetal assessments

2. Initiation of protocols used in patient care

3. All nursing and medical interventions and patient's response

4. Insulin dosage in units per hour

5. Initial and subsequent insulin dosages, as well as times of dosage changes

6. Time, indication, and results of glucose monitoring

7. Physician notification including indication and response.

REFERENCES

1. American College of Obstetricians and Gynecologists: Management of diabetes mellitus in pregnancy. *ACOG Tech Bull* 92, 1988.

2. Caplan RH, Pagliara AS, Beguin EA, et al: Constant intravenous insulin infusion during labor and delivery in diabetes mellitus. *Diabetes Care* 5(1):6–10, 1982.

3. Golde SH, Good-Anderson B, Montoro M, Artal R: Insulin

requirements during labor: A reappraisal. *Am J Obstet Gynecol* 144:556–559, 1982.

4. Miodovnik M, Mimouni F, Tsang RC, et al: Management of the insulin-dependent diabetic during labor and delivery. *Am J Perinatol* 4:106–114, 1987.

5. NAACOG, The Organization for Obstetric, Gynecologic, and Neonatal Nurses: *Standards for the Nursing Care of Women and Newborns* (4th ed.). Washington, DC, NAACOG, 1991.

6. Thurkauf G: How do you manage DKA with continuous IV insulin? *AJN:* 727–732, May 1988.

7. NAACOG, The Organization for Obstetric, Gynecologic, and Neonatal Nurses: *Practice Competencies and Educational Guidelines for Nurse Providers of Intrapartum Care.* Washington, DC, NAACOG, 1988.

Protocol for the Nursing Management of the Obstetric Patient Requiring Mechanical Ventilation

PURPOSE

To outline the nursing management of the obstetric patient requiring mechanical ventilation.

LEVEL

Interdependent

SUPPORTIVE DATA

A variety of complications during pregnancy including severe pregnancy-induced hypertension, trauma, sepsis, pneumonia, pulmonary embolism, disseminated intravascular coagulation, drug overdose, or aspiration of gastric secretions may result in the need for mechanical ventilatory support. The presence of maternal hypoxemia and acidemia also influences fetal well-being. Therefore, thorough maternal–fetal assessment followed by prompt administration of appropriate ventilatory support promotes optimal perinatal outcome in patients with pulmonary compromise.

CONTENT

Intubation

1. Assist during intubation as necessary.
2. Assess for correct placement of endotracheal tube:
   a. Feel for air movement through tube opening.
   b. Watch for bilateral chest excursion during inspiration and expiration.
   c. Auscultate both sides of chest and over stomach for breath sounds.
   d. Anticipate order for chest x-ray to confirm placement.
3. Suction as necessary after placement is confirmed.
4. Secure airway.
   a. Bite block or oral airway.
   b. Tape securely, allowing for turning of head.
   c. Note size of endotracheal tube and level of placement, and mark for future assessment of position.
   d. Restrain patient as necessary to prevent self-extubation.

Cuff Volume Pressure

1. Verify use of high-volume, low-pressure cuff.
2. Monitor cuff pressure using cuff pressure monitoring gauge.
   a. Cuff pressure >15 mmHg to prevent aspiration
   b. Cuff pressure <25 mmHg to prevent tracheal injury
3. Deflate and inflate cuff only to maintain appropriate pressure.

Ventilator Assessment

1. Verify initial ventilator settings.
2. Set alarms. *Immediately investigate any alarm.*
3. Ensure that equipment for manual ventilation with 100% oxygen is at bedside.
4. Check ventilator equipment every 2 hours.
   a. Verify settings with orders.
   b. Check tubing and connections for leaks or obstructions.
   c. Verify appropriate use of humidifier and temperature settings (95° to 100°F).

Respiratory Assessment

1. Auscultate breath sounds every 2 hours.
   a. Rate

b. Quality

c. Adventitious sounds

d. Bilateral, symmetrical excursion

2. Assess for signs and symptoms of respiratory distress.

a. Increased heart rate

b. Cyanosis

c. Diaphoresis

d. Agitation

3. Assess for signs and symptoms of barotrauma (especially with positive end-expiratory pressure)

a. Sudden extreme dyspnea

b. Distended neck veins

c. Pain on affected side

d. Sharp increase in ventilator pressures

e. Decreased breath sounds on affected side

f. Bradycardia and hypotension

g. Notify physician, remove patient from positive end-expiratory pressure, manually ventilate and anticipate need for chest decompression.

Assessment of Oxygenation

1. Assess arterial blood gases and arterial oxygen saturation (Sao_2) after stabilization on ventilator.

2. Assess Sao_2 continuously

3. Assess blood gases after each ventilator change

4. If pulmonary artery catheter is used, assess venous oxygen saturation (Svo_2) after changes in positive end-expiratory pressure.

5. Perform oxygen calculations as indicated including Cao_2, o_2AV (Do_2), Cvo_2, $avDo_2$, Vo_2, and O_2ER.

6. Notify physician of abnormal findings.

Hemodynamic Assessment

1. Assess heart rate, rhythm, and presence of dysrhythmias using electrocardiographic monitor.

2. Evaluate vital signs at least hourly (more frequently if indicated by patient status or protocol).

3. Assess pedal and radial pulses at least every 4 hours.

4. Evaluate invasive hemodynamic parameters as per protocol.

5. Assess for signs and symptoms of decreased cardiac output including the following:

a. Elevated heart rate

b. Decreased blood pressure

c. Abnormal arterial blood gas findings or Sao_2

d. Change in level of consciousness

e. Decreased urine output

f. Cyanosis

Fetal Monitoring

1. Initiate protocol for "Fetal Heart Rate Monitoring" (page 305).

2. Encourage lateral recumbent position to increase uterine perfusion

Precautions for Infection

1. Wash hands frequently and between "clean" and "dirty" procedures.

2. Ensure that ventilator tubing is changed every 24 to 72 hours or per hospital protocol.

3. Drain condensed water in ventilator tubing away from ventilator and humidifier.

4. Oral hygiene every shift.

5. Note color and consistency of sputum and secretions.

6. Monitor patient's temperature every 4 hours or more frequently if indicated.

Suctioning

1. Suction only when necessary as evidenced by the following:

a. Coarse adventitious breath sounds

b. Rhonchi

c. Increasing inspiratory pressures

2. Hyperoxygenate prior to closed suctioning; hyperventilate and hyperoxygenate prior to open suctioning

3. Suction pressures not to exceed 100 to 120 mmHg.

4. Maintain sterile technique.

5. Auscultate breath sounds after suctioning.

6. Sterile saline lavage if secretions are tenacious.

Fluid Volume Assessment

1. Infuse all intravenous fluids per infusion pump.
2. Urinary catheter to urimeter; notify physician of urine output <30 cc/hour.
3. Check hourly intake and output.
4. Check for skin turgor and edema.
5. Take daily weight.
6. Auscultate breath sounds for crackles and wheezes every 2 hours.
7. Evaluate invasive hemodynamic parameters per protocol.

Gastrointestinal Assessment

1. Auscultate bowel sounds every shift.
2. Assess for abdominal distention every shift.
   a. Anticipate need for nasogastric tube.
   b. Take *p*H of nasogastric aspirate.
3. Monitor hemoglobin and hematocrit levels.
4. Administer antacids as ordered.
5. Check stool for occult blood.

Comfort Measures

1. Make frequent position changes; avoid compression of vena cava.
2. Maintain tubing position to prevent pulling of endotracheal tube.
3. Reposition endotracheal tube to opposite side of mouth daily.
4. Assess level of consciousness and pain and medicate as ordered.

Psychologic Assessment and Interventions

1. Explain all procedures and equipment.
2. Provide information regarding current fetal and pregnancy status.
3. Verify call bell within reach.
4. Reassure patient that speech will return after extubation.
5. Ask yes and no questions.
6. Provide writing materials.
7. Provide family and significant others with information and support.

Documentation

1. Pertinent maternal and fetal assessments
2. Initiation of protocols used in patient care
3. All nursing and medical interventions and patient's response
4. Initial and subsequent ventilator settings and times
5. Physician notification including indication and response

REFERENCES

1. Alspach JC, Williams SM: *Core Curriculum for Critical Care Nursing.* Philadelphia, Saunders, 1985.
2. Berkowitz RL (ed.): *Critical Care of the Obstetric Patient.* New York, Churchill Livingstone, 1983.
3. Hudak CM, Gallo BM, Benz JJ: *Critical Care Nursing: A Holistic Approach.* Philadelphia, Lippincott, 1990.
4. Millar S, Sampson LK, Soukup SM: *AACN Procedure Manual for Critical Care.* Philadelphia, Saunders, 1985.
5. Zschoche DA: *Mosby's Comprehensive Review of Critical Care.* St. Louis, Mosby, 1986.

Protocol for the Nursing Management
of the Obstetric Trauma Patient

◆ ◆ ◆

PURPOSE

To outline a systematic approach for the initial assessment of the obstetric trauma patient.

LEVEL

Interdependent

SUPPORTIVE DATA

Trauma accounts for 22% of nonobstetric-related maternal deaths. The purpose of trauma assessment is to identify life-threatening injuries and begin appropriate interventions. Trauma assessment consists of the primary and secondary surveys. The primary survey prioritizes care by simultaneously assessing and intervening for life-threatening injuries. After the patient is stabilized, a secondary survey for assessment of less critical injuries is conducted. This method provides an organized and systematic approach for immediate resuscitation and stabilization procedures after which other protocols for specific care management may be initiated.

CONTENT

Primary Survey

Assessment

I. Airway
   A. Assess airway for patency; look, listen, and feel for air movement.
   B. Use modified jaw thrust maneuver to open airway and assess for obstruction or foreign matter.
   C. Do *not* turn patient's head to assess or open airway.
   D. Assume potential for cervical spine injury until proved otherwise.
II. Breathing
   A. Assess ventilatory and respiratory function noting the following:
      1. Rate and quality of respirations
      2. Signs and symptoms of respiratory distress
         a. Inability to move air despite presence of open airway
         b. Asymmetric chest excursion
         c. Shallow or painful respirations
         d. Dyspnea
         e. Use of accessory muscles
         f. Tachypnea
         g. Bradycardia
   B. Assess trachea noting the following:
      1. Position
      2. Deviation from midline (indicative of possible tension pneumothorax or massive hemothorax)
   C. Visually inspect chest noting the following:
      1. Contusions
      2. Asymmetric excursion
      3. Paradoxical breathing (indicative of possible flail chest)
      5. Open sucking wounds (indicative of possible open pneumothorax)
   D. Auscultate breath sounds bilaterally noting the following:
      1. Hyperresonance (indicative of possible pneumothorax).
      2. Dullness (indicative of possible hemothorax), if decreased or absent breath sounds noted, percuss thorax.
   E. Palpate thorax noting the following:
      1. Presence of pain
      2. Rib instability

3. Subcutaneous emphysema (indicative of possible flail chest)

F. Auscultate heart sounds noting the following:
  1. Distant heart sounds
  2. Muffled heart sounds (indicative of possible cardiac tamponade)

III. Circulation
  A. Assess cardiac output.
    1. Palpate pulses to estimate blood pressure:
      a. Carotid: systolic pressure ≥60 mmHg
      b. Femoral: systolic pressure ≥70 mmHg
      c. Radial: systolic pressure ≥80 mmHg
    2. Assess neck veins for flatness or distention.
      a. Flatness may indicate hypotension secondary to hypovolemia.
      b. Distention may indicate tension pneumothorax or cardiac tamponade.
    3. Assess capillary bed refill.
    4. Note skin color and temperature.
  B. Assess for bleeding.
    1. External
    2. Evidence of internal

IV. Neurologic status
  a. Assess level of consciousness.
  B. Determine Glasgow coma score.

Eye opening	Spontaneously	4
	To verbal command	3
	To pain	2
	None	1
Best verbal response	Oriented	5
	Confused	4
	Inappropriate words	3
	Incomprehensible sounds	2
	None	1
Best motor response	Follows commands	6
	Localizes pain	5
	Withdraws from pain	4
	Flexor posturing (decorticate)	3
	Extensor posturing (decerebrate)	2
	None	1
	Total	**3–15**

Interventions

I. Airway access and maintenance
  A. Maintain cervical alignment at all times.
  B. Immobilize cervical spine with collar or other device.
  C. Clear airway of foreign matter using forceps, suction, or finger sweep.
  D. Use nasopharyngeal or oropharyngeal airway to maintain airway patency.
  E. Anticipate and assist with endotracheal intubation as necessary.
  F. Avoid nasal intubation.
  G. Place nasogastric tube to prevent aspiration and relieve abdominal distension.
  H. Use "log rolling" or tilting of spine board to turn patient for airway management.

II. Respiratory interventions
  A. Administer oxygen at 12 liters/minute by tight nonrebreather mask.
  B. Anticipate need for mechanical ventilation if per minute respiratory rate is >25 or <12.
  C. Obtain arterial blood gases as ordered.
  D. Apply petrolatum gauze or airtight dressing to any open sucking chest wound.

III. Circulatory interventions
  A. Initiate cardiopulmonary resuscitation as indicated, with lateral uterine displacement.
  B. Apply direct pressure or pressure bandages to control external bleeding.
  C. Obtain peripheral intravenous access using large bore catheter(s). Two lines may be necessary.
  D. Obtain appropriate blood specimens as ordered.
  E. Infuse fluids as ordered.
  F. Apply pneumatic antishock garment as indicated. Abdominal compartment may be left uninflated.

Secondary Survey

I. Reassess neurologic status noting the following:
  A. Level of consciousness
    1. **A**—**a**lert and oriented
    2. **V**—responds to **v**erbal stimulus

3. **P**—responds only to **p**ain
4. **U**—**u**nresponsive
  B. Sensorimotor function
    1. Response to painful stimuli
    2. Presence of flaccid paralysis
    3. Glasgow coma scale
II. Examine head noting the following:
  A. Contusions, lacerations, and bony deformities
  B. Signs and symptoms of basilar skull fracture
    1. Check for bleeding from ear or nose.
    2. Check for Battle's sign: postauricular swelling and discoloration.
    3. Check for "raccoon eyes": periorbital edema and ecchymosis.
    4. Anticipate order for portable x-ray for evaluation of cervical spine.
III. Reassess chest and circulation.
IV. Anticipate order for x-ray of thorax.
V. Make abdominal assessment noting the following:
  A. Pain and tenderness
  B. Distention
VI. Assess musculoskeletal status noting the following:
  A. Soft tissue injury
  B. Skeletal injury
  C. Neurovascular function of affected extremity
    1. Sensation
    2. Movement
    3. Color
    4. Swelling
    5. Capillary refill
    6. Distal pulses

Uterine Assessment

1. Assess uterine activity.
  a. Contraction frequency, intensity, and duration
  b. Resting tone
2. Assess fundal height for approximation of gestational age.
3. Inspect perineum for presence of bleeding or leakage of amniotic fluid.
4. Perform vaginal exam (if bleeding absent).
  a. Cervical status
  b. Status of amniotic membranes

c. Fetal station, lie, presentation
d. Presence or absence of prolapsed cord
5. Assess for signs and symptoms of placental abruption.
  a. Presence of uterine contractions and/or irritability
  b. Vaginal bleeding or increasing fundal height
  c. Evidence of fetal hypoxemia
  d. Maternal hemodynamic instability

Fetal Assessment and Interventions

1. Reassess fetal heart activity (as appropriate for gestational age).
  a. Baseline rate
  b. Presence or absence of accelerations or decelerations
  c. Evidence of decreased variability
  d. Presence or absence of reassuring characteristics
2. Promote adequate uteroplacental perfusion.
  a. Displace uterus laterally and avoid supine positioning.
  b. Correct hypovolemia with fluid resuscitation.
  c. Administer O_2 as indicated.

Psychosocial Assessment and Interventions

1. Identify patient's support persons. Allow for contact as soon as acute resuscitative measures are completed.
2. Inform patient and family of status of baby and mother.
3. Allow expression of fear and anxiety.
4. Provide support and reassurance.

Documentation

1. Pertinent maternal and fetal assessment
2. Initiation of protocols used in patient care
3. All medical and nursing intervention and patient's response
4. Resuscitation measures
5. Physician notification including indication and response

REFERENCES

1. Bremer C, Cassata L: Trauma in pregnancy. *Nurs Clin N America* 21:706–716, 1986.
2. Baker DD: Trauma in the pregnant patient. *Surg Clin N America* 62(2):275–289, 1982.
3. Smith CV, Phelan JD: Trauma in pregnancy, in Clark SL, Phelan JD, Cotton DB (eds.): *Critical Care Obstetrics*. Oradell, NJ, Medical Economics Books, 1987.
4. Daddario JB: Trauma in pregnancy. *J Perinat Neonat* 3(2):14–22, 1989.
5. American College of Obstetricians and Gynecologists: Trauma in Pregnancy. *ACOG Update Ser* 12:4, 1986.
6. Smith LG: The pregnant trauma patient, in Cardona VD, et al. (eds.): *Trauma Nursing: From Resuscitation through Rehabilitation*. Philadelphia, Saunders, 1988.

Protocol for the Nursing Management of the Obstetric Patient Requiring Transport

◆ ◆ ◆ _____

PURPOSE

To outline nursing care of the patient immediately prior to and during transport to an alternative facility.

LEVEL

Interdependent

SUPPORTIVE DATA

Maternal transport may become necessary for a variety of reasons including presence of obstetric or medical risk factors and access to specialized neonatal care. The primary goals of nursing care are to stabilize the patient prior to transport, assess maternal–fetal status during transport, and continue or implement appropriate nursing interventions. Specific nursing protocols related to the patient's condition should continue to guide care during transport. However, additional issues should be addressed as well.

CONTENT

Nursing Care Immediately Prior to Transport

General Assessment

 I. Reason for transport
 II. Reassess
   A. Respiratory function including the following:
     1. Patency of airway
     2. Rate and quality of respirations
     3. Signs and symptoms of respiratory compromise

   B. Hemodynamic function including the following:
     1. Blood pressure
     2. Cardiac rate and rhythm
     3. Intake and output
     4. Sign and symptoms of hemodynamic compromise
   C. Recent change in maternal condition

Labor Assessment

 I. Note estimation of gestational age.
 II. Note labor status.
   A. Contraction frequency, strength, and duration
   B. Uterine resting tone
   C. Cervical status
   D. Fetal station and presentation
   E. Note presence or absence of vaginal bleeding
   F. Status of membranes, if ruptured note the following:
     1. Date and time of rupture
     2. Presence or absence of meconium

Fetal Assessment

1. Baseline fetal heart rate
2. Reassuring or nonreassuring findings

Nursing Interventions

1. Assure patent intravenous access with appropriate gauge catheter.
2. Assure clear labeling of intravenous fluids including date and time of preparation.
3. Use plastic rather than glass containers for intravenous fluids.
4. Place all intravenous fluids on infusion pumps.
5. Anticipate need for indwelling urinary catheter for accurate output measurement.

6. Initiate protocols for care of specific maternal diagnosis as specified by receiving hospital.
7. Obtain alternative orders from primary physician for complications that may arise during transport.
   a. Treatment of seizures or life-threatening complications
   b. Additional or alternative medications for tocolytic therapy
8. Assign transport personnel as appropriate for patient's level of care.
9. Assure that all necessary equipment is available and in proper working condition including the following:
   a. Airway management kit, bag-valve ventilation unit, and portable suction equipment
   b. Necessary medications including intravenous fluids and supplies
   c. Infusion pumps for intravenous fluid administration
   d. Electrocardiographic monitor
   e. Blood pressure cuff, sphygmomanometer, and thermometer
   f. Fetoscope or Doppler
   g. Oxygen with manual control, adjustable flow meter with gauge, and humidification attachment
   h. Oxygen reserve calculated by multiplying the flow rate by the length of transport and adding enough for a 45-minute delay.
   i. Obstetric delivery kit, isolette with oxygen, and temperature control for emergency delivery en route

Psychosocial Assessment and Interventions

1. Explain to patient and support persons reasons for transport and transport process.
2. Allow for expression of anxiety concerning transport and answer all questions.
3. Continually update patient and family on maternal and fetal status.
4. Anticipate need for directions, transportation, and contact persons for patient's family at arrival to receiving hospital.

Documentation

1. Obtain copy of prenatal records including name and address of prenatal caregiver if different from referring physician and institution.
2. Obtain copies of obstetric information.
   a. Pertinent clinical information including admission history and physical and care rendered to date
   b. Treatments, laboratory tests, and results to date
   c. Ultrasound or other diagnostic tests and results to date
   d. Any clinically significant portions of previous fetal heart rate tracing
   e. Document information regarding previous obstetric history.
3. Initiate "Maternal Transport Form" (page 331).

Nursing Care during Transport

Maternal Care

1. Monitor blood pressure, pulse, respirations, and temperature every 30 minutes unless otherwise indicated.
2. Maintain continual intake and output measurements.
3. Assess deep tendon reflexes if patient receiving $MgSO_4$ every 30 minutes as indicated.
4. Monitor contractions by palpation noting frequency, strength, and duration.
5. Assess for vaginal bleeding or leaking of fluid.
6. Monitor fetal heart rate using fetoscope or Doppler every 30 minutes unless otherwise indicated.

Nursing Interventions

1. Position patient.
   a. Allow for clear view and access to patient at all times during transport.
   b. Avoid supine positioning which decreases uterine perfusion.
   c. Utilize approved safety restraints during transport.

2. Administer oxygen via face mask as indicated.
3. Continue care by utilizing protocols initiated prior to transport.
4. Initiate all necessary protocols for care as patient's condition dictates (*i.e.,* delivery and infant resuscitation).

Psychosocial Assessment and Interventions

1. Continue to update patient regarding status.
2. Explain all procedures and answer questions.
3. Allow for expression of anxiety during transport and give reassurance.
4. Support and encourage relaxation and controlled breathing techniques.

Documentation

1. Pertinent maternal and fetal assessments
2. Initiation of protocols used in patient care
3. All nursing and medical interventions and patient's response

4. Initial and subsequent medication dosages as well as time of dosage changes
5. Completed follow-up status report sent to referring physician and hospital

REFERENCES

1. Harris BA, Wirtschafter DP, Huddleston JF, et al: In utero versus neonatal transportation of high-risk perinates: A comparison. *Obstet Gynecol* 57(4):496–499, 1981.
2. Hudak CM, Gallo BM, Benz JJ: *Critical Care Nursing*. Philadelphia, Lippincott, 1989.
3. MacDonald MG: *Emergency Transport of the Perinatal Patient*. Boston, Little, Brown, 1989.
4. Mondanlou HD, et al: Perinatal transport to a regional perinatal center in a metropolitan area: Maternal versus neonatal transport. *Am J Obstet Gynecol* 138(8):1157–1164, 1980.
5. NAACOG, The Organization for Obstetric, Gynecologic, and Neonatal Nurses: Maternal–neonatal transport. *OGN Nurs Prac Resource*. June: 8, 1983.
6. Troiano NH: Applying principles to practice in maternal–fetal transport. *J Perinat Neonat Nurs* 2(3):20–30, 1989.

Protocol for Fetal Heart Rate Monitoring
◆ ◆ ◆

PURPOSE

To outline the nursing management of intrapartum patients requiring fetal heart rate (FHR) monitoring.

LEVEL

Interdependent

SUPPORTIVE DATA

Fetal heart rate monitoring is an important tool for assessment of the fetus during labor and delivery. Two available methods for monitoring FHR are auscultation and electronic fetal monitoring. Both methods have advantages as well as limitations. The decision as to which method is employed is ideally made collaboratively between physician, nurse, and patient. Patient–fetal risk factors, stage of labor, presence of a qualified nurse, and availability of equipment should be considered when selecting a method for FHR and uterine activity assessment.

CONTENT

Auscultation

Nursing Assessment

1. Frequency of assessment for low-risk patients
   a. Auscultate every 30 minutes during active phase of labor.
   b. Auscultate every 15 minutes during second stage of labor.
2. Frequency of assessment for high-risk patients
   a. Auscultate every 15 minutes during active phase of labor.

b. Auscultate every 5 minutes during second stage of labor.
3. Count baseline FHR between uterine contractions.
4. Note presence or absence of decelerations.
5. Uterine contractions are assessed by palpation when FHR is auscultated noting the following:
   a. Frequency
   b. Duration
   c. Strength
   d. Uterine resting tone
6. Assess FHR by auscultation prior to:
   a. Ambulation of patient
   b. Transfer or discharge of patient
7. Assess FHR by auscultation immediately following:
   a. Admission of patient
   b. Artificial or spontaneous rupture of membranes
   c. Vaginal examinations or fetal stimulation
   d. Ambulation of patient
   e. Abnormal uterine activity
   f. Any invasive procedure

Nursing Diagnosis

1. A reassuring audible FHR may be characterized by the following:
   a. Normal baseline rate of 110 to 160 beats per minute
   b. Absence of decelerations
2. A nonreassuring audible FHR may be characterized by the following:
   a. Abnormal baseline rate
   b. Presence of decelerations

Nursing Interventions

1. Nonreassuring audible FHR
   a. Reposition patient to increase uteroplacental perfusion or alleviate cord compression.
   b. Administer O_2 at 8 to 10 liters/minute via face mask.

c. Discontinue oxytocin infusion.

d. Correct maternal hypovolemia by increasing intravenous fluids.

e. Notify physician.

f. Vaginal exam is performed if indicated to assess for prolapsed cord or relieve cord compression.

g. Initiate electronic fetal monitoring to clarify and document components of the FHR.

2. Technically inadequate audible FHR

a. Initiate electronic fetal monitoring.

b. Notify physician.

Electronic Fetal Heart Rate Monitoring

Nursing Assessment

1. Frequency of assessment for low-risk patients

a. Interpret tracing every 30 minutes during active phase of labor.

b. Interpret tracing every 15 minutes during second stage of labor.

2. Frequency of assessment for high-risk patients

a. Interpret tracing every 15 minutes during active phase of labor.

b. Interpret tracing every 5 minutes during second stage of labor.

3. Interpretation of FHR includes the following parameters:

a. Baseline rate

b. Variability (as appropriate)

c. Presence or absence of decelerations

d. Presence or absence of accelerations

4. Interpretation of these parameters can be accomplished by using either internal or external fetal monitoring equipment with the exception of variability, which requires the use of a fetal spiral electrode for accurate evaluation.

5. Uterine activity is assessed concurrently with FHR activity noting the following:

a. Frequency of contractions

b. Duration of contractions

c. Intensity of contractions

d. Uterine resting tone

6. When using external monitoring equipment for

evaluation of uterine activity, evaluation of contraction intensity and uterine resting tone is done by palpation.

7. Assess FHR prior to the following:

a. Ambulation of patient

b. Transfer or discharge of patient

8. Assess FHR immediately following:

a. Artificial or spontaneous rupture of membranes

b. Vaginal examinations or fetal stimulation

c. Ambulation of patient

d. Abnormal uterine activity

Nursing Diagnosis

1. A reassuring FHR tracing is characterized by the following:

a. Baseline rate of 110 to 160 beats per minute

b. Minimal or greater variability (as appropriate)

c. Variability may be classified as follows:

• Absent: 0 to 2 beats per minute

• Minimal: 3 to 5 beats per minute

• Moderate: 6 to 25 beats per minute

• Marked: >25 beats per minute

2. A nonreassuring FHR tracing may be characterized by the following:

a. Abnormal baseline rate

b. Absent variability

c. Repetitive late decelerations or prolonged decelerations

3. The following are considered abnormal uterine activity characteristics:

a. Uterine resting tone ≥20 mmHg measured by intrauterine pressure catheter or nonrelaxed by palpation

b. Contractions occurring more frequently than every 2 minutes or lasting longer than 2 minutes

Nursing Interventions

1. Nonreassuring FHR tracing:

a. Notify physician and initiate interventions based on suspected mechanism of insult.

• Uteroplacental insufficiency

a. Reposition patient in lateral recumbent position.

b. Administer O_2 at 8 to 10 liters/minute via tight face mask.

c. Increase intravenous fluids.

d. Discontinue oxytocin infusion.

e. Assess for signs and symptoms of placental abruption.

• Umbilical cord compression

a. Reposition patient.

b. Perform vaginal exam to assess for funic presentation or prolapsed cord. Relieve cord compression by lifting presenting part if prolapsed cord is noted.

b. Evaluate fetal response to interventions.

c. Continue interventions based on fetal response.

d. Anticipate emergency preparations for surgical intervention if nonreassuring fetal responses persist despite interventions.

2. Fetal heart rate tracing inadequate for interpretation:

a. Ensure that paper speed is set and maintained at 3 cm/minute.

b. If external monitor is in use, reposition equipment to obtain a clear continuous signal.

c. If an intrauterine pressure catheter is utilized, flush catheter, zero, and calibrate transducer.

d. If a fetal spiral electrode is in place, check for disconnection from fetus or equipment.

e. Anticipate need for internal monitoring if unable to maintain a technically adequate tracing despite nursing interventions using external monitoring.

f. Anticipate need for replacing internal monitoring equipment, if unable to maintain a technically adequate tracing despite nursing interventions.

g. The nurse may apply fetal spiral electrode or insert intrauterine pressure catheter as indicated after successful completion of competency validation in these procedures.

h. Notify physician of technical or equipment problems if unable to remedy.

3. Abnormal uterine activity

a. Notify physician.

b. Discontinue oxytocin.

c. Assess for signs and symptoms of placental abruption.

d. Anticipate need for placement of intrauterine pressure catheter for additional evaluation and documentation of uterine activity.

e. Anticipate need for emergency preparations for surgical intervention in case of fetal or maternal intolerance of abnormal uterine activity.

Documentation

1. Auscultation

A. Documentation of FHR data is written in narrative format on the labor record using the following objective descriptions:

• Numerical baseline rate

• Rhythm: regular or irregular

• Presence or absence of decelerations

b. Uterine activity data obtained by palpation is documented in the labor record.

2. Continuous electronic fetal monitoring

a. Type of monitoring equipment

b. Any change or adjustment of equipment

c. Evaluation of FHR data on the labor record includes the following:

• Rate expressed as a numerical range

• Variability (as appropriate)

• Presence of periodic patterns

a. Early, late, or variable decelerations

b. Prolonged decelerations

c. Accelerations

d. All uterine activity data obtained by palpation, internal or external uterine monitoring, or a combination of methods

e. The following information is documented on the FHR tracing prior to storage in the patient's permanent medical record:

• Patient name, date of birth, and hospital identification number

• Time and date monitoring initiated and discontinued

f. Further information may be noted on the tracing:

• Invasive procedure and person performing procedure on FHR tracing and labor record

- Physician notification
- Events, procedures, assessments, and interventions
- Nurse's initials to document evaluation of tracing at appropriate intervals

REFERENCES

1. NAACOG, The Organization for Obstetric, Gynecologic, and Neonatal Nurses: Statement on nursing responsibilities in implementing intrapartum fetal heart monitoring. Washington, DC, NAACOG, October 1988.

2. NAACOG, The Organization for Obstetric, Gynecologic, and Neonatal Nurses: Fetal heart rate auscultation. *OGN Nurs Pract Resource,* March 1990.

3. NAACOG, The Organization for Obstetric, Gynecologic, and Neonatal Nurses: The nurse's role in electronic fetal monitoring. *NAACOG Tech Bull* 7, 1980.

4. NAACOG, The Organization for Obstetric, Gynecologic, and Neonatal Nurses: *Standards for Nursing Care for Obstetric, Gynecologic and Neonatal Nursing* (4th ed.). Washington, DC, NAACOG, 1991.

5. NAACOG, The Organization for Obstetric, Gynecologic, and Neonatal Nurses: *Electronic Fetal Monitoring: Nursing Practice Competencies and Educational Guidelines.* Washington, DC, NAACOG, 1987.

Procedure for Intravenous Ritodrine Administration

PURPOSE

To outline nursing responsibility in the safe administration of ritodrine for tocolytic therapy.

SUPPORTIVE DATA

Ritodrine is a betamimetic used in the treatment of preterm labor. Currently, ritodrine is the only drug with approval from the Food and Drug Administration for tocolytic use.

Betamimetic drugs stimulate beta$_1$ and beta$_2$ receptors. Stimulation of these receptors activates an enzyme that increases cyclic adenosine monophosphate within smooth muscle cells. Beta$_1$ receptors are located in the heart, liver, and pancreas and in intestinal and adipose tissue. Beta$_2$ receptors are located in the uterus, bronchioles, and vasculature. The increase in cyclic adenosine monophosphate within the uterine smooth muscle results in a decrease in both intracellular calcium for muscle contraction and in uterine smooth muscle activity. Maternal and fetal side effects result from stimulation of both the beta$_1$ and beta$_2$ receptors as ritodrine is not selective for uterine beta$_2$ receptors only. Ritodrine is metabolized in the liver and excreted in the urine.

EQUIPMENT

Intravenous fluids as prescribed
Ritodrine
Appropriate intravenous tubing
Infusion pump
Cardiac monitor
Propranolol

PROCEDURE	KEY POINTS
1. Prepare equipment.	
a. Check physician's order for correct drug, dosage, and route.	A physician's order is necessary to initiate the infusion.
b. A primary line for infusion of an appropriate intravenous maintenance solution should be established.	A primary line is necessary to maintain intravenous access should intravenous ritodrine be discontinued.
c. Obtain ritodrine from the pharmacy, add medication, and label intravenous bag with date, dosage, time, and signature of registered nurse.	The usual admixture consists of 150 mg of ritodrine added to 500 cc D5 ¼ NS.
d. Place ritodrine solution on an infusion pump. "Piggyback" ritodrine into primary intravenous line. Place primary intravenous line on an infusion pump.	An infusion pump is required to ensure accurate flow rate.
e. Ensure propranolol is at bedside, and a cardiac monitor is readily available.	Propranolol 1 mg intravenously is administered for the reversal of arrhythmias. Cardiac monitoring may be necessary due to ritodrine's effect on the beta$_2$ receptors located in the heart.

PROCEDURE	KEY POINTS
2. Prepare patient. a. Identify patient by name and identification band and check for allergies. b. Assess patient's level of understanding and acceptance of procedure. c. Explain procedure, equipment, and nursing care involved to the patient and significant others.	Individualized patient teaching is necessary to meet the needs of the patient and family for information and emotional support. The patient should understand the potential for side effects such as nervousness, fast heart rate, and shaking.
3. Perform baseline nursing assessments. a. Record patient's baseline temperature, pulse, respirations, and blood pressure. b. Monitor fetal heart rate and uterine activity. c. Review baseline laboratory evaluations. d. Anticipate orders for baseline electrocardiogram and continuous cardiac monitoring if complications occur.	Maternal and fetal baseline information is necessary to establish presence or absence of preexisting complications. Maternal continuous cardiac monitoring may be necessary, depending on past medical history, baseline electrocardiogram results, heart rate >120 beats per minute, or symptoms that suggest arrhythmias.
4. Begin primary intravenous fluid bolus.	Intravenous fluid bolus of 300 cc of maintenance fluid may be given over 15 minutes prior to the start of ritodrine infusion.
5. Begin ritodrine infusion.	The initial infusion is begun at 50 to 100 μg/minute. This is equal to 0.05 to 0.1 mg/minute.
6. Document primary and secondary intravenous infusions.	
7. Document initial dosage and time of ritodrine administration.	
8. Continue care by initiating "Protocol for the Nursing Management of the Patient in Preterm Labor Requiring Intravenous Tocolytic Therapy," page 283.	

REFERENCES

1. American College of Obstetricians and Gynecologists: Preterm labor. *ACOG Tech Bull* 133, 1989.
2. Aumann GM, Blake GD: Ritodrine hydrochloride in the control of premature labor: Implications for use. *J Obstet Gynecol Neonat Nurs* 75–79, Mar.–Apr. 1982.
3. Bardon TP, Peter JB, Merkatz I: Ritodrine hydrochloride: A betamimetic agent for use in preterm labor. Pharmacology, clinical history, administration, side effects and safety. *Am J Obstet Gynecol* 56(1):1–6, 1980.
4. NAACOG, The Organization for Obstetric, Gynecologic, and Neonatal Nurses: Labor and tocolytics. *OGN Nurs Pract Resource* 10, Sept. 1984.

Procedure for Intravenous Oxytocin Administration

PURPOSE

To outline nursing responsibility in the safe administration of oxytocin for induction and augmentation of labor.

SUPPORTIVE DATA

Oxytocin is a synthetic hormone used in the induction and augmentation of labor. Oxytocin, with an immediate onset of action, stimulates the smooth muscle of the uterus to produce rhythmic contractions. As pregnancy progresses, the uterine muscle becomes increasingly sensitive to the effects of oxytocin. Precise delivery of the drug is critical to avoid hyperstimulation of the uterus. Oxytocin also exhibits antidiuretic effects, which may lead to water intoxication.

EQUIPMENT

Intravenous fluids as prescribed
Synthetic oxytocin
Appropriate intravenous tubing
Infusion pump

PROCEDURE	KEY POINTS
1. Prepare equipment. a. Check physician's order for correct drug, dosage, and route.	A physician's order is necessary to initiate the infusion. A medical indication should be noted on the medical record and a cervical exam performed prior to the start of the infusion.
b. A primary line for infusion of an appropriate intravenous maintenance solution should be established.	A primary line is necessary to maintain intravenous access should intravenous oxytocin be discontinued.
c. Obtain synthetic oxytocin from pharmacy, add medication, and label intravenous bag with date, dosage, time, and signature of registered nurse.	Fifteen units of oxytocin added to 250 ml of a physiologic electrolyte-containing solution yields an administration ratio of 1 ml/hour = 1 mU/minute. Use of a pediatric infusion pump will permit administration of dosages less than 1 mU/minute
d. Place oxytocin solution on an infusion pump. "Piggyback" oxytocin into primary line at the port most proximal to the patient.	An infusion pump is required to ensure accurate flow rate. The proximal port is used for oxytocin administration to avoid a bolus dose of oxytocin should the primary rate be increased. Distal ports on the mainline intravenous may be used for administering other medications without affecting oxytocin delivery.

2. Prepare patient.
  a. Identify patient by name and identification band and check for allergies.
  b. Assess patient's level of understanding and acceptance of procedure.
  c. Explain procedure, equipment, and nursing care involved to patient and significant others.
	Individualized patient teaching is necessary to meet the needs of the patient and family for information and emotional support. The patient should understand that oxytocin will stimulate or augment contractions and that she will "feel" contractions soon initiation of the drug.

PROCEDURE	KEY POINTS
3. Perform baseline assessments. a. Record patient's baseline temperature, pulse, respirations, and blood pressure.	Maternal and fetal baseline information is necessary to establish presence or absence of preexisting complications.
b. Monitor fetal heart rate. If continuous electronic fetal monitoring is utilized, obtain 20-minute tracing to assess baseline fetal heart rate and uterine activity.	
4. Begin oxytocin infusion.	
5. Document initiation rate of primary line infusion.	
6. Document initial dosage and time of oxytocin infusion.	
7. Continue care by initiating "Protocol for the Nursing Management of the Patient Requiring Oxytocin for Induction and Augmentation of Labor," page 287.	

REFERENCES

1. American College of Obstetricians and Gynecologists: *ACOG Standards for Obstetric Gynecologic Services* (6th ed.). Washington, DC, ACOG, 1985.
2. American College of Obstetricians and Gynecologists. Induction and augmentation of labor. *ACOG Tech Bull* 157, 1991.
3. NAACOG, The Organization for Obstetric, Gynecologic, and Neonatal Nurses: *Practice Competencies and Educational Guidelines for Nurse Providers of Intrapartum Care.* Washington, DC, NAACOG, 1988.
4. NAACOG, The Organization for Obstetric, Gynecologic, and Neonatal Nurses: The Nurse's role in the induction/augmentation of labor. *OGN Nurs Pract Resource,* 1988.

Procedure for Intravenous Magnesium Sulfate Administration

◆ ◆ ◆

PURPOSE

To outline nursing responsibility in the safe administration of intravenous magnesium sulfate ($MgSO_4$).

SUPPORTIVE DATA

Magnesium sulfate is a medication frequently used in obstetrics. It may be given to inhibit contractions in patients diagnosed with preterm labor as well as to prevent or control seizure activity in the treatment of pregnancy-induced hypertension. The route of administration and concentration of the admixture are usually similar. The maintenance dosage may vary depending on the reason for administration.

In the treatment and control of seizure activity in pregnancy-induced hypertension, $MgSO_4$ competes with the calcium necessary for conduction of nerve impulses by blocking the release of acetylcholine at the synapses, thus decreasing neuromuscular irritability. The tocolytic effect of interfering with uterine smooth muscle contraction is not well understood. It is thought that $MgSO_4$ interferes with the transport of calcium so that less calcium is available for the actin–myosin coupling necessary for muscle contraction.

In both treatments, $MgSO_4$ may be administered for a prolonged period of time. The patient should be monitored for signs and symptoms of magnesium toxicity as respiratory depression and cardiac arrest can occur with serum magnesium levels ≥ 12 mEq/liter. Therapeutic levels are generally considered to be between 4 to 7 mEq/liter. Parenteral $MgSO_4$ is excreted through the kidneys, therefore urinary output must be monitored hourly.

EQUIPMENT

Intravenous fluids as prescribed
Magnesium sulfate
Infusion pump
Appropriate intravenous tubing
Calcium gluconate 1 g of 5% or 10% solution

PROCEDURE	KEY POINTS
1. Prepare equipment. a. Check physician's order for correct drug, dosage, and route.	A physician's order is necessary to initiate the infusion.
b. A primary line for infusion of an appropriate intravenous maintenance solution should be established.	A primary line is necessary to maintain intravenous access should intravenous $MgSO_4$ be discontinued.
c. Obtain $MgSO_4$ from the pharmacy, add medication, and label intravenous bag with date, dosage, time, and signature of registered nurse.	The usual admixture is 40 g of $MgSO_4$ in 1000 cc of 5% dextrose in lactated Ringer's solution. This yields 2 g $MgSO_4$ per 50 cc of solution.
d. Place $MgSO_4$ solution on an infusion pump. "Piggyback" $MgSO_4$ into primary intravenous line. Place primary intravenous line on an infusion pump.	An infusion pump is required to ensure accurate flow rate.
e. Ensure that calcium gluconate is at bedside.	Calcium gluconate is given for the reversal of $MgSO_4$. The usual dosage is 1 g of 5% or 10% solution admin-

PROCEDURE	**KEY POINTS**
	istered by intravenous push over 1 to 2 minutes. Blood pressure, pulse, respirations, deep tendon reflexes, and level of consciousness are monitored every 5 minutes until stable.
2. Prepare patient.	
a. Identify patient by name and identification band and check for allergies.	Individualized patient teaching is necessary to meet the needs of the patient and family for information and emotional support. The patient should understand the potential for side effects such as headache, visual blurring, sensations of heat or burning, lethargy, nausea and vomiting, and constipation.
b. Assess patient's level of understanding and acceptance of procedure.	
c. Explain procedure, equipment, and nursing care involved to the patient and significant others.	
3. Perform baseline nursing assessments.	
a. Record patient's baseline temperature, pulse, respirations, and blood pressure.	Maternal and fetal baseline information is necessary to establish presence or absence of preexisting complications.
b. Perform baseline deep tendon reflex assessment.	
c. Monitor fetal heart rate.	
d. Initiate hourly intake and output measurements. Anticipate need for indwelling urinary catheter for accurate output measurement if necessary.	
4. Initiate intravenous MgSO$_4$ loading dose as prescribed by physician.	Usual loading dose is 4 to 6 g given by infusion pump over 15 to 20 minutes.
5. Begin maintenance infusion.	After the loading dose is given, the maintenance infusion is begun. The usual dose is 2 to 3 g/hour if given as tocolytic therapy. If given for seizure prevention in treatment of pregnancy-induced hypertension, give 1 to 2 g/hour. The loading dose is usually the same regardless of reason for administration.
6. Document primary and secondary line infusions.	
7. Document loading and maintenance dosage and times.	Magnesium sulfate is always documented in grams per hour.
8. Continue care by initiating either "Protocol for Nursing Management of the Patient in Preterm Labor Requiring Intravenous Tocolytic Therapy" (page 283) or "Protocol for the Nursing Management of the Patient with Pregnancy-Induced Hypertension" (page 289).	

REFERENCES

1. American College of Obstetricians and Gynecologists: Management of preeclampsia. *ACOG Tech Bull* 91, 1986.
2. American College of Obstetricians and Gynecologists: Preterm labor. *ACOG Tech Bull* 133, 1989.
3. Alonso BK: Hypertensive disorders of pregnancy. *NAACOG Update* 3:3, 1985.
4. NAACOG, The Organization for Obstetric, Gynecologic, and Neonatal Nurses: Labor and tocolytics. *OGN Nurs Pract Resource* 10, Sept.: 1984.

Procedure for Intravenous Insulin Administration

PURPOSE

To outline nursing responsibility in the safe administration of insulin by continuous infusion.

SUPPORTIVE DATA

Infants of women with diabetes are at risk for development of neonatal hypoglycemia. Euglycemia during the intrapartum period may decrease the incidence and severity of neonatal hypoglycemia. Continuous insulin is titrated to the patient's blood glucose level during the intrapartum period. The usual dosage for intravenous insulin is 0.25 to 2 U/hour to maintain a blood glucose level of 60 to 110 mg/dl. Continuous insulin infusion is also administered for diabetic ketoacidosis. The usual insulin infusion rate is 2 to 10 U/hour with an initial bolus of 0.1 U/kg of body weight.

EQUIPMENT

Intravenous fluids as prescribed
Regular insulin
Infusion pump
Appropriate intravenous tubing

PROCEDURE	KEY POINTS
1. Prepare equipment.	
a. Check physician's order for correct drug, dosage, route, and intravenous fluid.	A physician's order is necessary to initiate the infusion.
b. A primary line for infusion of an appropriate intravenous maintenance solution should be established.	A primary line is necessary to maintain intravenous access should intravenous insulin be discontinued.
c. Obtain regular insulin from pharmacy, add medication, and label intravenous bag with date, dosage, time, and signature of registered nurse.	Regular insulin is added to normal saline to produce a concentration of 1 cc normal saline = 1 U regular insulin (*e.g.,* 100 U regular insulin added to 100 cc normal saline.)
d. Place insulin solution on an infusion pump and flush 50 cc of solution through cassette or tubing and discard.	An infusion pump is required to ensure accurate flow rate and precise titration of intravenous insulin. Flushing the tubing allows the insulin binding sites on the polyvinylchloride tubing to become saturated, preventing the admixture from being "robbed" of insulin during the infusion.
e. "Piggyback" insulin into primary intravenous line at the port most proximal to the patient.	Insulin is easily titrated according to blood glucose levels if administered via a secondary line, rather than added to the mainline intravenous solution. Other medications may be given through the distal port without altering the insulin flow rate.
f. Ensure that 50% dextrose is available at the bedside.	In the event severe hypoglycemia occurs, 50% dextrose is administered.

PROCEDURE	KEY POINTS
2. Prepare patient.	
a. Identify patient by name and identification band and check for allergies.	Individualized patient teaching is necessary to meet the needs of the patient and family for information and emotional support.
b. Assess patient's level of understanding and acceptance of procedure.	
c. Explain procedure, equipment, and nursing care involved to patient and significant others.	
d. Review signs and symptoms of hypo- and hyperglycemia and instruct patient to notify nursing staff of any of the following: shaking; numbness of the tongue or lips; severe hunger; lightheadedness; cold, clammy skin; and nausea or vomiting.	The pregnant woman with diabetes is at risk for both diabetic ketoacidosis and accelerated hypoglycemia.
3. Perform baseline nursing assessments.	
a. Record patient's baseline temperature, pulse, respirations, and blood pressure.	Maternal and fetal baseline information is necessary to establish presence or absence of preexisting complications.
b. Baseline laboratory evaluations: blood glucose, urine ketones.	
4. Begin insulin infusion.	
5. Document primary and secondary line infusions.	
6. Document initial dosage and time.	Insulin must be documented in units per hour.
7. Continue care by initiating "Protocol for the Nursing Management of the Intrapartum Patient with Insulin-Dependent Diabetes," page 291.	

REFERENCES

1. American College of Obstetricians and Gynecologists: Management of diabetes mellitus in pregnancy. *ACOG Tech Bull* May: 92, 1988.

2. Caplan RH, Pagliara AS, Beguin EA, et al: Constant intravenous insulin infusion during labor and delivery in diabetes mellitus. *Diabetes Care* 5(1):6–10, 1982.

3. Golde SH, Good-Anderson B, Montoro M, Artal R: Insulin requirements during labor: A reappraisal. *Am J Obstet Gynecol* 144:556–559, 1982.

4. Miodovnik M, Mimouni F, Tsang RC, et al: Management of the insulin-dependent diabetic during labor and delivery. *Am J Perinatol* 4:106–114, 1987.

5. NAACOG, The Organization for Obstetric, Gynecologic, and Neonatal Nurses: *NAACOG Standards for the Nursing Care of Women and Newborns* (4th ed.). Washington, DC, NAACOG, 1991.

6. Thurkauf G: How do you manage DKA with continuous IV insulin? *AJN* 727–732, May: 1988.

7. NAACOG, The Organization for Obstetric, Gynecologic, and Neonatal Nurses: *Practice Competencies and Educational Guidelines for Nurse Providers of Intrapartum Care.* Washington, DC, NAACOG, 1988.

Procedure for Assisting with Invasive Hemodynamic Monitoring in Obstetrics

◆ ◆ ◆ ———————————————————————————————————

PURPOSE

To outline nursing care of the obstetric patient requiring invasive hemodynamic monitoring via an intraarterial or pulmonary artery catheter.

SUPPORTIVE DATA

An intraarterial catheter connected to a pressure monitoring system permits continuous arterial blood pressure assessment and withdrawal of arterial blood samples. Catheters are usually 20 or 22 gauge and are inserted under sterile conditions into the radial artery by a physician. Complications include trauma during insertion and infection.

A pulmonary artery catheter is a balloon-tipped, flow-directed catheter inserted into the heart via an introducer placed in the central venous circulation. Catheters used in obstetrics range in size from 7.0 to 8.5 French and may have a variety of optional capabilities. Four ports are common to all pulmonary artery catheters.

The pulmonary artery, or distal, port opens into the pulmonary artery and records pulmonary artery systolic, diastolic, and mean pressures. The central venous pressure, or proximal, port opens into the right atrium and records central venous pressure. It is used intermittently as an injectate port during thermodilution cardiac output assessment and may also be used to infuse fluids or medications. The balloon port is used for intermittent inflation of the balloon during catheter insertion and to obtain pulmonary capillary wedge pressures. The thermistor port connects to a cardiac output computer and records blood temperature during thermodilution cardiac output assessment. Additional information may be derived using hemodynamic formulas once baseline data are obtained.

The catheter is usually inserted through a 7.5 to 8.5 French introducer under sterile conditions by a physician. The insertion site usually preferred in obstetrics is the right internal jugular vein. Complications include trauma during insertion of the introducer, infection, and arrhythmias. Rare complications include catheter knotting, pulmonary artery rupture, thromboembolism, and balloon rupture.

EQUIPMENT

500 cc of 0.9% normal saline
Heparin (2 to 10 U/ml intravenous fluid)
Disposable pressure lines
  IV tubing
  Pressure transducers
  Pressure extension (noncompliant) tubing
Pressure bag(s) with 300 mmHg inflation marking
Intravenous pole and transducer manifold
Hemodynamic monitor and cables
Nonvented stopcock caps
Appropriate invasive hemodynamic catheters

PROCEDURE	KEY POINTS
Pressure lines I. Add heparin to 0.9% normal saline as prescribed by physician.	Usual preparation for nonobstetric critical care patients is 1 U of heparin per 1 cc of normal saline. Additional heparin may be utilized in obstetric critical

PROCEDURE	**KEY POINTS**
	care because of the hypercoagulability of pregnancy. Continuous heparin flush is used to prevent clotting.
II. Place solution in pressure bag.	
III. Flush tubing and transducer using gravity to remove air and prime with heparin.	
IV. Replace all stopcock ports with nonvented caps. Ensure that system is free of air and that there are no leaks.	
V. Inflate pressure bag to 300 mmHg.	Pressure is maintained at 300 mmHg to ensure an infusion rate to each pressure line of 3 to 5 ml/hour.
VI. Zero each pressure line to the patient's phlebostatic axis.	
VII. Calibrate the transducer.	

Intraarterial Catheter

I. Prepare pressure line as previously described	
II. Prepare patient.	
A. Ensure that a signed consent form for procedure is in patient's chart.	Placement of an intraarterial catheter is an invasive procedure that requires informed consent.
B. Perform the Allen test prior to radial artery catheterization.	
1. Instruct patient to close hand tightly.	The Allen test assesses collateral circulation of hand when radial artery is occluded.
2. Occlude patient's ulnar and radial arteries until blanching occurs.	
3. Ask patient to open fist while the ulnar artery is released.	
4. Examine palm for color and refill time to determine ulnar artery patency.	Refill in <5 seconds is normal.
5. Do not perform radial artery puncture if the Allen test is nonreassuring.	
C. Assess patient's level of understanding and acceptance of procedure.	
D. Answer any questions concerning the procedure, equipment, or related nursing care.	
III. Assist physician with insertion of catheter.	
IV. Apply dressing to insertion site. Utilize dressing that allows site to be visualized at all times.	Estimated blood loss of patient may be 300 to 500 cc/minute if catheter becomes disconnected. Patient may need a reminder that catheter is in place.
V. Immobilize site of insertion by placing patient's arm on an armboard.	
A. Do not dorsiflex wrist.	Dorsiflexion of wrist may cause median nerve damage.
B. Place restraints (if utilized) on armboard rather than patient's wrist.	
VI. Rezero after connecting patient to system.	
VII. Set alarms.	
VIII. Nursing care.	
A. Rezero the pressure line and calibrate the transducer every shift and as necessary.	
B. Verify alarm settings every shift.	

PROCEDURE	**KEY POINTS**

C. Do not give medication, blood or intravenous fluid other than continuous flush solution through intraarterial catheter.

D. Ensure that reserpine is at bedside for arterial spasm.

    Reserpine 0.5 to 1.0 mg is given for arterial spasm.

E. Obtain cuff pressure every shift for comparison or when acute changes in blood pressure occur.

F. Assess extremity for adequate perfusion every 2 hours by noting presence or absence of the following:
  1. Pain
  2. Pallor
  3. Paresthesia
  4. Ischemia

G. Assess for evidence of tissue damage every 2 hours as evidenced by the following;
  1. Blanching
  2. Coldness
  3. Cyanosis

H. Check nailbeds for capillary refill every 2 hours.

  I. Check all connection sites every 2 hours.

  J. Sterile dressing change every 24 hours.

  K. Change heparin flush bag and pressure line every 24 to 48 hours or as indicated by hospital infection control policy using aseptic technique.

IX. Removal of arterial catheter.

A. After removal apply direct pressure to site for 5 to 10 minutes.

B. Apply pressure dressing to site and leave in place 30 to 60 minutes.

C. Check site for any bleeding, oozing, or hematoma formation.

D. Assess collateral circulation.

E. Check quality of pulses bilaterally.

F. Check site every 2 hours after removal of pressure dressing.

X. Documentation.

A. Date, time, site of insertion, and physician who performed procedure

B. Results of Allen test

C. Type and gauge of catheter, number of attempts, and patient's tolerance of procedure

D. Time of zeroing and calibration of transducer and verification of alarms

E. Cuff pressure (when obtained)

F. Sterile dressing and pressure line changes

G. Removal of intact catheter, date, time, and related nursing care

PROCEDURE	**KEY POINTS**

H. Pertinent nursing assessments, interventions, and patient response

I. All protocols initiated in conjunction with patient care

Pulmonary Artery Catheter

I. Prepare two pressure lines (as described earlier) for central venous pressure and pulmonary artery ports.

II. Prepare patient.

    A. Ensure that a signed consent form for procedure is in patient's chart.

    B. Assess patient's level of understanding and acceptance of procedure. Answer any questions concerning the procedure, equipment, or related nursing care.

    C. Initiate continuous electrocardiographic monitoring.

IV. Test balloon patency prior to insertion.

V. Nursing management during insertion.

    A. Monitor the electrocardiogram for ventricular dysrhythmias as catheter passes through right ventricle and ensure lidocaine bolus is at bedside.

    B. Observe and record pressures as catheter is passed through the chambers of the heart.

    C. Anticipate orders for chest x-ray to confirm correct placement after catheter is inserted.

    D. Ensure balloon is deflated. Always allow balloon to deflate passively. Do not withdraw air from balloon.

    E. Apply dressing after physician secures catheter.

    F. Ensure that a continuous reading of pulmonary artery tracing is on monitor.

VI. Nursing assessments.

    A. Assess insertion site for evidence of bleeding or infection

    B. Check all connection sites every 2 hours and monitor system for presence of air or blood clots.

    C. Verify that alarms are set at all times.

    D. Record hemodynamic parameters as indicated by patient status and care protocols. When obtaining pulmonary capillary wedge pressure, do the following:

        1. Inflate balloon slowly.

KEY POINTS

Placement of a pulmonary artery catheter is an invasive procedure that requires informed consent.

Ventricular ectopy may occur when the catheter enters the right ventricle. Less than 1% of patients require suppression with lidocaine 1 mg/kg.

PROCEDURE   **KEY POINTS**

    2. Note amount of air necessary for pulmonary artery waveform to change to pulmonary capillary wedge pressure waveform on tracing. Do not inflate balloon beyond amount necessary to obtain pulmonary capillary wedge pressure. Never inflate beyond balloon capacity.

    3. Assess for feeling of resistance during balloon inflation.

    4. Do not leave balloon inflated for more than 30 seconds.

    5. Allow balloon to deflate passively, do not aspirate air from syringe.

    6. Note return of pulmonary artery waveform to monitor after deflation of balloon.

  E. Monitor heparinized pressure flush for correct pressure (300 mmHg).

  F. Assess equipment for proper functioning.

    1. Rezero and calibrate transducer every shift and as necessary.

VII. Nursing interventions for the following:

  A. Spontaneous wedging

    1. Determine if balloon is completely deflated.

    2. Reposition patient and have patient cough and breathe deeply.

    3. If catheter remains wedged, notify physician immediately for repositioning of catheter.

    4. Monitor for return of pulmonary artery waveform.

  B. Backward migration of catheter into right ventricle as evidenced by right ventricle tracing on monitor.

    1. Notify physician immediately for repositioning of catheter.

    2. Monitor for premature ventricular contractions.

  C. Suspected balloon rupture as evidenced by absence of resistance felt when inflating balloon and inability to obtain reading of pulmonary capillary wedge pressure.

    1. Attach syringe and slowly withdraw plunger.

    2. If able to aspirate fluid or blood, balloon rupture is confirmed. Do not inject any air.

    3. Label catheter inflation port, "balloon rupture."

    4. Notify physician.

PROCEDURE	KEY POINTS

   D. Change pressure transducer system every 24 to 48 hours or as indicated by hospital infection control policy.
   E. Perform site care daily.
VIII. Nursing care during catheter removal.
   A. Obtain vital signs and electrocardiographic tracing.
   B. Monitor for arrhythmias during removal of catheter.
   C. After removal, apply direct pressure for 5 minutes. Ensure that bleeding has stopped completely.
   D. Apply pressure dressing to site.
   E. Pressure dressing to remain in place for 8 hours.
 IX. Documentation
   A. Date, time, site of insertion, and name of physician who performed procedure
   B. Type of pulmonary artery catheter, number of attempts, confirmation of placement by x-ray, and patient's tolerance of procedure
   C. Pertinent nursing assessments and medical and nursing care
   D. Zeroing and calibration of transducers and verification of alarm settings
   E. Date and time of removal of intact catheter
   F. Nursing care and assessments after removal
   G. Site care
   H. Transducer system changes
    I. All protocols initiated in conjunction with patient's care

REFERENCES

1. Alspach JC, Williams SM: *Core Curriculum for Critical Care Nursing.* Philadelphia, Saunders, 1985.
2. Berkowitz RL (ed.): *Critical Care of the Obstetric Patient.* New York, Churchill Livingstone, 1983.
3. Hudak CM, Gallo BM, Benz JJ: *Critical Care Nursing: A Holistic Approach.* Philadelphia, Lippincott, 1990.
4. Miller S, Sampson LK, Soukup SRM: *AACN Procedure Manual for Critical Care.* Philadelphia, Saunders, 1985.
5. Pursley PM: Arterial catheters: Nursing management to decrease complication. *Crit Care Nurse* July/Aug. 1981.
6. Zschoche DA: *Mosby's Comprehensive Review of Critical Care.* St. Louis, Mosby, 1986.

APPENDIX
INTRAPARTUM NURSING FORMS
AND FLOWSHEETS

♥ Vanderbilt University Medical Center
L & D FLOWSHEET

DATE	SIGNATURE	INT.	SHIFT

Date of Service

Div or Clinic

Pt

Unit No.

DTR'S
0 - Absent
1+ - Present c Hammer
2+ - Present c Fingertips
3+ - Brisk c Fingertips
4+ - Clonus Present

LOC
1 - Alert/Oriented
2 - Disoriented

BREATHSOUNDS
C - Clear
Cr - Crackles
Wh - Wheezes

BINDING LINE

DATE											
ASSESSMENT	1 Protocol										
	2 Temp.										
	3 BP Systolic										
	4 Diastolic										
	5 Pulse										
	6 Resp Rate										
	7 Breathsounds L										
	8 Breathsounds R										
	9 SOB										
	10 Chestpain										
	11 DTR's										
	12 HA										
	13 RUQ Pain										
	14 Visual Changes										
	15 LOC										
	16 Blood Glucose										
	17 V. E. (examiner)										
	18 Scalp Stim.										
	19										
	20										
MATERNAL/FETAL MONITORING	21 Monitor Mode										
	22 Baseline Low										
	23 Baseline High										
	24 BTBV										
	25 Accels										
	26 Decels										
	27 Nsg. Diagnosis										
	28										
	29 Monitor Mode										
	30 Freq. (q min.)										
	31 Duration (sec.)										
	32 Intensity										
	33 Resting Tone										
	34 MVU's										
	35										
IV MEDICATIONS	36 Oxytocin mU/Min.										
	37 MgSO4 Gm/Hr.										
	38 Ritodrine mg/min.										
	39 Insulin U/Hr.										
	40										
	41										
	42										
	43 See Nurse's Notes										
	44 O2 L/Min.										
	45 Position										
	46										
	47										
	48										
	49										
	50										
	51 Initials										

This is page 1 of 3 (front pages) within a trifold format. Front pages 2 and 3 are continuation sheets to provide 24 columns for patient data entry.

Form No.
60-001-290 (Rev. 12/90) - Page 1 of 3 (back)

❂ Vanderbilt University Medical Center

L & D FLOWSHEET

LABOR CURVE

Date of Service		Div or Clinic

Pt

Unit No.

DATE/TIME	PROGRESS NOTES

TIME					
MARK •	10	8	6	4	2
MARK X					

CERVICAL DILATION

	-2	0	+2	+4	

STATION

EFFACEMENT %

HOUR OF LABOR

AM PM (00 15 30 45) — repeated vertical time columns

Page 1 of 3 (back) of a trifold format.

Form No.
60-001-290 (Rev. 12/90) - Page 2 of 3 (back)

✪ Vanderbilt University Medical Center

L & D FLOWSHEET

DATE/TIME	NURSING PROGRESS NOTES

Date
of
Service

Div
or
Clinic

Pt

Unit No.

BINDING LINE

Page 2 of 3 (back) of a trifold format.

Form No.
60-001-290 (Rev 12/90) - Page 3 of 3 (back)

Vanderbilt University Medical Center

L & D FLOWSHEET

DATE	SIGNATURE	INT.	SHIFT

Date of Service

Div or Clinic

Pt

Unit No.

YESTERDAY'S INTAKE ____________

YESTERDAY'S OUTPUT ____________

TODAY'S WEIGHT ____________

YESTERDAY'S WEIGHT ____________

TIME	INITIALS	INTAKE: I.V. Fluids									P. O.		OUTPUT: URINE					OTHER OUTPUT	IV Site
			Amount Infused		Amount Infused		Amount Infused		Amount Infused	Total IV	Type	Volume	Protein	Ketones	Glucose	Sp. Gr.	Volume		
12 HOUR TOTAL																			
PREVIOUS 12 HOUR TOTAL																			
24 HOUR TOTAL																			

BINDING LINE

Page 3 of 3 (back) of a trifold format.

OB-ICU
SUPPLEMENTAL FLOWSHEET

DATE														
TIME														

CARDIOVASCULAR	Art. Line: Sys														
	Dia														
	Mean														
	HR														
	Rhythm														
	PA: Sys														
	Dia														
	Mean														
	PCWP														
	CVP														
	C.O.														
HEMO CALCS	SV														
	SVR														
	PVR														
	LCW														
	LVSW														
	RCW														
	RVSW														
	BSA														
RESPIRATORY	FiO_2														
	Mode														
	T. Vol.														
	Rate: Total/Set														
	PSV/PEEP														
	P.I.P.														
	SaO_2														
	SvO_2														
O_2 CALCS	CaO_2														
	CvO_2														
	$avDO_2$														
	O_2AV (DO_2)														
	VO_2														
	O_2ER														
	$AaDO_2$														
	Qs/Qt														

OB-ICU
LABORATORY RESULT FLOWSHEET

DATE TIME											
PT											
PTT											
FSP											
Platelets											
Fibrinogen											
BLD TIME											
HCT											
HGB											
WBC											
BUN											
NA											
CR											
K											
CL											
CO_2											
GLU											
Magnesium											
Uric Acid											
SGOT											
SGPT											
LDH											
Total Protein											
PHOS											
CPK											
Other											
Other											
Other											
PH											
PCO_2											
PO_2											
HCO_3											
COP											
PLASMA OSM											
URINE NA											
URINE CR											
URINE OSM											
URINE SP G											
URINE CR CL											

MATERNAL TRANSPORT FORM

To Accompany Patients
Transported To

❤ Vanderbilt University Medical Center
Department of Obstetrics and Gynecology
Maternal-Fetal Division

Note: Please complete both sides of this form and send, along with photocopies of pertinent clinical records (prenatal record, hospital chart, labwork, FHR monitor tracing, etc.), with patient.

GENERAL INFORMATION

Patient's Name: _____ Date: _____

Age: _____ Gravida: _____ Para: _____ AB: _____

LMP: _____ EDC: _____ Estimated Gestational Age: _____

Blood type/RH: _____ Allergies: _____

County of Patient's Residence: _____

Referring MD: _____ Phone #: _____

Referring Hospital: _____

Transport Accepted By: _____ (M.D. - Vanderbilt)

REASON FOR REFERRAL

_____ Diabetes Mellitus   _____ Preeclampsia/Eclampsia

_____ Fetal Demise   _____ Preterm Labor

_____ Multiple Gestation   _____ Preterm Rupture of Membranes

_____ Post-Term Pregnancy   _____ Vaginal Bleeding

          _____ Other (specify)

          _____

          _____

          _____

TRANSPORT MODE

_____ Ambulance   _____ Private Auto   _____ Air Transport

Accompanied By: _____

          _____ M.D.   _____ R.N.   _____ L.P.N.

          _____ E.M.T.   _____ Paramedic   _____ Other

MATERNAL TRANSPORT WORKSHEET
(To Be Used En Route)

1. CARE AT REFERRING HOSPITAL

A. Labor Assessment:

Onset of contractions: _____ / _____ at _____ AM/PM
month   day

Membranes: _____ intact

_____ ruptured (_____ / _____ at _____ AM/PM)
month   day

Fetal monitor used?

_____ no

_____ yes (_____ internal _____ external)

B. Cervical Exam:

	On admission to referring hospital	Last exam at referring hospital
Cm. dilation		
Position		
Consistency		
% Effacement		
Presentation/Station		

C. Meds and IVF previous 24 hours

_____
_____
_____

2. CARE EN ROUTE

A. Time of departure: _____ AM/PM

B. Patient position during transport: _____

C. Assess pertinent info below at least q 30 min.

Time	B/P	P	R	Contraction Freq	Int.	Dur	FHR	DTR	IV/Count

Additional Comments:

3. DELIVERY (If occurred en route)

Date: _____ Time: _____ AM/PM

Apgar: _____ 1 min. _____ 5 min Sex: _____

Resuscitation: _____ stimulation _____ IPPB

_____ 0 to face

Comments:

4. ARRIVAL AT REFERRAL CENTER

Time of departure: _____ AM/PM

Report given by: _____

Report received by: _____

Pertinent patient records sent with patient: _____ yes _____ no

Index